Springer
Berlin
Heidelberg
New York
Barcelona
Hong Kong
London
Milan
Paris
Singapore
Tokyo

J. Bogaert · A. J. Duerinckx · F. E. Rademakers (Eds.)

Magnetic Resonance of the Heart and Great Vessels

Clinical Applications

With Contributions by

J. Bogaert · H. Bosmans · P. Croisille · J. F. Debatin · A. De Roos · A. J. Duerinckx
S. Dymarkowski · G.G. Hartnell · W. A. Helbing · S. Neubauer · Y. Ni · R. A. Niezen
D. J. Pennell · T. Pfammatter · F. E. Rademakers · D. Revel · A. M. Taylor · S. Wildermuth

Foreword by
A.L. Baert

With 188 Figures in 445 Separate Illustrations, Some in Color

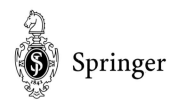

Springer

JAN BOGAERT, MD, PhD
Department of Radiology
University Hospitals Gasthuisberg
Catholic University of Leuven
Herestraat 49
B-3000 Leuven
Belgium

ANDRÉ J. DUERINCKX, MD, PhD
Radiology Service (Mail route: W114), MRI Clinik, Bld #507
West Los Angeles Veterans Affairs Medical Center (VAMC)-Wadsworth
11301 Wilshire Blvd.
Los Angeles, CA 90073
USA

FRANK E. RADEMAKERS, MD, PhD
Department of Cardiology
University Hospitals Gasthuisberg
Catholic University of Leuven
Herestraat 49
B-3000 Leuven
Belgium

MEDICAL RADIOLOGY · Diagnostic Imaging and Radiation Oncology

Continuation of
Handbuch der medizinischen Radiologie
Encyclopedia of Medical Radiology

ISSN 0942-5373
ISBN 3-540-63448-7 Springer-Verlag Berlin Heidelberg New York

Library of Congress Cataloging-in-Publication Data. Magnetic resonance of the heart and great vessels : clinical applications / J. Bogaert, A. J. Duerinckx, F. E. Rademakers (eds); with contributions by J. Bogaert ... [et al.] ; foreword by A. L. Baert   p. cm. -- (Medical radiology)   Includes bibliographical references and index.   ISBN 3-540-63448-7 (alk. paper)   1. Cardiovascular system--Diseases--Magnetic resonance imaging. 2. Heart--Diseases--Magnetic resonance imaging. I. Bogaert, J. (Jan) , 1964- . II. Duerinckx, Andre J. III. Rademakers, F. E. (Frank E.), 1955- . IV. Series   [DNLM: 1. Cardiovascular Diseases--diagnosis. 2. Magnetic resonance imaging. WG 141 M1965 1999] RC670.5.M33C55 1999 616.1'07548--DC21   DNLM/DLC   for Library of Congress   98-24570   CIP

Printed in Germany

The use of general descriptive names, registered names, trademarks, etc. in this publication does not imply, even in the absence of a specific statement, that such names are exempt from the relevant protective laws and regulations and therefore free for general use.

Product liability: The publishers cannot guarantee the accuracy of any information about dosage and application contained in this book. In every individual case the user must check such information by consulting the relevant literature.

Typesetting: Best-set Typesetter Ltd., Hong Kong

SPIN: 10546228   21/3135 – 5 4 3 2 1 0 – Printed on acid-free paper

To Brigitte
Christophe, Sébastien and Julie

To David

To Karin
Frederik and Emilie

Foreword

Magnetic resonance imaging (MRI) is a rapidly evolving technique and new MR sequences and applications are still being developed at an astonishing rate. This statement is particularly true for cardiovascular MRI. In itself this would have been a sufficient reason to publish a new volume on the current clinical applications of MRI of the heart and the great vessels. But for radiologists, involvement in cardiovascular MRI offers a unique opportunity to become more active again in an organ area where their role has tended to decrease. Indeed, because of the excellent ability of ultrasound, which is performed in most instances by cardiologists, to display morphological and functional changes of the cardiovascular system and the rather limited applications of computed tomography in this organ area, the role of the radiologist as a consultant for the cardiologist is frequently limited to interpretation of standard chest roentgenograms. A radiologist able to combine his specific technical expertise in MRI with knowledge in cardiology should be able to contribute substantially to the clinical management of heart diseases.

This book both provides a description of the essential features of cardiovascular MRI and covers all aspects of morphological and functional pathology of the heart and the great vessels in a clear and didactic fashion.

As one of the editors of this book series I do hope that this volume will inspire radiologists to overcome their traditional reluctance to enter the field of cardiac radiology and that they will find this book a useful practical tool in their daily clinical activity. In addition this book will serve very well the needs of cardiologists and cardiac surgeons willing to integrate cardiovascular MR into their clinical practice.

On behalf of the editors of this book series I would like to express my sincere gratitude to the editors of this volume for their enormous efforts in planning, preparing, and writing this book with the help of a select group of international experts in the field.

Leuven   ALBERT L. BAERT

Preface

Since its introduction in the medical field in the early 1980s, magnetic resonance (MR) has become an increasingly important imaging modality with which to study the human body. It combines superior contrast and spatial resolution with multiplanar imaging capability in a fast and totally noninvasive manner. Magnetic resonance is probably the most rapidly evolving technique in the cardiovascular domain, and further MR sequences and applications will no doubt soon become available. Against this background of rapid progress, it remains the intention of this book to provide the reader with a comprehensive survey of all clinical applications of MR in the study of the heart and graet vessels, to discuss its limitations, and to compare this technique with the other cardiac imaging modalities. Since many of our readers may not yet be familiar with cardiovascular MR, a discription is provided of its more essential features including a chapter on technical aspects of cardiovascular MR and a chapter on the normal cardiovascular anatomy with MR. In the following chapters, all facets of cardiovascular MR are discussed using an anatomical rather than a disease-oriented approach, e.g. pericardial disease, myocardial disease, valvular heart disease, coronary artery disease, and great vessels.

One of the major strengths of cardiac MR is unquestionably the potential to study ventricular function, myocardial perfusion, and myocardial metabolism very accurately. These topics are therefore discussed in separate chapters. Moreover, an entire chapter is devoted to the increasing role of MR (and specific MR contrast agents) in the assessment of myocardial viability in ischemic heart disease. The non invasive character of MR and the potential not only to visualize cardiac morphology but also the evaluate cardiac function and flow patterns make this technique very appealing in the assessment and follow-up of patients with congenital heart disease. A specific chapter is dedicated to congenital heart disease. Finally, the availability of active multi device MR-tracking must be considered a significant step towards the clinical realization of interventional MR angiography. Therefore, the preliminary results in this fascinating domain are discussed in a separate chapter.

We gratefully thank all those who were involved in the preparation of this book. Without their help and expertise it would not have been possible to achieve our goal. This book is offered in the hope that the reader will be convinced of the huge potential of MR in the study of the heart and great vessels.

Leuven   JAN BOGAERT
Los Angeles   ANDRÉ J. DUERINCKX
Leuven   FRANK E. RADEMAKERS

Contents

1 Techniques for Cardiac MRI

H. BOSMANS

CONTENTS

1.1
Basic Principles of Cardiac MRI

1.1.1
Introduction

Cardiac magnetic resonance imaging (MRI) relies on exactly the same basic principles as other MRI techniques (RAJAN 1997). During an examination, the patient is brought into a huge static magnetic field that aligns the spins of the human body. These spins can be excited and subsequently detected with coils. Their signal is influenced by two relaxation times (T1 and T2), proton density, flow and motion, changes in susceptibility, molecular diffusion, magnetization

H. BOSMANS, PhD, Department of Radiology, University Hospitals Gasthuisberg, Catholic University of Leuven, Herestraat 49, B-3000 Leuven, Belgium

transfer, etc. The timing of the excitation pulses and the successive magnetic field gradients determine the image contrast.

1.1.2
Basic Characteristics of the Spins

The nucleus of a proton is sensitive to the presence of a magnetic field. Its interaction with this field can be described via a property that has been called a "spin." This spin or magnetic moment precesses with a specific frequency, the Larmor frequency, around the magnetic field. The larger the magnetic field strength, the higher will be the precessional frequency. Considering a large group of spins, such as present in any tissue sample, the net effect is an alignment of these spins with the magnetic field. A radiofrequency (RF) pulse whose frequency matches with the Larmor frequency can destroy this alignment. Quantum electrodynamics is required for a thorough description of this resonance phenomenon. For MRI techniques, the important thing is that after the RF pulse, the tissue has a net magnetic moment that is no longer aligned with the field. The magnetic moment of the tissue can be considered to be the sum of a small magnetic moment that is still aligned with the field, the so-called longitudinal magnetization, and a component perpendicular to the field, the transverse magnetization. The angle between the magnetic field and the spin is called the "flip angle" (Fig. 1.1). The flip angle is small after a short, low-energy RF pulse. In most traditional acquisition techniques, the flip angle is 90°. A 180° pulse inverts the net magnetic moment. It is called an inversion recovery (IR) pulse if it is the purpose to invert the magnetization with regard to the static magnetic field. The same pulse applied to spins in the transverse plane acts as a refocusing pulse.

After excitation, the spins will gradually return to their original position, aligned with the field, as this is energetically the most favorable situation. Therefore, their magnetic component along the magnetic

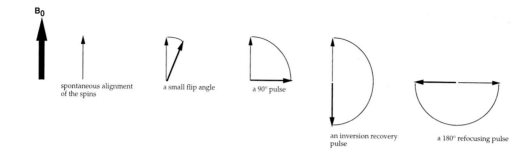

Fig. 1.1. The effect of resonant radiofrequent pulses on a spin system

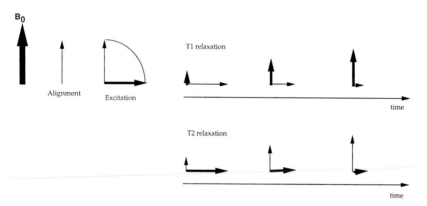

Fig. 1.2. The T1 and T2 relaxation times. The T1 relaxation time describes the relaxation of the longitudinal magnetization after an RF pulse. T2 describes the relaxation of the transverse component

field has to increase; the component in the transverse plane has to gradually disappear (Fig. 1.2). The first process is described by a T1 relaxation time. A tissue with a long T1 recovers slowly after an RF pulse; the spins of tissues with short T1 align very quickly with the magnetic field. The component in the transverse plane disappears after the excitation pulse. Tissues in which the transverse magnetization is rapidly lost are said to have a short T2. The T1 and T2 relaxation processes have a major influence on the image contrast in most MR images.

The proton density of the spins is related with the net magnetic moment of the tissues due to the presence of the static field. Tissues with low proton density have a smaller net magnetic moment than tissues with a very dense distribution of protons.

1.1.3
Measurement Schemes of Proton Density, T1-, and T2-Weighted Images

The proton density of the tissues can be measured in a straightforward way: with all the spins maximally aligned with the magnetic field, a 90° RF excitation

pulse is applied. The signal in the transverse plane is measured as soon as possible, before any relaxation phenomenon can have an influence (Fig. 1.3a). The time in between the RF pulse and the measurement is defined as "echo time" (TE). For proton density weighted measurements, the TE is as short as possible. This type is only seldom used in cardiac MRI.

T1-weighted images show the differences in T1 relaxation between adjacent pixels. A T1-weighted measurement therefore starts with an RF excitation pulse of, as an example, 90°. After a period of typically 500 ms, the differences in longitudinal components are largest. At that moment, a new RF pulse is given to tilt the spins into the transverse plane and make them visible for the measuring coils. The measurement is then performed as soon as possible, before the T2 effect changes the signal in the transverse plane (Fig. 1.3b). T1-weighted measurements also require a short TE.

As the T2 effect manifests itself in the transverse plane, the detector can readily measure the T2-weighted signals (Fig. 1.3c). Typical echo times in cardiac MRI are 40–120 ms.

The information in T1- and T2-weighted acquisitions is often complementary, as illustrated in Fig.

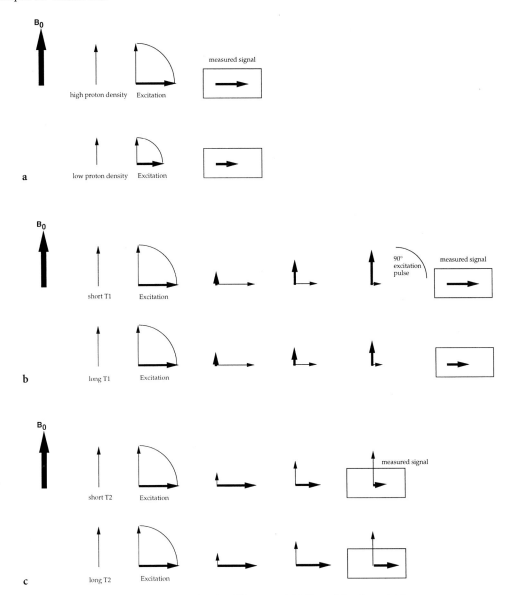

Fig. 1.3. Measurement schemes for (**a**) proton density, (**b**) T1-, and (**c**) T2-weighted acquisitions

1.4. Proton density weighted images are usually not part of a routine cardiac protocol.

1.1.4
MR Sequences

A single measurement of proton density, T1-, or T2-weighted signals does not provide enough information to reconstruct a complete image, as the detector as such cannot correlate the signal with the position where it originated from. A detailed discussion on how the spatial encoding is performed is beyond the scope of this text, but can be found in any basic MR textbook (RAJAN 1997). The procedure is based on the Larmor equation, namely that the precessional frequency of the spins is proportional to the magnetic field at the location of the spin. In practice, magnetic field gradients are applied over the patient. Along a certain direction, e.g., from caudal to cranial, the precessional frequency of the spins then changes (Fig. 1.5a). As an RF pulse with a specific RF frequency will excite only the spins with the corresponding precessional frequency, the use of a magnetic field gradient makes it possible to selectively excite only the spins of a thin slice (Fig. 1.5b).

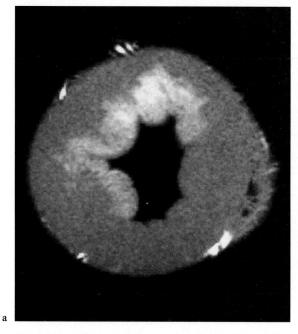
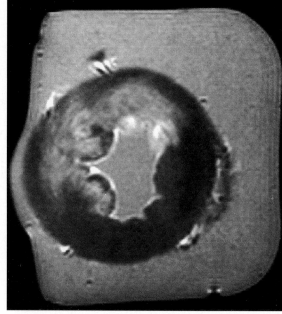

Fig. 1.4 a,b. The complementary nature of T1- and T2-weighted acquisitions is illustrated in the postmortem study of a dog with a myocardial infarct following a 2-h occlusion of the left anterior descending coronary artery. **a** T1-weighted acquisition, after injection of an infarct-avid contrast agent that shortens the T1, nicely shows the infarcted tissue. **b** The T2-weighted acquisition shows hyperintense signal intensities in edematous tissue

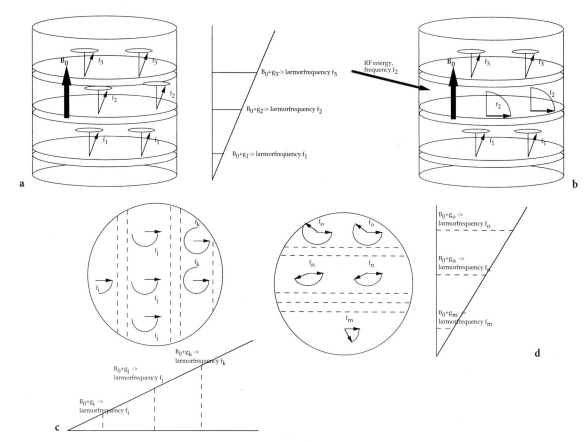

Fig. 1.5 a–d. Techniques for position encoding. **a** A magnetic field gradient induces different Larmor frequencies in the tissues. **b** A radiofrequent pulse with frequency f_2 excites only the spins with frequency f_2. **c** The in-plane position encoding for the columns is performed with a magnetic field gradient during the measurement. **d** The position encoding for the rows in the image is performed with a magnetic field gradient along this direction, in between excitation and signal measurement

During the measurement of the signal, another magnetic field gradient is applied along another direction in the excited slice, e.g., from left to right, and defined as the read-out direction. As a consequence, spins of different columns in the excited image precess with a different frequency and the measured signal consists of magnetic moments with different frequency (Fig. 1.5c). If this particular signal is measured during N successive time points, it is possible to redistribute the signals afterwards over N different columns. The necessary mathematical technique to perform this "column reconstruction" technique is the well-known Fourier transform.

In order to create differences between the different rows in an image, an encoding scheme has to be used for this direction too. A third magnetic field gradient is applied between RF excitation pulse and signal read out. It forces the spins of different rows onto a different frequency during a certain time (Fig. 1.5d). The result of this magnetic field gradient will be another phase for spins of different rows. This technique is called "phase encoding." In practice, if an image of M rows × N columns is required, M different phase encoding gradients have to be applied on the same group of spins. A series of successive measurements is therefore necessary. The time in between successive RF excitation pulses is called the repetition time (TR). All the measurements are written in the raw data plane and two-dimensional (2D) Fourier transform of these data is performed.

Because of the common mathematical use of the parameter "k" in Fourier calculations, the raw data space is often called the "k-space."

In a conventional MR acquisition technique, the total measurement time for an image with matrix M × N is M × TR, occasionally further multiplied by the number of signal averages or number of excitations (NEX). The total series of excitation pulses, magnetic field gradients, and measurements is defined as the "MR sequence" (Fig. 1.6).

In three-dimensional (3D) acquisition techniques, a very thick slice or slab is being excited. A phase encoding technique similar to the in-plane phase encoding scheme is used to encode different slices ("partitions") within this slab. If P partitions have to be reconstructed, M × N × P measurements have to be performed. If no signal averaging is used, the total measurement for this 3D acquisition technique is M × P × TR.

The k-space has a very crucial role in MRI. The total amount of data in the k-space determines the image matrix. In principle, a raw data space of M × N pixels gives rise to an image with matrix M × N. A 3D k-space leads to a 3D image set. If an M × N k-space is only partially filled with data, high-quality M × N images can occasionally be obtained using dedicated reconstruction schemes. This is the case in half Fourier acquisition schemes, such as in HASTE (half Fourier single shot turbo spin-echo) (STEHLING et al. 1996).

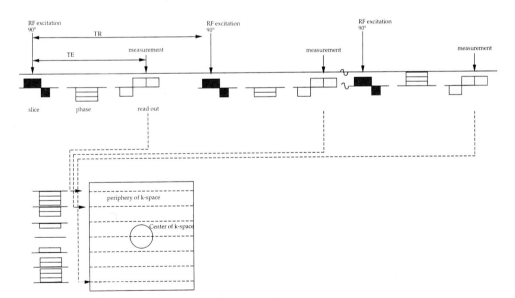

Fig. 1.6. Overview of an MR sequence: a series of slice selective excitation, phase encoding, and signal read-out is performed, filling the raw data space line by line

All data in k-space have experienced another amount of phase encoding and read out gradients. Those which have experienced the strongest gradients are written near the periphery of the k-space; it are these which make the greatest contribution to the final image resolution. The data samples acquired with the weakest gradients are saved in the center of k-space. They have a major influence on the image contrast. The relative gray values in the images reflect the contrast present during the acquisition of the center of k-space data.

1.1.5
Gradient Echoes and Spin Echoes

A maximal net signal of a group of spins occurs when all the individual spins are well aligned or "in phase." Misalignment or "dephasing" occurs due to differences in precessional frequency. Some of the dephasing effects are strictly desirable and necessary, such as the T2 effect (which is a dephasing effect at the microscopic level) and dephasing due to encoding gradient. Local inhomogeneities in the magnetic field, however, also manifest themselves as incoherence in the phase behavior, a phenomenon called the T2* effect. In cardiac MRI, this is most obvious at the lung–heart tissue transitions or in the neighborhood of metallic implants. Flowing blood in the great vessels and in the cavity is also subject to large phase variations. This type of phase effect is discussed in the next section.

Unfortunately, the detector cannot differentiate between the influence of the phase encoding schemes and these other factors. The best technical solution to get rid of the effects of local inhomogeneities is the acquisition of "spin echoes" (SE). In these MR schemes, a 180° (refocusing) pulse is applied exactly halfway between the RF pulse and signal acquisition. Spins with the largest phase angle due to a slightly higher local magnetic field acquire the largest negative phase angle after the 180° pulse. However, as the enlarged magnetic field is still present after this pulse, these spins still have a faster precessional frequency. At the echo time, the effect of the slightly enlarged magnetic field is overcome (Fig. 1.7).

In gradient-echo (GE) acquisitions, the 180° refocusing pulse is not applied. Therefore the TE can be much shorter. Keeping the TE very short is another means to reduce dephasing effects. GE techniques play an important role in cardiac MRI because they can be used to depict dynamic phenomena such as

myocardial contraction, motion of valve leaflets, and blood flow.

1.1.6
Flow Effects

Most MR sequences presume that the spins in the tissues do not move during the procedure. As an example, it is considered that a positive magnetic field gradient can be compensated by a negative magnetic gradient with the same gradient amplitude and the same duration (Fig. 1.8a). For flowing spins, such as those in the great vessels or in the coronary arteries, this assumption is not valid. Spins moving along the direction of a magnetic field gradient ac-

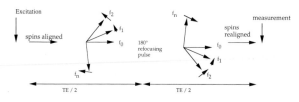

Fig. 1.7. An SE acquisition uses a 180° refocusing pulse to compensate for differences in Larmor frequencies induced by inhomogeneities in the magnetic field

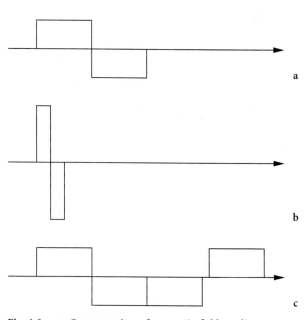

Fig. 1.8 a–c. Compensation of magnetic field gradients can be performed with: **a** regular bipolar pulses, which gives rise to flow-induced phase artifacts; **b** ultrashort bipolar pulses, which suppresses phase artifacts; **c** flow-compensated gradients, which refocuses the phase of spins flowing with a constant velocity

quire a phase angle that depends on the magnetic field and on their flow. Therefore, a simple negative pulse does not compensate for a positive gradient. In most sequences, this effect causes an incomplete visualization of the vessels, and ghost images can be observed of the great vessels and of the cavity along the phase-encoded direction. The following techniques are known to overcome flow-induced phase effects: shortening of the pulses and consequently also of TE (Fig. 1.8b) and the application of three dedicated magnetic field gradients instead of bipolar pulses (Fig. 1.8c).

A paradoxical signal enhancement of flowing blood is observed in GE acquisitions whenever the spins experience only a restricted number of RF excitation pulses and then disappear from the imaged volume. Hence, the continuous refreshment or inflow of the spins ensures a maximal alignment of spins with the external field prior to the excitation pulses. Compared with the partially relaxed signals in the stationary tissues, subjected to a long series of RF pulses, the signal in the vessel can therefore be very strong (Fig. 1.9a). This characteristic is the basis for "time-of-flight" (TOF) MR angiography acquisitions. Even without the use of contrast agents, these images show hyperintense signals in the vessels. This principle is robust as long as the spins in the blood experience only a few pulses before being refreshed. In practice, images are acquired perpendicular to the vessels. To visualize the aortic dissection in Fig. 1.9b, TOF images were acquired perpendicular to the

aorta. Vessels with a long segment in the slice show a gradual signal decrease due to saturation.

For some applications, flow-induced phase effects caused by extra bipolar pulses are exploited to study the flow. Due to a bipolar pulse, flowing spins acquire a phase angle that is, in a first approach, proportional to the amplitude of the gradients, the time between the onset of the first and the second pulse, and, most importantly, the velocity of the spins (whenever their motion can be described by a constant velocity flow during the application of the gradients). Under well-controlled conditions, the velocity of the spins can thus be measured from the phase angles. A typical flow-encoded phase image is shown in Fig. 1.10a. Measuring the phase angle over the cardiac cycle permits the calculation of the mean flow over, for example, the descending aorta, as shown in Fig. 1.10b. This phase effect is used to study the flow patterns (see also Chap. 11). The range of velocities that can be measured is determined by the gradients and generally described by the VENC (the strength of the velocity encoding bipolar pulse).

Using the same type of bipolar pulses, angiographic images can be made. Four measurements are usually performed: a normal (phase compensated) acquisition and phase encoded acquisitions with bipolar pulses along the x, the y, and the z direction. After subtracting the measured magnetic vectors induced by the spins in an encoded series from the spin vectors of a compensated series, there is, in theory,

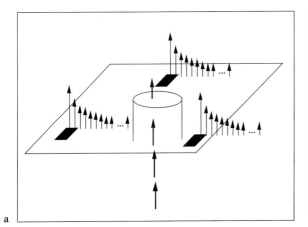

a

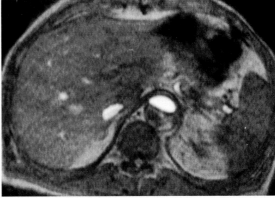

b

Fig. 1.9 a,b. The inflow effect can be exploited to visualize the vessels. **a** The signal intensity is hyperintense in the vessels due to a continuous inflow of spins with fully aligned magnetization. The signal in the stationary tissue saturates gradually and therefore has a low steady state value during the larger part of the acquisition. **b** A 2D TOF acquisition in a patient with a dissection of the thoracoabdominal aorta shows a high signal in the patent true lumen and a low signal in the obliterated false lumen

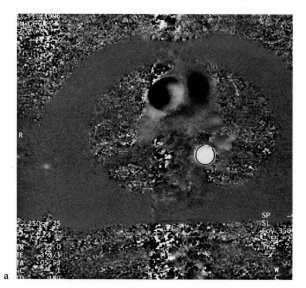

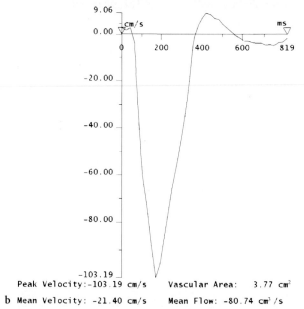

Peak Velocity: -103.19 cm/s   Vascular Area: 3.77 cm²

b Mean Velocity: -21.40 cm/s   Mean Flow: -80.74 cm³/s

Fig. 1.10 a,b. Flow-induced phase shifts can be evaluated in the phase images. **a** A flow-encoded phase image at the level of the descending thoracic aorta shows the lumen with hyperintense signal intensity. **b** From successive flow-encoded and rephased phase images, the flow in the vessel can be estimated over the cardiac cycle. The flow curve obtained in the descending aorta is negative because the blood flow is directed craniocaudally

1.1.7
Fast MRI Techniques

Magnetic resonance imaging is intrinsically a time-consuming process as it visualizes a relaxation behavior. For instance, T2-weighted SE measurements require a time in between RF pulse and signal read out of approximately 60 ms for optimal contrast. In a conventional T2-weighted SE measurement, a time delay of at least 2 s is required before the next excitation and signal read out can be performed. T2-weighted SE measurements that take 10 min are not an exception. The TR could be significantly shortened, only 1 NEX could be used, and the matrix could be reduced. However, both the contrast-to-noise ratios and the image resolution would be decreased. Gradient-echo acquisitions are another way to cope with the long acquisition times. Images are then T1 and T2* weighted.

Therefore, a better approach to increase the speed of SE techniques is to acquire a series of echoes per excitation pulse (ATKINSON and EDELMAN 1991). All of these echoes require another phase encoding such that they can be saved in the appropriate row of the k-space (Fig. 1.11). The group of lines acquired per RF pulse is usually called a k-space segment. Whenever N echoes are read out per pulse, the total imaging time reduces with N. It can be argued that these echoes are obtained at different echo times and that therefore an image with a strange mixture of image contrast will result. In practice, segmented k-space techniques acquire the k-lines belonging to the center of the k-space at a fixed TE time. As these lines have the major impact on the image contrast, the effective echo time of the sequence is defined as the time between the RF pulse and the acquisition of the raw data lines through the center of the k-space. Currently, many clinical trials are studying the performance of new fast acquisition schemes.

The same approach can be used to speed up GE acquisitions. Single shot echo planar imaging (EPI) is the fastest possible technique: it acquires the whole train of echoes after a single excitation pulse (Fig. 1.12) (EDELMAN et al. 1994; DAVIS et al. 1995).

1.1.8
Preparation Pulses

A preparation pulse creates a certain condition in the spin population prior to an RF pulse with signal read out. This notion is not new in MRI. Typical examples are saturation pulses and fat suppression pulses.

only signal left in the vessels. This MR angiographic technique is called "phase contrast imaging." Compared with a normal MR measurement, it takes 4 times longer, but it is a very efficient way to suppress the signal of the stationary tissues and therefore improve the contrast to noise ratios in the vessels.

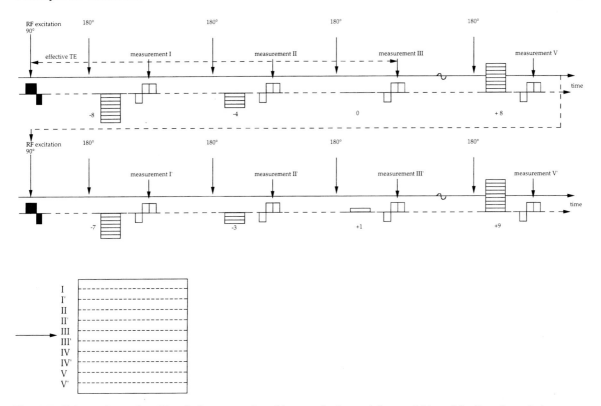

Fig. 1.11. Using turbo or fast SE techniques, a series of k-space lines (a so-called echo train) is acquired per excitation pulse. The effective echo time is defined as the time between excitation and the acquisition of the lines through the center of k-space

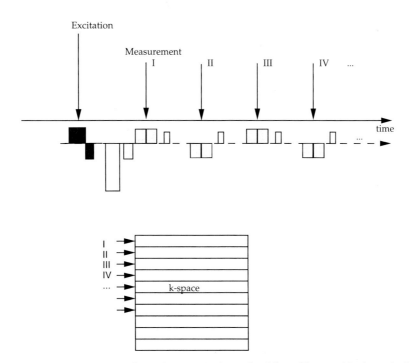

Fig. 1.12. The basic EPI acquisition consists of a single RF excitation pulse followed by a rapid echo train that fills the k-space completely

Other types of preparation pulse have been introduced, such as magnetization transfer pulses, vessel tracking pulses, etc. They are beyond the scope of this chapter.

1.1.8.1
Inversion Recovery Based Fat Suppression

The classical inversion recovery (IR) sequence starts with a 180° RF pulse that inverts the magnetization. After this pulse, the spin population relaxes: it realigns its magnetization with the external magnetic field. This relaxation behavior is, by definition, described by the T1 relaxation time. A time constant "inversion time" (TI) is associated with the use of this pulse: it defines the time in between the IR pulse and the actual measuring process. This sequence parameter could be set to optimize the T1-weighted contrast. Fat suppression is achieved with a TI of about 120 ms (Fig. 1.13). After this TI, the signal of the fat crosses the zero point. As the spins of the fat cannot be excited, they are absent in the subsequent image. An IR pulse can precede not only T1-weighted but also T2-weighted acquisitions. Usually, the IR pulse is repeated before each RF pulse. An exception is the turboFLASH measurement, where only one IR pulse is used, followed by a very fast (complete) GE acquisition (Fig. 1.14). The function of the IR pulse in this acquisition is to increase the image contrast. EPI acquisitions that consist basically of one (or a few) RF pulses followed by a fast

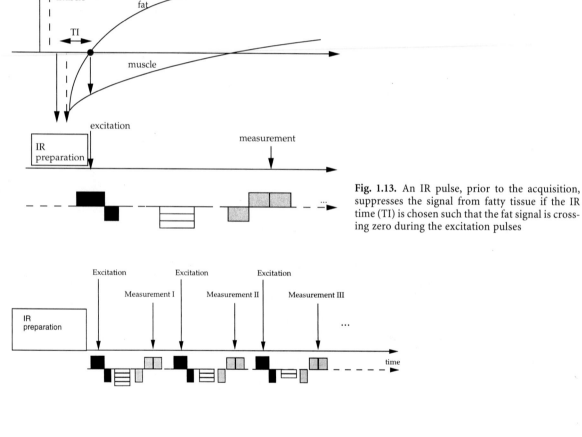

Fig. 1.13. An IR pulse, prior to the acquisition, suppresses the signal from fatty tissue if the IR time (TI) is chosen such that the fat signal is crossing zero during the excitation pulses

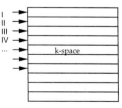

Fig. 1.14. A turboFLASH measurement consists of a single IR preparation pulse, followed by an ultrashort GE acquisition

train of GE acquisitions also use only one (or a few) IR pulses.

1.1.8.2
Chemical Shift Based Fat Suppression

Another technique for fat suppression consists of a 90° preparation pulse with a frequency that exactly matches with the Larmor frequency of the fat. Hence, under identical conditions, the Larmor frequencies of water and fat differ by a value that is called the chemical shift. In order to maximally suppress the fatty tissue signal, the time in between the fat saturating pulse and the regular RF excitation pulse has to be as short as possible.

1.1.8.3
Saturation Pulses

Saturation pulses are normal 90° RF excitation pulses that are applied on tissues prior to the measurement, thereby avoiding interference of their signal with the images. This is an efficient way to suppress image artifacts originating from a traceable source that does not have to be visualized in the image. A current limitation consists in the shape of these saturation pulses: only the signal in thin or thick "planes" can be suppressed. A very interesting application of these saturation pulses is the selective saturation of parts of the myocardium, as first described by ZERHOUNI et al. (1988). The saturated tissues can be used as noninvasive markers or "tags" to study the myocardial deformation and motion during the heart cycle (see Sects. 1.3.3.3 and 6.6).

1.2
Typical Aspects of Cardiac MRI

1.2.1
Introduction

Compared with other anatomical regions, the heart and great vessels present with specific characteristics, such as cardiac motion, respiratory motion, etc. Dedicated tools are required to cope with these peculiarities. During recent years, many conventional MR sequences have been adjusted for use in cardiac MRI (HIGGINS 1986). In this section, we discuss a series of tools that can be used in practice.

1.2.2
Cardiac Motion

The contraction of the heart muscle is a major determining factor in cardiac MRI. The straight application of a routine MRI protocol, such as a T2-weighted fast SE technique as used in neuroradiological applications, would result in unreadable images due to overwhelming motion artifacts.

1.2.2.1
Cardiac Gating Techniques

The devastating effects of cardiac contraction on the image quality can be significantly reduced by coupling the data acquisition to the cyclic motion of the heart, i.e., gating or triggering. Different methods are currently available. Acquisition of gated cardiac MR images is most commonly accomplished with electrocardiographic gating. Imaging is then performed after a fixed delay following the R wave of the surface electrocardiogram (ECG) (LANZER et al. 1985). However, it is important to consider that the surface electrodes also measure other electrical currents, such as those induced by the magnetic field on the blood flow in the cardiac chambers and vessels, i.e., magneto-hydrodynamic effects. The large flow of blood in the aorta during systole, for example, creates a relatively large electrical pulse, particularly at higher field strengths of 1.5 T. This pulse is superimposed on the normal T wave of the ECG. The degree of electrical potential produced by the magneto-hydrodynamic effect on the T wave can reach levels comparable to the R wave, and can be misinterpreted by the trigger device. Therefore, other triggering techniques such as pressure gating and pulse oximetry have been developed (PIROLO et al. 1992; DENSLOW and BUCKLES 1993), but these are less frequently used in clinical practice than the commercially available ECG triggering. ECG electrodes and leads made of carbon fiber minimize distortion and artifacts on MR images obtained during ECG gating. These materials cause no image degradation and, because the leads are reinforced with plastic, they are less vulnerable to bending than leads made of graphite (VAN GENDERINGEN et al. 1989).

Three ECG electrodes are placed ventrally or dorsally on the patient's skin close to the position of the heart. Special care needs to be taken to achieve best positioning of the electrodes. They should be on those parts of the body least prone to motion (such as respiratory motion), for example on the patient's back when in the supine position. For a normally positioned heart, electrodes are placed on the patient's back along the middle of the shoulder, parallel to the spine. The longer electrode is placed just below the shoulder, and both of the shorter leads lower down, thereby forming a triangle. To reduce the induction of artifact potentials in the electrodes, each lead should be fully extended in its fixed position. In pathological conditions, the electrical axis of the heart can differ widely from the normal anatomical axis, and repositioning of the electrodes can be necessary. Furthermore it is important to note that a good contact between the electrodes and the surface of the skin is important.

1.2.2.2
Multislice and Multiphase Acquisition

The generally used approach to acquire a set of tomographic (2D) images covering the heart and great vessels is an ECG-triggered multislice acquisition (AMPARO et al. 1984). Most frequently, a SE technique is used with the TR adjusted to the length of the RR interval. A set of parallel images is acquired through the heart: the data for the most basal slice are acquired always immediately after the trigger pulse, followed by a more apical slice. The position encoding must be performed properly: in a conventional SE acquisition, the phase encoding gradient is incremented after each ECG pulse (Fig. 1.15a). Per heart cycle, one echo is acquired per image. This signifies that each image is acquired during a different period of the cardiac cycle (Fig. 1.15b,c). In other words, some of the images will be acquired during systole, others during diastole. It is therefore more appropriate to excite the series of slices in descending or ascending order rather than in an interleaved way, which is otherwise common practice in MR to reduce the cross-talk effect.

Another way to acquire the data is to excite and measure always the same slice at different time points during the cardiac cycle, i.e., the single slice multiphase approach (Fig. 1.16a). The multiphase approach is typically performed with GE acquisitions as they can be run with short TR times in between successive excitations. They are generally used to study dynamic phenomena of the heart such as the myocardial contraction (Fig. 1.16b,c) or the valve function. The number of phases that can be acquired over the heart cycle is calculated from the acquisition time per phase and the averaged RR interval. The

entire set of images can be loaded into an endless cine loop providing information on dynamic cardiac processes similarly to other cardiac imaging techniques such as echocardiography, however taking into account the fact that the MR images are not real-time images but are acquired over several heart beats.

Using faster acquisition schemes, a few k-lines can be acquired per image and per heart cycle. The k-space corresponding to one particular image is then filled with a fixed number of k-lines per heartbeat. This part of k-space is defined as a "segment," and the corresponding technique is a "segmented acquisition." Multiphase measurements of successive images can even share some data, which further shortens the acquisition time. Many of these techniques can therefore be run in breath hold (Fig. 1.16d,e).

1.2.2.3
Timing of the Acquisition During the Cardiac Cycle

Some MR techniques are very sensitive to motion artifacts and for this reason they should not be applied during systole and early diastole, when motion of the heart muscle is maximal. Using a time delay constant, it is possible to postpone the acquisition process over a certain period, for instance to mid-diastole, when the heart motion is minimal.

The minimal time between successive measurements of an identical cardiac phase is one heartbeat. For some applications, this time constant is too short. Most T2-weighted SE acquisitions require a time between successive excitations of about 2 s to allow for complete relaxation of the spins. For many T2-weighted SE acquisitions, the trigger signal should only activate the measurement after two or three heartbeats. This parameter of the MR sequence has to be specified in practice. T1-weighted SE acquisitions should be performed with a TR of about 500 ms. Currently no technique is available to shorten the effective TR using ECG triggering. In practice, T1-weighted acquisitions are often acquired with new acquisition schemes that have slightly different parameters (GE acquisitions, turboFLASH measurements, etc).

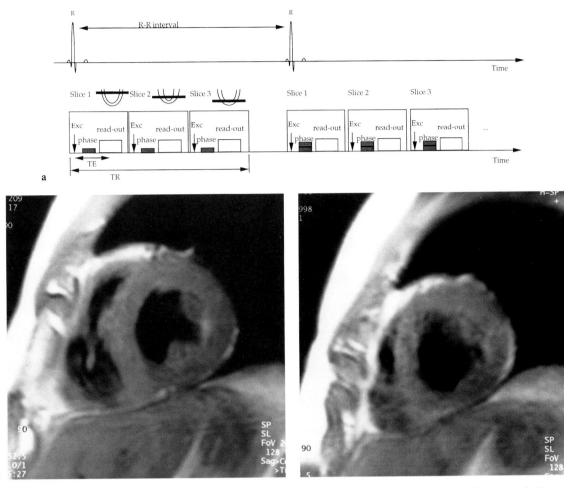

Fig. 1.15 a–c. Multislice acquisitions provide images of different positions, each acquired at a different cardiac phase. Their most common use is to study the cardiac or great vessel anatomy; **a** Measurement scheme; **b** T1-weighted SE image near the base of the heart; **c** T1-weighted SE image closer to the apex

1.2.2.4
Prospective Versus Retrospective Triggering

Both prospective and retrospective cardiac triggering can be used. The first technique is the more traditional approach: after each trigger pulse, phase encoding tables are incremented and an otherwise identical series of measurements is performed. The total acquisition time is equal to the averaged RR interval, multiplied by the number of lines in the image and the number of signal averages (divided by the echo train length or the number of k-space lines per segment, if applicable). For most acquisitions, the changes in effective TR due to changes in RR interval do not lead to artifacts. There are, however, exceptions. Retrospective gating enables a continuous succession of excitation and data read out. Phase encoding tables are incremented after a fixed time,

calculated a priori from an estimated averaged RR interval. The ECG is recorded during the measurement, and after this measurement, signals are redistributed over the k-space according to their timing over the cardiac cycle. The total acquisition time is necessarily longer, to ensure the complete coverage of the heartbeat for each phase encoding increment. Usually, image quality is similar to that of prospectively gated acquisitions (Fig. 1.16f,g).

1.2.3
Respiratory Motion

Respiration and the associated motion of the organs in the thorax and the abdomen are well-known problems in MRI. This kind of motion superimposes on

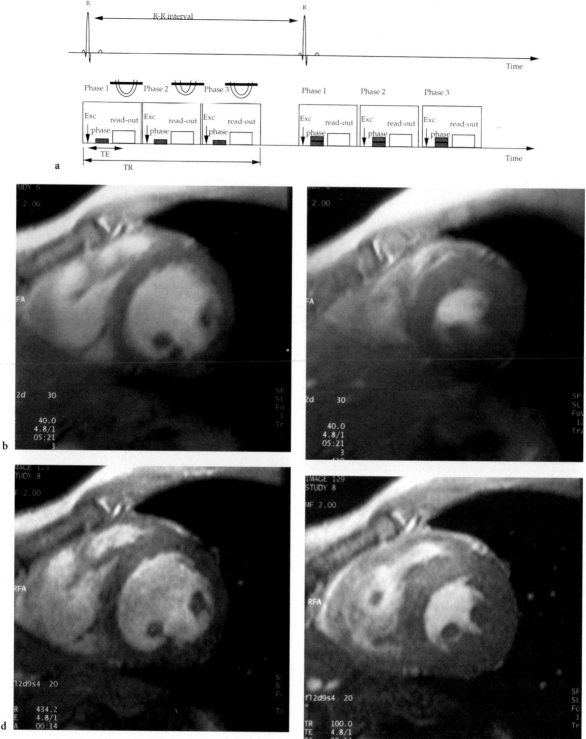

Fig. 1.16 a–g. Multiphase acquisitions acquire a series of images of the same position over the cardiac cycle. They allow study of the function of the heart. In practice, they can be shown with cine viewing. **a** Measurement scheme. **b, c** Study in a normal volunteer. End-diastolic (**b**) and systolic (**c**) images acquired with a conventional GE acquisition (TR/TE/Fl 40 ms/ 4.8 ms/30°, 3 Nex, acquisition time: 5 min 21 s). **d, e.** End-diastolic (**d**) and systolic (**e**) images acquired with a segmented GE acquisition (lines per segment: 9, echo sharing, acquisition time: 14 s). **f, g** Identical to **b** and **c**, but acquired using retrospective gating and 1 Nex (acquisition time: 3 min 26 s)

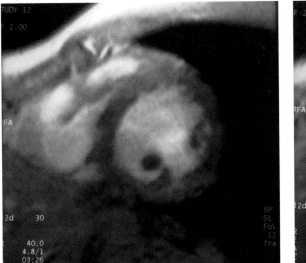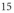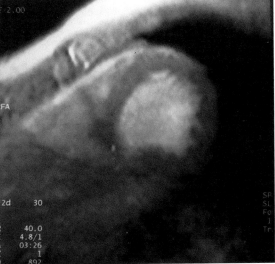

f   g

Fig. 1.16. *Continued*

the cardiac contraction and is of approximately equal importance for image quality.

1.2.3.1
Signal Averaging

From early experience with MRI, it is known that increasing the number of signal averages decreases motion artifacts in the images. However, as the total acquisition time is proportional to this number, this approach can be very time-consuming. In addition, even for properly adjusted T1-weighted SE techniques, good results cannot be guaranteed.

1.2.3.2
Respiratory Gating

Similar to cardiac triggering, acquisitions can be triggered by the respiratory cycle. Hence, use of a device that indicates expiration or inspiration, excitation and signal read out can be performed during a certain phase only. In practice, such pulses can be obtained from measuring the expansion of a belt during respiration. Cardiac and respiratory gating may even be combined. There is, however, one serious disadvantage of this procedure, namely that acquisitions become very long. As one respiratory cycle easily takes about 5 s, the minimal effective TR for this acquisition would be 5 s.

1.2.3.3
Cardiac MRI During a Single Breath Hold

Many developments in MRI have gone in the direction of techniques that can be acquired during a single breath hold. Gradient-echo acquisitions are frequently used as an alternative to T1-weighted SE acquisitions. However, as increasing the number of lines per excitation pulse increases the total acquisition window per heart cycle, but reduces the acquisition time, a compromise is required in practice. Typically nine lines and echo sharing can be acquired per heartbeat (Fig. 1.16d,e).

A turboFLASH or fast-FLASH acquisition is a single shot technique with TR/TE minimal and an IR preparation pulse to improve the image contrast (Fig. 1.14). A typical example is shown in Fig. 1.17a. For some applications, this total acquisition window is too long or constraints may arise from the ultrashort TR/TE, such as poor signal-to-noise ratios (SNRs) and large fields of view (MATSUDA et al. 1994). Segmented turboFLASH techniques have been developed based on the same schemes as the turboFLASH technique, but filling only a part of the k-space per heart cycle (Fig. 1.17b). These acquisitions can still be performed during a breath hold.

T2-weighted acquisitions can also be performed with fast acquisition schemes. Both fast SE (Fig. 1.17c) and EPI-based techniques have been explored. The echo train length that can be accepted for T2-weighted imaging is subject to the same type of compromise as segmented FLASH acquisitions. There is

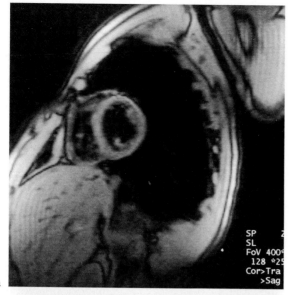

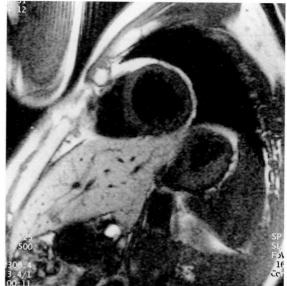

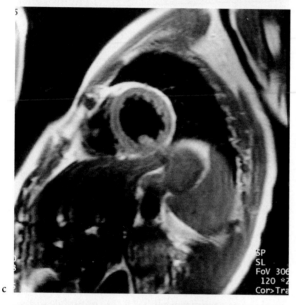

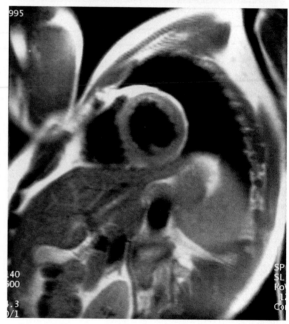

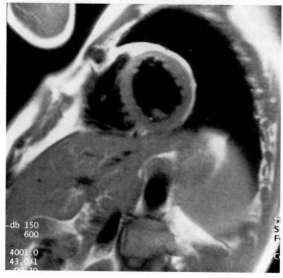

Fig. 1.17 a–e. Overview of rapid acquisition techniques in a normal volunteer. **a** TurboFLASH acquisition, TE 2.3 ms, Fl 15°, dark blood preparation pulse, acquisition time 1 s, no breath hold required. **b** Segmented turboFLASH acquisition, 33 lines per segment, TE 4.8 ms, TI 450 ms, acquisition time 15 s, breath holding required. **c** Turbo or fast SE acquisition with black blood preparation pulse, echo train length 15, TE 57 ms, effective TR 210 ms, total acquisition time 24 s, acquisition during breath holding. **d** Single shot HASTE with black blood preparation pulse, TE 43 ms, total acquisition time <300 ms, no breath holding. **e** Segmented HASTE with black blood preparation pulse, TE 43 ms, total acquisition time 3 s

a trade-off between total acquisition time and image sharpness. A single shot version of the fast (turbo) SE acquisition that fills only half of the k-space yields high-quality images (with the use of a black blood preparation pulse, see Sect. 1.2.4.5). The total acquisition window is currently still about 400 ms for a 160 × 256 matrix (Fig. 1.17d). A segmented HASTE acquisition fills only part of the k-space per heartbeat and requires breath holding (Fig. 1.17e). EPI acquisitions can be run as a single shot, taking approximately 100 ms, or the acquisition can be spread over a few heartbeats (Davis et al. 1995).

1.2.3.4
Navigator Echo Acquisitions

The ultimate goal for cardiac MRI could be the acquisition of snapshot images with high spatial and/or temporal resolution, in which breath holding is no longer a prerequisite. A few 2D sequences show promising results, but the resolution cannot be further increased because of intrinsic limitations even on state of the art equipment. For 3D imaging or time-consuming 2D acquisitions, automatic techniques have therefore been developed to track the position of the diaphragm and then perform acquisitions during specific phases of the respiratory cycle, without any need for patient cooperation. A noninvasive MR tool to provide this information consists of one signal read out of a sagittal slice through the thorax and the diaphragm, but not including the heart. This one line in k-space reflects the sagittal projection of the slice. Due to contrast differences between the diaphragm (liver) and the lungs, the level of the diaphragm can be determined from this one line. Successive measurements of this type show the motion of the diaphragm (Fig. 1.18a). A specific part of the respiratory cycle can be determined via a threshold value. Once the threshold value is reached, a trigger pulse can be generated and a regular acquisition scheme starts, until a second threshold value terminates the acquisition window. In practice, such extraordinary acquisitions are performed intermittently, during the regular acquisition. The normal data are continuously generated, but at a trigger signal determined from the navigator echo technique, and during a user-defined interval, phase encoding is incremented and the signals are written to the k-space for further reconstruction. This acquisition mode takes more time than regular schemes. Respiratory motion is usually frozen, which results in high-quality images (Fig. 1.18b). This particular technique has been developed for applications that are not feasible during a breath hold, in regular acquisitions where there is a need for a better resolution and/or SNR, and in patients who cannot cooperate. This technique is being investigated to better visualize the coronary arteries (Muller et al. 1997).

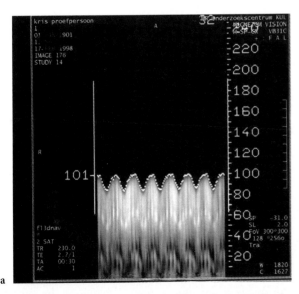

a

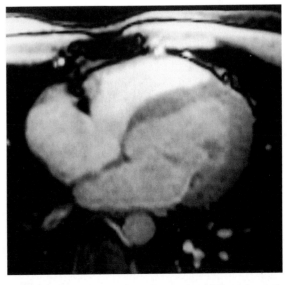

b

Fig. 1.18 a,b. 3D GE acquisition with respiratory gating by means of the acquisition of navigator echoes. **a** Position of the diaphragm as obtained with the navigator echo technique.

b The 3D GE acquisition shows images in which motion artifacts are absent

1.2.4
Flow in the Cavity

The pumping action of the heart is the cause of high velocities and accelerations or decelerations in the blood pool. As in other regions of the body where large arteries produce ghost artifacts in certain acquisitions, dedicated approaches are necessary for cardiac MRI.

1.2.4.1
Spin-Echo Acquisitions with Extra Bipolar Pulses

In some SE acquisitions, extra, bipolar magnetic field gradients are applied to increase the phase incoherence of flowing spins and in this way destroy any signal in the cavity. This is a practical application of the basic MR principle that states that artifacts can be avoided by nulling the signal of the disturbing tissue prior to signal read out.

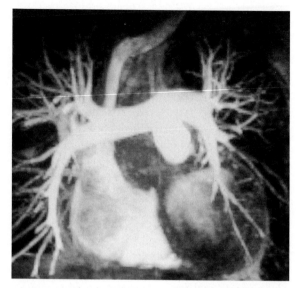

Fig. 1.19. Ultrafast contrast-enhanced MR angiography acquisition, TR/TE/Fl 3.8 ms/1.3 ms/25°, 42 partitions, total acquisition time only 16 s, is a robust and noninvasive technique to visualize the great vessels such as the pulmonary arteries

1.2.4.2
Saturation Pulses

Another way to null the signal is by using saturation pulses. However, the blood in the cavity cannot be completely saturated with the currently available shapes of saturation pulses. Saturation pulses parallel to the imaged slice could be considered for short-axis acquisitions.

1.2.4.3
Flow-Compensating Gradients

Another approach consists in the use of flow-compensated magnetic field gradients. In a particular sequence, every couple of a negative and a positive magnetic field gradient is then replaced by three dedicated new gradients. In some sequences, spins flowing with a constant velocity in between excitation and signal read out then remain in phase. The signal even becomes bright and the cavity does not provoke artifacts, as there is no dephasing.

1.2.4.4
Ultrashort Echo Times

An ultrashort time between excitation and signal read out prevents the development of dephasing problems. On state of the art MR systems, TEs as short as 1–2 ms can be obtained. Ghost artifacts and even flow-induced dephasing are then absent. These types of acquisition are the basis of current (contrast-enhanced) MR angiography acquisitions (Fig. 1.19).

1.2.4.5
Black Blood Preparation or PRESTO Pulses

Recently, a new preparation pulse has been developed that suppresses the signal in the cavity (Fig. 1.20) (STEHLING et al. 1996). It consists of a 180° (inversion) pulse applied over a large part of the heart, including the slice to be imaged. A slice-selective 180° pulse immediately follows this pulse. This sequence is called preceding inversion recovery preparing pulse pair (PRESTO). This pulse cancels the effects of the first pulse in the stationary tissues in the particular slice. In the ideal situation, there is no net effect for the spins in the myocardium. Most spins in the blood pool and especially those with high velocity experience only parts of the two pulses. Their signal is significantly reduced and/or partly inverted. A black signal in the cavity will occur with the image acquisition process starting at the time when the spins in the cavity have no net magnetization. The optimal TI between the preparation pulses

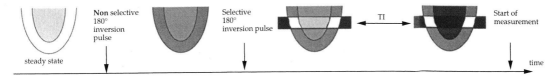

Fig. 1.20. A black blood preparation pulse consists of (1) a nonselective 180° pulse that inverts the signal of all the tissues, (2) a slice selective 180° pulse that reinverts the signal of the particular slice, as well as some signal in the cavity, (3) a time delay to further null the signal of the blood in the cavity

and image acquisition is patient and flow dependent. Usually a TI of about 600 ms is a good compromise. In practice, the pulse is used prior to single shot techniques or acquisitions with a long echo train length, in which it is a very helpful and robust technique, not only to suppress the artifacts from the cavity but also to better delineate the myocardium. In acquisitions with a short TR, such as segmented FLASH acquisitions for dynamic studies, these pulses would prolong the total acquisition time too much.

Disadvantages of this pulse are that slowly flowing blood near the myocardium can be incompletely suppressed, and may appear hyperintense. Furthermore, parts of the myocardium can be partially suppressed, which would result in hypointense regions.

1.2.5
Poor Signal-to-Noise Ratios

Magnetic resonance imaging is intrinsically a technique providing very weak signals that furthermore depend on many parameters.

1.2.5.1
Acquisition Parameters

The type of acquired image determines the global SNR in the image. As an example, conventional T1-weighted SE measurements are known to provide stronger signals than T2-weighted SE techniques. Reducing the TE or increasing the flip angle, while keeping the TR sufficiently long, is also beneficial for the SNR. The recently developed T1-weighted acquisitions with extremely short TR/TE for contrast-enhanced MR angiography purposes are characterized by extremely poor SNR (except for SNR in the vessels as a result of the T1 shortening following bolus administration of paramagnetic contrast agents). A lower external magnetic field strength also gives rise to lower SNR and there exist many other factors that influence the SNR and therefore the choice of an appropriate image protocol.

Practical constraints with regard to image resolution or total acquisition time often originate from signal-to-noise considerations, as the SNR is proportional to (1) the voxel sizes and (2) the square root of the product of the number of phase encoding increments and the signal averages. A poor SNR may require the use of large voxel sizes or multiple signal averages.

The bandwidth that defines the gradient strength during the signal acquisition is a more hidden parameter. The higher the bandwidth, the quicker the read out, and the shorter can be the TE. Increasing the bandwidth, however, reduces the SNR.

1.2.5.2
Detector Efficiency

The efficiency of the detector is a coil parameter. The rule of thumb is to always choose the smallest possible coil with good characteristics. However, as the imaged volume may be large (a complete thorax), the largest coil is usually chosen: a body phased array coil or a (built in) circularly polarized coil (SAKUMA et al. 1996). Smaller surface coils can be used to image the parts of the heart closest to the chest wall. The patient has to be in the prone position in the magnet, which makes the examination rather uncomfortable. A major application for this approach is the visualization of the free wall of the right ventricle in patients suspected of having arrhythmogenic right ventricular dysplasia. Other applications include visualization of the left anterior descending coronary artery by means of 2D MR coronary angiography. Visualization of other parts of the coronary artery tree such as the left circumflex artery may be hampered by the insufficient penetration of the coil.

1.3
Protocols

In the following sections, the most frequently used cardiac MR protocols are considered. Each of these protocols is discussed from a technical point of view, mentioning the strengths and limitations of the MR sequences. Some of these protocols are discussed in more detail in the other chapters of this book. A routine cardiac MR study is always started with one or a series of scout images. Next, depending on the clinical question, different protocols are available to obtain accurate information on cardiac morphology, function, perfusion, etc.

1.3.1
Scout Image

Since the axes of the heart do not correspond to the body axes (see Chap. 2), one or a series of localizers or scout images is necessary to search for the anatomical plane best fitting the cardiac axis of interest. The first requirement for these acquisitions is that anatomical structures are recognized. Secondly, the acquisition should be as short as possible. Single shot techniques, preferably preceded by a black blood pulse (such as HASTE), can be used.

1.3.2
Cardiac Morphology

High image contrast and a sufficient spatial resolution characterize anatomical images of high quality. As explained in detail above, image contrast can be based on several parameters, of which T1 and T2 are the most frequently studied. The required weighting is in practice application dependent. For instance, the visualization of myocardial edema is optimal with a T2-weighted acquisition, whereas other lesions such as pericardial thickening benefit from T1-weighted measurements. The visualization of a lesion after an intravenous injection of a currently available gadolinium chelate also requires a T1-weighted approach.

1.3.2.1
T1-Weighted Acquisitions

Conventional T1-weighted SE techniques may suffer from disturbing motion artifacts, even when per-

formed with many signal averages and a long TE with extra bipolar pulses. Black blood pulses cannot be used, as the effective TR would increase beyond the limitations for T1-weighted imaging. Fast SE techniques, even when acquired during a breath hold, suffer from the same type of artifact (SEMELKA et al. 1992). Although very often used in literature, there is in practice no guarantee of reliable image quality. GE acquisitions with flow-compensating gradients or with ultrashort TE are quite robust with regard to motion artifacts. A first GE acquisition with a good T1-weighting is a multislice technique with a 90° flip angle and a very short TE. The measurement time would be equal to the averaged RR interval multiplied by the number of lines and the number of signal averages. Using a segmented GE approach can significantly reduce the acquisition time. A turboFLASH acquisition with a black blood preparation pulse is a single shot T1-weighted acquisition that is also free of motion artifacts. The spatial resolution of this type of acquisition can be improved with the segmented turboFLASH version. The delineation of the endocardium frequently benefits from contrast enhancement (Fig. 1.21).

1.3.2.2
T2-Weighted Acquisitions

T2-weighted sequences used to be very difficult for cardiac imaging. SE acquisitions completed with any

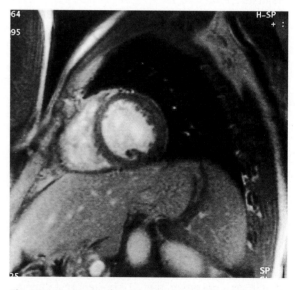

Fig. 1.21. Contrast-enhanced segmented turboFLASH acquisition shows hyperintense signals in the cavity, making delineation of the endocardium easier

possible tool to suppress motion artifacts are often of no clinical use. A breakthrough came with fast SE acquisitions using long echo trains and in which a black blood pulse suppresses the artifacts from the cavity (SEELOS et al. 1993). They are performed during a moderate to long breath hold and are run as single slice techniques. More recently, the single shot HASTE technique became available. It can be run without patient cooperation and is very robust with regard to motion artifacts. The segmented HASTE version again requires a minimum of breath holding (approximately 4 s). EPI provides T2*-weighted images. After careful shimming and fat suppression techniques, the total acquisition time is very short (LAMB et al. 1996).

1.3.3
Cardiac Function

As will be discussed more extensively in Chap. 6, accurate assessment of cardiac function remains one of the main goals of each technique dealing with cardiac imaging. Cardiac function can be assessed on different levels. The pump activity of the heart is usually expressed by the global (left or right) ventricular function (e.g., stroke volume, ejection fraction, cardiac output). The underlying mechanisms of this pump activity, i.e., myocardial contraction and relaxation, are expressed by regional functional parameters such as wall thickening and wall motion. Finally, while the basic element of myocardial contraction, i.e., sarcomere shortening, cannot be measured in vivo, information on fiber shortening can be obtained by means of MR myocardial tagging.

1.3.3.1
Global Ventricular Function

Several approaches are at present available to assess global ventricular function (see Chap. 6). Essentially, the volume of the ventricle has to be quantified at end diastole and end systole, i.e., end-diastolic and end-systolic volume. Subtraction of the two volumes yields the stroke volume. Other parameters such as cardiac output and ejection fraction can be calculated from these data. Usually single slice, multiphase GE acquisitions with small flip angle are used for this purpose. This acquisition is robust with regard to motion artifacts; the myocardium can be delineated due to hyperintense signals in the cavity

and has a sufficiently high temporal resolution to catch end diastole and end systole. In order to speed up this type of acquisition and perform it during a breath hold, segmented GE acquisitions can be used (BOGAERT et al. 1995; BLOOMGARDEN et al. 1997). The acquisition window per reconstructed cardiac phase then defines the temporal resolution of the images. k-Space segments of 9 lines per heartbeat are not uncommon. However, one has to realize that the longer the acquisition window, the more the images will be blurred by cardiac motion and the higher the risk that end diastole and/or end systole will be missed. Sharing of the measured raw data reduces these problems at least to a certain extent.

1.3.3.2
Regional Ventricular Function

Assessment of regional function relies on the same principles as assessment of global ventricular function, but rather than looking at changes in ventricular volumes, the myocardial deformation and wall motion are assessed throughout the cardiac cycle. Regional ventricular function can be assessed at rest or during stress conditions (e.g., exercise or dobutamine induced). Single slice, multiphase GE acquisitions are used for this purpose. A temporal resolution as low as 10 ms can be obtained. For most purposes, however, a time resolution of 10 ms is not required. For instance with a temporal resolution of 40 ms and a heart rhythm of 60 beats per minute, 25 images are obtained during the cardiac cycle. Next, the entire set of images can be loaded in an endless cine loop, providing dynamic information on the myocardial contraction and relaxation. In this way, wall motion and/or thickening can be qualitatively assessed (VAN RUGGE et al. 1993). A quantitative evalution of regional ventricular function is also feasible and can be based on the centerline method (VAN RUGGE et al. 1994). Segmented GE techniques can also be used to study the regional ventricular function. They are attractive since they can be performed during breath hold, which is appealing when one would like to evaluate the regional ventricular function during stress. As mentioned in the preceding section on the assessment of global ventricular function, the same limitations for segmented GE sequences remain valid.

1.3.3.3
MR Myocardial Tagging

Ultrasmall saturation pulses can be applied immediately after the ECG trigger signal and prior to a multiphase acquisition scheme. This RF excitation pulse tags specific parts of the myocardium by nulling the magnetization. The so-called tagged tissue will produce markedly decreased signal intensity during a certain period after the application of the saturation pulse. In a multiphase acquisition, the position of this tag can be traced.

Different types of tagged sequences have been developed (Zerhouni et al. 1988; Axel and Dougherty 1989;). The first uses normal saturation pulses, applying one RF pulse per tagging line. Tagging in the short-axis plane is then performed with a series of radial tagging lines through the center of the myocardium (Fig. 1.22). Parallel lines can be used on long-axis views of the heart. It is possible to merge the information of two such data sets to calculate the true 3D positions of the myocardium over the cardiac cycle. In a next step, it is possible to track the contraction of the left ventricle to calculate the strains in the ventricle and to estimate the related wall stress in particular regions.

Other centers apply a grid of tag lines on the image. Saturation is typically achieved with a series of flip angles, e.g., 30°, −60°, +60°, and −30°. A magnetic gradient modulates the phases of the spins, such that spins in a first series of lines end up with a 0° flip angle, and others, in other lines, experience effectively 90°. The latter are saturated. This technique is known as "SPAMM" (see Fig. 6.8). The acquisitions are straightforward, but post-processing (and in particular the 3D analysis) is more difficult.

1.3.4
Myocardial Perfusion

Perfusion measurements visualize the uptake of a contrast agent in the parenchyma (see also Chap. 8). The basic theory behind this is that, after the injection of a gadolinium chelate, the T1 and the T2 relaxation times of the perfused tissues shorten and that this shortening correlates with the uptake of the agent (Muhler 1995). Quantification of this uptake is difficult. First, using extracellular contrast agents there is a significant leakage of the agent to the extracellular tissues during the first-pass through the myocardium. As a result, the amount of contrast agent in the tissue is not proportional to the blood flow into the tissue. A second restriction results from the MR acquisition technique itself. Signal intensities are not necessarily proportional to the local concentrations of the contrast agent. Calibration curves that link the concentration of gadolinium chelates to the SNR have to be acquired. It is not appropriate to acquire data at fixed time points, due to variations in the heart cycle. Triggered acquisitions may induce signal changes in the images due to variations in the RR interval. Aside from a strict mathematical analysis, a more modest purpose can be to visualize regional differences in tissue perfusion. Figure 1.23 shows a perfusion study obtained in a dog during the intracoronary delivery of the 0.01 mmol/kg of Gd-DTPA and nicely shows the region of the myocardium perfused by the right coronary artery.

High image quality is not a basic requirement for perfusion studies. Hence, in principle, perfusion data could be matched with high-quality anatomical images. The major prerequisites for perfusion acquisitions are a short acquisition time and an adequate T1 or T2 weighting. In practice, ultrafast (subsecond) T1- and T2-weighted sequences have been used for perfusion measurements. The turboFLASH technique is a rapid GE technique that is very sensitive to small changes in T1 relaxation time. Theoretical problems may arise in the case of quantification. The heart beat of the patient can be very irregular, which is reflected in changes in the total relaxation behavior prior to a new 180° pulse of the turboFLASH measurement, and therefore slightly different signals can result. "Saturation-recovery fast FLASH" techniques, which start with a 90° pulse, overcome this problem, as the 90° pulse guarantees the nulling of the entire signal prior to the effective acquisition.

T2-weighted single shot techniques can have a GE or SE nature. In the literature, evidence is provided that the EPI approach is feasible for perfusion measurements (Saeed et al. 1994). Rigorous quantification of the tissue perfusion is difficult for the same reasons as in the case of turboFLASH measurements.

1.3.5
Flow Quantification

The insertion of a bipolar pulse into any normal sequence induces flow-related phase shifts in the acquired data. This characteristic, which is usually unwanted, is exploited in flow quantification tech-

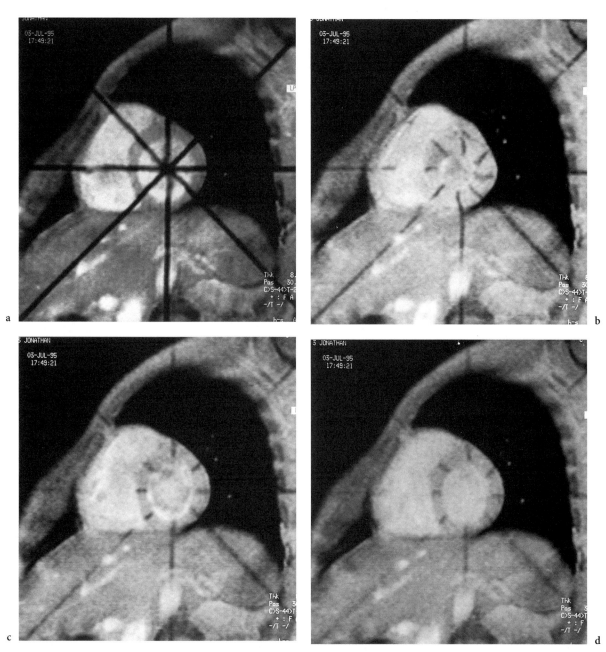

Fig. 1.22 a–d. In a tagging experiment, tissues are saturated and then measured to show the strain in the left ventricle. The example shows an example with radial tag lines: an end-diastolic (**a**), a systolic (**b**), an early diastolic image (**c**), and a late diastolic image (**d**)

niques. Magnetic field gradients applied in the through-plane direction require that the image be positioned perpendicular to the vessel. Gradients along the in-plane directions quantify the flow in the plane (LEE et al. 1997).

Data are known at discrete time points only. The more images that are acquired per heart cycle, the better will be the temporal resolution. Encoded and rephased images, necessary for good subtraction, are performed intermittently. The shorter the TR, the better can be the temporal resolution. Sometimes echo sharing is used to increase the temporal resolution and segmented GE techniques are applied to shorten the total acquisition time.

Flow quantification techniques do not require the injection of a contrast agent. Limitations can be summarized as follows:

- Optimal sequences have to be chosen for each specific clinical application (the VENC has to be chosen such that the majority of the spins will acquire a phase shift of about 180°).
- The examination is performed slice by slice.
- Quite long acquisition times are required for a sufficient spatial resolution.
- It is difficult to assess the flow in small and tortuous vessels such as in the coronaries (DAVIS et al. 1997).

1.3.6
MR Angiography

Until recently, the majority of the angiographic protocols for the great vessels of the chest were based on 2D TOF acquisitions (SEELOS et al. 1994). A similar approach has been used to visualize the proximal parts of the coronary arteries (BOGAERT et al. 1994). An acceptable image quality of the coronary arteries can be obtained if a series of measures is taken: the use of a small coil with the patient in the prone position; good cooperation of the patient concerning breath holding; adequate fat suppression; the use of dedicated acquisitions (special flip angles, etc); the use of carefully adjusted sequence parameters, such as delay times after the trigger pulse to ensure a mid-diastolic acquisition, etc. (Fig. 1.24).

Ultrafast 3D contrast-enhanced MR angiography has recently become a first choice for the visualization of the great vessels of the chest (LEUNG and DEBATIN 1997). Imaging of the vessels relies on a T1 shortening of the blood following a bolus injection of gadolinium chelates. Since the acquisition of the k-space (especially the central k-lines) has to take place at the time of the bolus passage inside the vessel of interest, a test bolus is strongly advisable to calculate the peak enhancement time in this vessel. Moreover, since the time between the arterial enhancement and the venous filling is extremely short, the acquisitions have to be well timed to avoid venous overlap (see Fig. 13.1). The total acquisition time, which relies mainly on the number of partitions acquired, varies in clinical practice between 7 and 27 s, and can be performed during breath hold. Furthermore, sequential angiographic measurements allow visualization of the passage of contrast medium in the thoracic vessels following injection in a cubital vein (e.g., first the pulmonary arteries and veins, followed by the thoracic aorta and its branches, and then, finally, the systemic venous return). Although many topics such as total dose, injection scheme, and total acquisition time are still under study, this ultrafast 3D angiographic acquisition is quite robust and very promising. Post-processing of the 3D data includes multiplanar reformatting (MPR) (Fig. 1.25a), maximum intensity projection (MIP) (Fig. 1.25b),

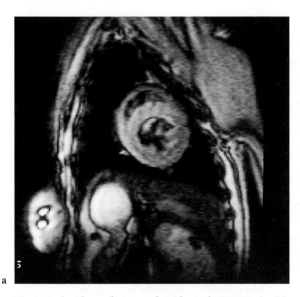

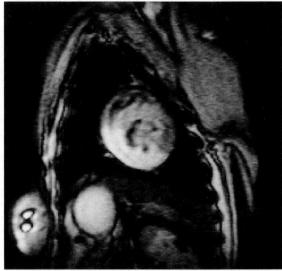

a   b

Fig. 1.23 a,b. The perfusion study with a turboFLASH acquisition, at a rate of one image per second, was performed in a dog model after an intracoronary injection of 0.01 mmol/kg of Gd-DTPA. **a.** Acquisition prior to the injection. **b** Acquisition during peak enhancement of the inferior left ventricular myocardial wall after selective injection of Gd-DTPA in the right coronary artery. This perfusion study demonstrates very nicely the vascular territory of this coronary artery

and virtual intra-arterial endoscopy. MPR provides tomographic images of the vessels in virtually any desired plane while MIP provides projections similar to conventional contrast angiography. Rotating these MIP images provides a 3D view of the thoracic vasculature. Virtual intra-arterial endoscopy is a form of "virtual reality" image processing capable of rendering internal views of the vessel walls.

1.3.7
MR Spectroscopy

Magnetic resonance spectroscopy (MRS) is another interesting application of the MR phenomenon. The basic characteristics that are exploited in MRS are differences in Larmor frequency due to the structure of molecules. MRS acquires the resultant magnetic signal of the spins after an excitation pulse. The signal is not position encoded in the usual way as in MRI. This so-called free induction decay (FID) is, however, a spectrum consisting of tissues with different Larmor frequencies. The goal is to characterize and to quantify metabolites. The techniques that can be used for cardiac MRS are explained in detail in Chap. 9.

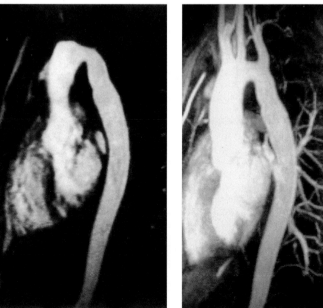

Fig. 1.24. ECG triggered 2D MR coronary angiography of the right coronary artery, using fat suppression. The total acquisition time is 16 s and acquisition is performed during breath hold. To improve image sharpness, the k-lines are acquired during diastasis (or mid-diastole), when the cardiac motion is minimal

1.4
Contraindications to Cardiac MRI

There are possible hazards associated with MRI. An MR system consists of a huge, static magnetic field in

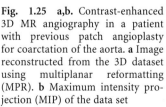

Fig. 1.25 a,b. Contrast-enhanced 3D MR angiography in a patient with previous patch angioplasty for coarctation of the aorta. **a** Image reconstructed from the 3D dataset using multiplanar reformatting (MPR). **b** Maximum intensity projection (MIP) of the data set

a

b

which, periodically during the measurements, RF energy is released. As electrically stimulated or ferromagnetic implants may interact with these components, it is absolutely necessary to carefully interview a patient prior to an MRI examination.

Ferromagnetic materials are, by definition, attracted by a magnetic field. Depending on the field strength, on the one hand, and on the size, shape, and orientation of the ferromagnetic material, on the other, huge forces can be exerted. As a result, ferromagnetic implants or devices (such as some valves and clips) may move in the magnetic field and potentially even dislodge with possible injury to the patient. In overview books of different implants, it is reported whether a particular material is attracted by static magnetic fields (SHELLOCK and KANAL 1994). These lists should be consulted for every implant of which the ferromagnetic characteristic is unknown. Another approach consists in an ex vivo test with the same type of material, measuring whether the magnetic field has any influence (SHELLOCK and MORISOLI 1994). However, it can be said that almost all cardiac valve prostheses (an exception being the Star-Edwards pre-6000 series) can be considered safe for an examination in an MR unit with a field strength not higher than 1.5 T (SHELLOCK et al. 1993).

Patients with electrically activated implants or devices should not undergo MR procedures because electromagnetic fields may interfere with the operation of these devices. The presence of a cardiac pacemaker is currently a strict contraindication (ACHENBACH et al. 1997). Recently, however,

GIMBEL et al. (1996) reported on their experience of MRI in five patients with a pacemaker. They concluded that, under these conditions, MRI could only be performed in experienced centers with pacing facilities and under a series of very strict conditions.

Image artifacts due to (nonferromagnetic) metallic implants are caused by a failure of the position encoding schemes. These implants induce local changes in the magnetic field, which affects the precessional frequencies of the spins. The 1:1 relation between the position of the spin and its frequency is then no longer valid. Paradoxical hypo- or hyperintense signals result (Fig. 1.26). The image is distorted to a certain degree. The acquisition of SE images using the highest possible bandwidth is recommended in these situations.

References

Achenbach S, Moshage W, Diem B, Bieberle T, Schibgilla V, Bachmann K (1997) Effects of magnetic resonance imaging on cardiac pacemakers and electrodes. Am Heart J 1997 134:467–473

Amparo EG, Higgins CB, Farmer D, Gamsu G, McNamara M (1984) Gated MRI of cardiac and paracardiac masses: initial experience. Am J Roentgenol 143:1151–1156

Atkinson DJ, Edelman RR (1991) Cineangiography of the heart in a single breath hold with a segmented turboFLASH sequence. Radiology 178:357–360

Axel L, Dougherty L (1989) Heart wall motion: improved method for spatial modulation of magnetization for MR imaging. Radiology 172:349–350

Bloomgarden DC, Fayad ZA, Ferrari VA, Chin B, Sutton MG, Axel L (1997) Global cardiac function using fast breath-hold MRI: validation of new acquisition and analysis techniques. Magn Reson Med 37:683–692

Bogaert J, Duerinckx AJ, Baert AL (1994) Coronary MR angiography: a review. J Belge Radiol-Belg Tijdschr Radiol 77:255–261

Bogaert JG, Bosmans H, Rademakers F, et al. (1995) Left ventricular quantification with breath-hold MR imaging: comparison with echocardiography. MAGMA 3:5–12

Davis CP, McKinnon GC, Debatin JF, Duewell S, von Schulthess G (1995) Single-shot versus interleaved echo-planar MR imaging: application to visualization of cardiac valve leaflets. J Magn Reson Imaging 5:107–112

Davis CP, Liu PF, Hauser M, Gohde SC, von Schulthess GK, Debatin JF (1997) Coronary flow and coronary flow reserve measurements in humans with breath-held magnetic resonance phase contrast velocity mapping. Magn Reson Med 37:537–544

Denslow S, Buckles DS (1993) Pulse oximetry-gated acquisition of cardiac MR images in patients with congenital cardiac abnormalities. Am J Roentgenol 160:831–833

Edelman RR, Wielopolski PP, Schmitt F (1994) Echo planar MR imaging. Radiology 192:600–612

Gimbel JR, Johnson D, Levine PA, Wilkoff BL (1996) Safe performance of magnetic resonance imaging on five patients with pemanent cardiac pacemaker. PACE 19:913–919

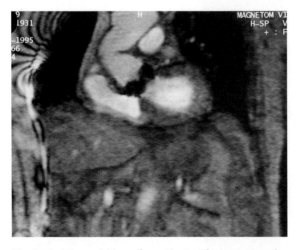

Fig. 1.26. GE acquisition of a patient with an aortic valve prosthesis. Signal void is observed in the neighborhood of the valve prosthesis

Higgins CB (1986) Overview of MR of the heart. Am J Roentgenol 146:907–918

Lamb HJ, Doornbos J, van der Velde EA, Kruit MC, Reiber JH, de Roos A (1996) Echo planar MRI of the heart on a standard system: validation of measurements of left ventricular function and mass. J Comput Assist Tomogr 20:942–949

Lanzer P, Barta C, Bovinick EH, et al. (1985) ECG-synchronized cardiac MR imaging: method and evaluation. Radiology 155:681–686

Lee VS, Spritzer CE, Carroll BA, et al. (1997) Flow quantification using fast cine phase-contrast MR imaging, conventional cine phase-contrast MR imaging, and Doppler sonography: in vitro and in vivo validation. Am J Roentgenol 169:1125–1131

Leung DA, Debatin JF (1997) Three-dimensional contrast-enhanced magnetic resonance angiography of the thoracic vasculature. Eur Radiol 7:981–989

Matsuda T, Yamada H, Kida M, Sasayama S (1994) Is 300 msec too long for cardiac MR imaging? Feasibility study demonstrating changes in left ventricular cross-sectional area with use of single-shot turboFLASH imaging. Radiology 190:353–362

Muhler A (1995) Assessment of myocardial perfusion using contrast-enhanced MR imaging: current status and future developments. MAGMA 3:21–33

Muller MF, Fleisch M, Kroeker R, Chatterjee T, Meier B, Vock P (1997) Proximal coronary artery stenosis: three-dimensional MRI with fat saturation and navigator echo. J Magn Reson Imaging 7:644–651

Pirolo JS, Branham BH, Creswell LL, Perman WH, Vannier MW, Pasque MK (1992) Pressure-gated acquisition of cardiac MR images. Radiology 183:487–492

Rajan SS (1997) MRI: a conceptual overview. Springer, Berlin Heidelberg New York

Saeed M, Wendland MF, Yu KK, et al. (1994) Identification of myocardial reperfusion with echo planar magnetic resonance imaging: discrimination between occlusive and reperfused infarctions. Circulation 90:1492–1501

Sakuma H, Globits S, Bourne MW, Shimakawa A, Foo TK, Higgins CB (1996) Improved reproducibility in measuring LV volumes and mass using multicoil breath-hold cine MR imaging. J Magn Reson Imaging 6:124–127

Seelos KC, von Smekal SA, Vahlensieck M, Gieseke J, Reiser M (1993) Cardiac abnormalities: assessment with T2-weighted turbo spin-echo MR imaging with electrocardiogram gating at 0.5 T. Radiology 189:517–522

Seelos KC, Von SA, Steinborn M, et al. (1994) MR angiography of the heart and thoracic vessels: application of fast ECG-gated techniques with multiplanar reconstruction capability. Radiologe 34:454–461

Semelka RC, Shoenut JP, Wilson ME, Pellech AE, Patton JN (1992) Cardiac masses: signal intensity features on spin-echo, gradient-echo, gadolinium-enhanced spin-echo, and TurboFLASH images. J Magn Reson Imaging 2:415–420

Shellock FG, Kanal E (1994) Guidelines and recommendations for MR imaging safety and patient management. III. Questionnaire for screening patients before MR procedures. The SMRI Safety Committee. J Magn Reson Imaging 4:749–751

Shellock FG, Morisoli SM (1994) Ex vivo evaluation of ferromagnetism and artifacts of cardiac occluders exposed to a 1.5-T MR system. J Magn Reson Imaging 4:213–215

Shellock FG, Morisoli S, Kanal E (1993) MR procedures and biomedical implants, materials, and devices: 1993 update. Radiology 189:587–599

Stehling MK, Holzknecht NG, Laub G, Bohm D, von Smekal A, Reiser M (1996) Single-shot T1- and T2-weighted magnetic resonance imaging of the heart with black blood: preliminary experience. MAGMA 4:231–240

Van Genderingen HR, Sprenger M, De Ridder JW, Van Rossum AC (1989) Carbon-fiber electrodes and leads for electrocardiography during MR imaging. Radiology 171:852

van Rugge FP, van der Wall EE, de Roos A, Bruschke AV (1993) Dobutamine stress magnetic resonance imaging for detection of coronary artery disease. J Am Coll Cardiol 22:431–439

van Rugge FP, van der Wall EE, Spanjersberg SJ, et al. (1994) Magnetic resonance imaging during dobutamine stress for detection and localization of coronary artery disease. Quantitative wall motion analysis using a modification of the centerline method. Circulation 90:127–138

Zerhouni EA, Parish DM, Rogers WJ, Yang A, Shapiro EP (1988) Human heart: tagging with MR imaging – a new method for noninvasive assessment of myocardial motion. Radiology 169:59–63

2 Cardiac Anatomy

F.E. Rademakers and J. Bogaert

CONTENTS

2.1
Introduction

The major advantage magnetic resonance imaging (MRI) has over other imaging techniques is the ability to visualize the heart in every imaginable plane and to give a full three-dimensional (3D) insight into cardiac structure and anatomy (Longmore and Forbat 1992). With the first generation of scanners only the three intrinsic axes of the body could be used, i.e., transverse, sagittal, and coronal, but with the advent of double oblique scanning, use of the true cardiac axes, short and long, became feasible as well as any other imaging plane necessary to obtain an optimal view of a normal or pathological structure. The most recent MR machines have added higher spatial resolution and shorter imaging times to these features so that a comprehensive anatomical study of the heart and its surrounding structures can be obtained with multiple breath-hold sequences in 10–15 minutes. In this context the transverse plane remains a good starting point, with other, more appropriate imaging planes being chosen for specific indications and pathologies. This chapter describes

F.E. Rademakers, MD, PhD, Department of Cardiology, University Hospitals Gasthuisberg, Catholic University of Leuven, Herestraat 49, B-3000 Leuven, Belgium
J. Bogaert MD, PhD, Department of Radiology, University Hospitals Gasthuisberg, Catholic University of Leuven, Herestraat 49, B-3000 Leuven, Belgium

the different imaging planes and the structures in them, as well as the specific uses for each plane.

2.2
Body Axes

Spin-echo (SE), turbo SE and Haste sequences can be used to study cardiac anatomy in the transverse, sagittal, and coronal or frontal planes. The transverse or axial plane (Fig. 2.1) is very appropriate for study of the morphology and relationships of the four cardiac cavities and the pericardium. Sagittal images (Fig. 2.2) allow one to study the connections between the ventricles and the great vessels, while frontal or coronal images (Fig. 2.3) are most interesting for investigation of the left ventricular (LV) outflow tract, the left atrium, and the pulmonary veins. The optimal planes also depend on the global positioning of the heart in the thorax, which is more vertical in the young individual and more diaphragmatic in the elderly. It has to be stressed that while these images are appropriate for evaluation of the overall morphology of the heart, quantitative measurements of wall thickness, cavity dimensions, and functional data cannot be obtained accurately since the planes are not perpendicular to the wall or the cavity with the consequence that partial volume effects and obliqueness can introduce a large overestimation of the true dimensions. The cardiac imaging planes are more suitable for this purpose (Longmore et al. 1985).

2.3
Cardiac Axes

To obtain the correct inclinations for imaging in the cardiac axes one starts with a transverse or axial scout view at the level of the left ventricle (Burbank et al. 1988). On this image a new plane is chosen running through the apex and the middle of the atrioventricular junction. This yields a vertical

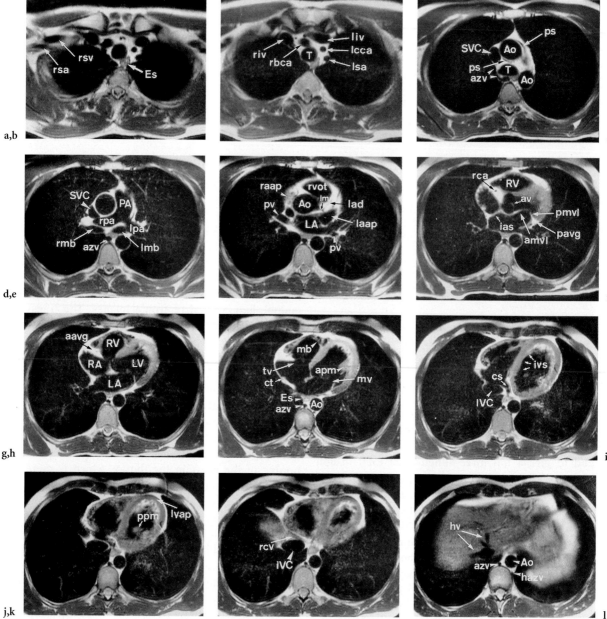

Fig. 2.1 a–l. Transverse images. *aavg,* Anterior atrioventricular groove; *amvl,* anterior mitral valve leaflet; *Ao,* aorta; *apm,* anterior papillary muscle; *av,* aortic valve; *azv,* azygos vein; *cs,* coronary sinus; *ct,* crista terminalis; *Es,* esophagus; *hazv,* hemiazygos vein; *hv,* hepatic vein; *ias,* interatrial septum; *IVC,* inferior vena cava; *ivs,* interventricular septum; *LA,* left atrium; *laap,* left atrial appendage; *lad,* left anterior descending coronary artery; *lcca,* left common carotid artery; *liv,* left innominate, (or brachiocephalic) vein; *lm,* left main coronary artery; *lmb,* left main stem bronchus; *lpa,* left pulmonary artery; *lsa,* left subclavian artery; *LV,* left ventricle; *lvap,* left ventricular apex; *mb,* moderator band; *mv,* mitral valve; *PA,* pulmonary artery; *pavg,* posterior atrioventricular groove; *pmvl,* posterior mitral valve leaflet; *ppm,* posterior papillary muscle; *ps,* pericardial sac; *pv,* pulmonary vein; *RA,* right atrium; *raap,* right atrial appendage; *rbca,* right brachiocephalic artery; *rca,* right coronary artery; *rcv,* right coronary vein; *riv,* right innominate (or brachiocephalic) vein; *rmb,* right main stem bronchus; *rpa,* right pulmonary artery; *rsa,* right subclavian artery; *rsv,* right subclavian vein; *RV,* right ventricle; *rvot,* right ventricular outflow tract; *SVC,* superior vena cava; *T,* trachea; *tv,* tricuspid valve

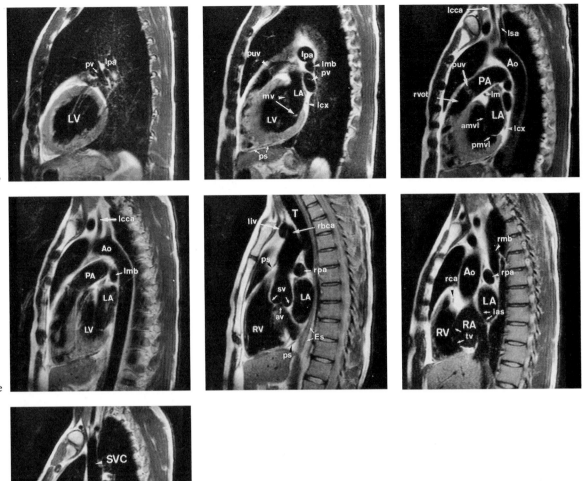

Fig. 2.2 a–g. Sagittal images. *lcx*, Left circumflex artery; *puv*, pulmonary valve; *SV*, sinus of Valsalva; other abbreviations as in Fig. 2.1

long-axis plane on which a position is chosen transecting the LV apex and the middle of the mitral ring. One then obtains a horizontal long-axis plane close to the echocardiographic four-chamber or five-chamber view, on which parallel short-axis images (Fig. 2.4) can be positioned. The inclination of these short-axis slices is not always easy since the anterior and inferior walls of the left ventricle are not exactly parallel with the result that no single plane is absolutely perpendicular to both walls; a compromise is necessary: sometimes the short-axis planes can be oriented parallel to the mitral valve ring, which is

usually more perpendicular to the inferior than to the anterior LV wall. If absolute reproducibility of the orientation of the imaging planes is required, the true four-chamber plane or horizontal long-axis plane (Fig. 2.5) can then be obtained on the short-axis slices by choosing a plane transecting the interventricular septum exactly in the middle between the insertions of the right ventricle. The two-chamber plane or vertical long-axis plane (Fig. 2.6) is perpendicular to the former and also passes through the middle of the LV cavity. Another caveat has to be mentioned here, i.e., the somewhat "banana-shaped"

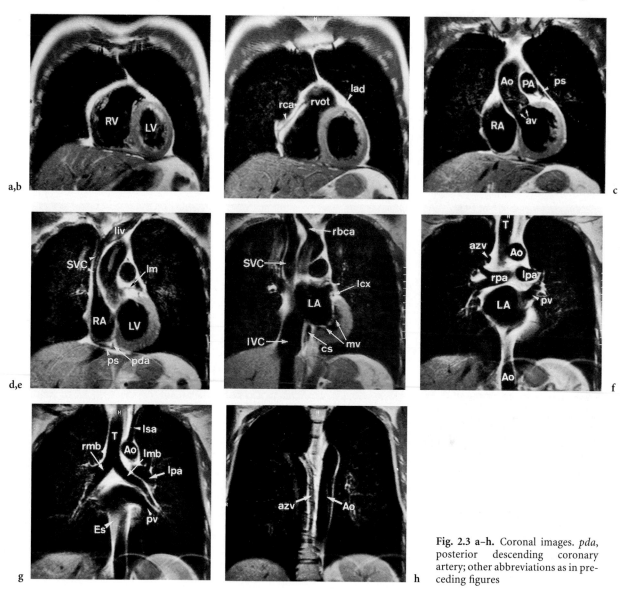

Fig. 2.3 a–h. Coronal images. *pda*, posterior descending coronary artery; other abbreviations as in preceding figures

left ventricle: on a stack of short-axis images the middle of the LV cavity at a more basal location does not correspond to the middle of the cavity at a more apical location, sometimes necessitating slight readjustment of the inclination of the short-axis planes so that the centers of the cavity on these short-axis images are exactly superimposed from base to apex. While this is unimportant for measurements of cavity dimensions and volumes or for wall thickness, it can be critically important for 3D reconstruction algorithms and stress-strain calculations (see Chap. 6).

Beside these standard cardiac imaging planes, specific planes can be chosen depending on the pathology under study. Especially in congenital heart disease it may be necessary to obtain multiple nonclassical imaging planes to achieve optimal visualization. Also imaging of the coronary arteries requires nonclassical imaging planes, as discussed in Chap. 12.

In each of the cardiac planes information can be gained with regard to cardiac dimensions, wall thickness, and function (when cine images in those planes are acquired) but attention has to be paid to the exact timing of the images. While data can be obtained at each phase of the cardiac cycle, often one is most interested in end-diastolic and end-systolic frames to measure dimensions and wall thickness and to calculate systolic deformation. True end diastole

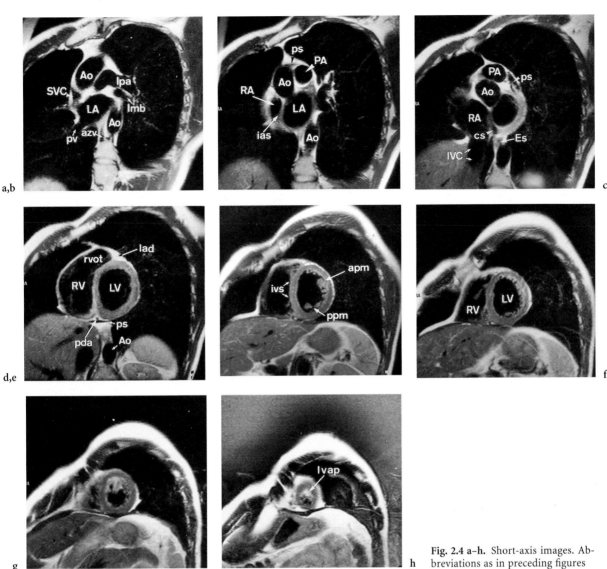

Fig. 2.4 a–h. Short-axis images. Abbreviations as in preceding figures

occurs at mitral valve closure when ventricular pressure starts to rise and exceeds left atrial pressure. This time point has a variable relation to the QRS complex depending on many variables, e.g., heart rate, conduction (bundle branch block, pacing), contractility, and end-diastolic pressure. Furthermore the exact point on the QRS complex for the triggering of the MR sequence differs from one manufacturer to another, as does the time between the beginning of the sequence and acquisition of the actual image. Therefore the exact timing of the "diastolic" image, usually the first image acquired after the trigger without delay, does not always coincide with mitral valve closure. In most circumstances this will not make much difference, but when exact strain analyses are required it can be necessary to take this into account; in particular errors may be introduced for images acquired "too late," since substantial deformation and reshaping of the ventricles occurs during the isovolumic contraction phase. Sometimes it can be helpful to acquire a fast cine image through the mitral valve plane to ascertain the exact timing of mitral valve closure with respect to the QRS complex and the trigger.

While dimensions, volumes, and function can be studied in all cardiac planes, a 3D reconstruction would be most appropriate. While this is possible in a research setting, at present most commercial cardiac analysis packages only allow semiautomated contouring of a limited set of images with calculations of dimensions and volumes. More precise information can be extracted when all acquired images

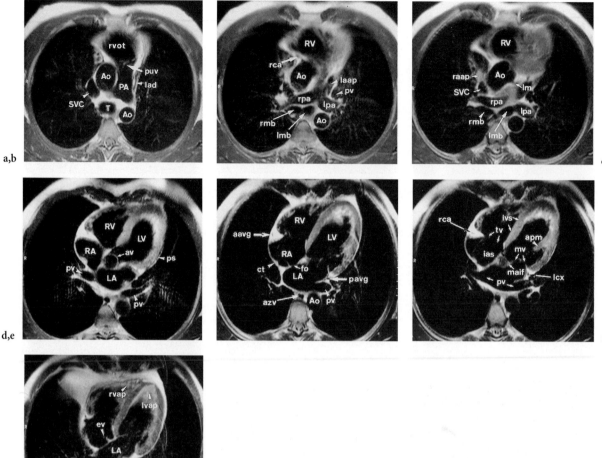

c

d,e

f

g

Fig. 2.5 a–g. Horizontal long-axis images. *ev*, Eustachian valve; *fo*, fossa ovalis; *maif*, mitral-aortic intervalvular fibrosa; *rvap*, right ventricular apex. Other abbreviations as in preceding figures

are used to create a full 3D reconstruction of the entire heart.

2.4
Cardiac Structures

2.4.1
Atria

The left and right atrium can be nicely visualized and measured on the transverse or axial images. The right atrium can be identified by its broad, triangular appendage (Fig. 2.5c), which has a wide connection to the main chamber, containing the prominent crista terminalis (Fig. 2.1h). In most cases the interatrial septum (Fig. 2.1f) can be seen as a thin line

separating the two atria except at the level of the foramen ovale, which is often too thin to be seen (Fig. 2.5e). Sometimes a fatty infiltration of the interatrial septum is observed, which can be easily differentiated from pathological masses by the characteristic signal intensity corresponding to the subcutaneous fat (see Sect. 10.4.4.4 and Fig. 10.18). It is a mostly benign, usually asymptomatic condition, with a low frequency on autopsy series. The veins (superior and inferior vena cava for the right atrium and the four pulmonary veins for the left atrium) are easily visualized in multiple views (Mohiaddin et al. 1991; Galjee et al. 1995). The eustachian valve (guarding the orifice of the inferior vena cava) (Figs. 2.2g, 2.5g), the thebesian valve (protecting the coronary sinus opening), and Chiari's network can be identified in the right atrium and differentiated from

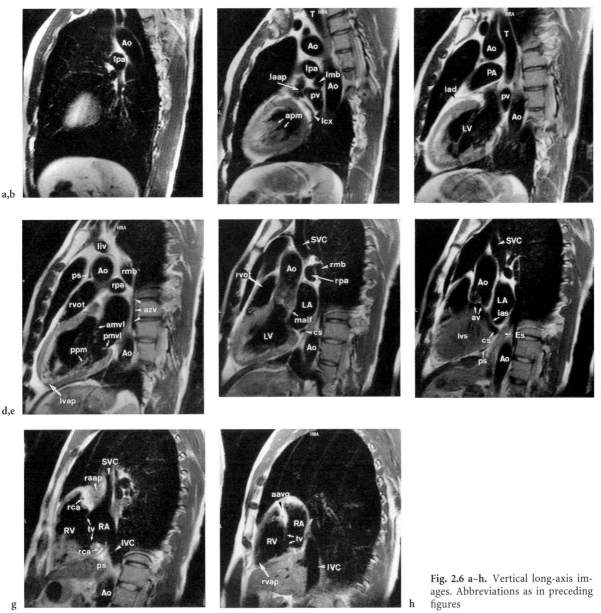

Fig. 2.6 a–h. Vertical long-axis images. Abbreviations as in preceding figures

thrombi or tumors (MENEGUS et al. 1992; MEIER and HARTNELL 1994; MIROWITZ and GUTIERREZ 1992). The left atrial appendage is, in comparison to the right, long and tubular with a narrow junction to the main chamber (Fig. 2.5b). Pectinate muscles, prominent in the right atrium, can only be found in the appendage on the left. The coronary sinus in the posterior atrioventricular groove can be seen opening in the right atrium (Fig. 2.1i). Sometimes, the right coronary vein, also draining in the right atrium, is visible in the anterior atrioventricular groove (Fig. 2.1k).

2.4.2
Ventricles

The myocardium and its trabeculation, coarser on the right side, can be easily appreciated (Fig. 2.4e,f). Intracavitary muscular bands are always present on the right as the moderator band and sometimes also on the left, where they are called false tendons. The interventricular septum can be identified except at the level of the membranous part, where it is sometimes too thin to be seen. As with the interatrial septum, a diagnosis of septal defect cannot be made on the basis of this morphological (i.e., SE measurement) finding alone and additional cine and flow measurements should be obtained to make a definite diagnosis.

Myocardial thickness can be measured on long- and short-axis images but towards the apex the wall is somewhat tilted and no longer exactly perpendicular to the parallel short-axis images; some degree of partial volume effect and overestimation therefore comes into play and only a 3D reconstruction can completely compensate for this deviation and deliver an exact wall thickness (AURIGEMMA et al. 1991, 1992, 1995; LIMA et al. 1993; FORBAT et al. 1994). Another method is the use of the epicardial and endocardial contours to define wall thickness, either by using perpendicular lines between the two contours or by using segmental areas divided by the length of the segment, yielding mean thickness values. Both give better results than simple measurements of wall thickness, but remain inferior to the 3D method.

For calculation of ventricular mass a stack of adjacent short-axis images is used on which the epicardial and endocardial contours are delineated with inclusion of the papillary muscles (AURIGEMMA et al. 1991, 1992, 1995; LIMA et al. 1993; FORBAT et al. 1994; GERMAIN et al. 1992). Taking into account slice thickness and interslice distance, LV mass can be obtained by multiplication of the volume with the specific density of myocardium, $1.05\,g/cm^3$. Since the ventricle shortens from base to apex during ejection and lengthens during the subsequent filling, these images should all be acquired at the same time during the cardiac cycle, whenever that is (ROGERS et al. 1991). For practical purposes, to be able to acquire multiple slices during the same cardiac cycle, the phase of diastasis, after fast filling but before atrial contraction, is most appropriate. With fast acquisition during breath-hold, end-diastolic or end-systolic images can also be used. Some differences in mass (or myocardial volume) between end diastole and end systole can be seen, which may be attributable to differences in coronary blood volume or the more extensive inclusion of endocardial trabeculae at end systole, but the results (mostly not published, personal communication) are not consistent.

In an identical way LV volumes can be obtained by using only the endocardial contour and usually excluding the papillary muscles. An added difficulty is the delineation of the ventricle towards the left atrium, since it is not always possible to accurately identify the mitral valve; often the mitral valve ring plane is used, which overestimates LV volumes. Another difficulty, when using a stack of short-axis

slices, is the partial volume effect towards the apex, which renders accurate definition of the cavity nearly impossible. On long-axis images, by contrast, the apical region is easy to delineate, again showing the advantage of combining short- and long-axis imaging in a 3D approach with reconstruction of the entire volume from all the available information. Right ventricular mass and volumes are obtained in a similar way but in the non-hypertrophied right ventricle it can be difficult to assess wall thickness accurately.

2.4.3
Valves

Closed valves are usually seen on SE images (Fig. 2.2b,c,e,f; Fig. 2.3c; Fig. 2.5f) but appreciation of small changes in thickness, structure, and integrity are difficult to appreciate. Abnormal valve opening and valve calcifications can be appreciated on cine MRI sequences (DE ROOS et al. 1995) (see Chap. 11).

2.4.4
Coronary Arteries

Segments of coronary arteries can often be seen on good SE images; this is especially true of the right coronary artery in the anterior atrioventricular groove (Fig. 2.3b), the left coronary artery at its origin (Fig. 2.3d), and the bifurcation into the left anterior descending artery (Figs. 2.5a, 2.6c) and the circumflex artery. Special techniques that attempt to compensate for cardiac and diaphragmatic motion are now being used to improve image quality and to obtain larger segments of the coronaries (EDELMAN et al. 1991; HOLMAN et al. 1995; WANG et al. 1992; PENNELL et al. 1993). Chapter 12 is entirely dedicated to the current status of MR coronary angiography. Coronary bypass grafts can also be visualized and the flow evaluated (GALJEE et al. 1996). In future it may also be possible to evaluate plaque composition in order to assess the risk of instability (MOHIADDIN and LONGMORE 1993).

2.4.5
Pericardium

The pericardium envelops the heart and the origin of the great vessels (Fig. 2.1c, 2.6d) and consists of serous visceral and parietal layers and a fibrous outer layer. This fibrous part is attached to the sternum and diaphragm. The pericardial cavity between the serous layers normally contains 15–50 ml of fluid. Two serosal tunnels can be identified: the transverse sinus, posterior to the great arteries and anterior to the atria and the superior vena cava, and the oblique sinus, posterior to the left atrium. The fibrous pericardium can be visualized in the normal subject as a curvilinear structure of low signal intensity on SE images (SECHTEM et al. 1986; PROTOPAPAS and WESTCOTT 1995; HIGGINS 1988). It is surrounded by the high-intensity mediastinal and epicardial fat. On MRI the normal pericardium has a thickness of less than 4 mm (Fig. 2.6g), which is more than the true thickness of the fibrous pericardium (1–1.5 mm); this is due to the absence of signal from the moving fluid between the two layers of the serous pericardium. MRI thus measures both the fibrous pericardium and the thin layer of fluid in the pericardial cavity. In the absence of pericardial fat, certainly at the free LV border juxtaposed to the low-intensity lungs, identification of the normal thin epicardium can be difficult.

2.5
Great Vessels

The right ventricular outflow tract, the pulmonary artery, and its bifurcation are readily seen on the transverse images and specific imaging planes in a parasagittal plane through the left and right pulmonary branches can be used for cine and flow measurements (PAZ et al. 1993; MURRAY et al. 1994; TARDIVON et al. 1995; BOUCHARD et al. 1985). The thoracic aorta can be visualized over its entire course (FRIEDMANN et al. 1985; BYRD et al. 1985; GULISANO et al. 1992; HIGGINS and HRICAK 1987; DINSMORE et al. 1986) but it is not always possible to achieve this in a single plane because usually the aortic arch does not fall in the same plane as the ascending and descending parts. To obtain accurate dimensions, an image plane perpendicular to the long axis of the vessel should be used.

References

Aurigemma G, Reichek N, Venugopal R, Trivedi S, Herman G (1991) Automated left ventricular mass, volume, and shape from three-dimensional magnetic resonance imaging: In vitro validation. Am J Card Imaging 5:257–263

Aurigemma G, Davidoff A, Silver K, Boehmer J (1992) Left ventricular mass quantitation using single-phase cardiac magnetic resonance imaging. Am J Cardiol 70:259–262

Aurigemma GP, Gaasch WH, Villegas B, Meyer TE (1995) Noninvasive assessment of left ventricular mass, chamber volume, and contractile function. Curr Probl Cardiol 20:361–440

Bouchard A, Higgins CB, Byrd BF, Amparo EP, Osaki L, Axelrod R (1985) Magnetic resonance imaging in pulmonary hypertension. Am J Cardiol 56:938–942

Burbank F, Parish D, Wexler L (1988) Echocardiographic-like angled views of the heart by MR imaging. J Comput Assisted Tomogr 12:181–195

Byrd FB, Schiller NB, Botvinick EH, Higgins CB (1985) Normal cardiac dimensions by magnetic resonance imaging. Am J Cardiol 55:1440–1442

de Roos A, Doornbos J, van der Wall EE, van Voorthuisen AE (1995) Magnetic resonance of the heart and great vessels. Nat Med 1:711–713

Dinsmore RE, Liberthson RR, Wismer GL, et al. (1986) Magnetic resonance imaging of the thoracic aorta in long and short axis planes: comparison with other techniques in patients with aortic aneurysms. Am J Roentgenol 146:309–314

Edelman RR, Manning WJ, Burstein D, Paulin S (1991) Coronary arteries: breath-hold MR angiography. Radiology 181:641–643

Forbat SM, Karwatowski SP, Gatehouse PD, Firmin DN, Longmore DB, Underwood SR (1994) Technical note: rapid measurement of left ventricular mass by spin echo magnetic resonance imaging. Br J Radiol 67:86–90

Friedmann BJ, Waters J, Kwan OL, De Maria AN (1985) Comparison of magnetic resonance imaging and echocardiography in determination of cardiac dimensions in normal subjects. J Am Coll Cardiol 5:1369–1376

Galjee MA, Van Rossum AC, van Eenige MJ, et al. (1995) Magnetic resonance imaging of the pulmonary venous flow pattern in mitral regurgitation. Independence of the investigated vein. Eur Heart J 16:1675–1685

Galjee MA, Van Rossum AC, Doesburg T, Hofman MBM, Falke THM, Visser CA (1996) Quantification of coronary artery bypass graft flow by magnetic resonance phase velocity mapping. Magn Reson Imaging 14:485–493

Germain P, Roul G, Kastler B, Mossard JM, Bareiss P, Sacrez A (1992) Inter-study variability in left ventricular mass measurement. Comparison between M-mode echography and MRI. Eur Heart J 13:1011–1019

Gulisano M, Bandiera P, Montella A (1992) La dimensioni dell'arco aortico e dell' aorta toracica umani studiate mediante rizonanza magnetica nucleare (RMN). Boll Soc It Biol Sper 6:351–357

Higgins CB (1988) MR of the heart: anatomy, physiology, and metabolism. Am J Roentgenol 151:239–248

Higgins CB, Hricak H (1987) Magnetic resonance of the body. Raven Press, New York

Holman MB, Paschal CB, Li D, Haacke M, Van Rossum AC, Sprenger M (1995) MRI of coronary arteries: 2D breath-hold vs 3D respiratory-gated acquisition. J Comput Assist Tomogr 19:56–62

Lima JA, Jeremy R, Guier W, et al. (1993) Accurate systolic wall thickening by nuclear magnetic resonance imaging with tissue tagging: correlation with sonomicrometers in normal and ischemic myocardium. J Am Coll Cardiol 21:1741–1751

Longmore D, Forbat S (1992) Studies of the heart using magnetic resonance. J Cardiovasc Pharmacol 5:S87–S111

Longmore DB, Underwood SR, Hounsfield GN, et al. (1985) Dimensional accuracy of magnetic resonance in studies of the heart. Lancet I:1360–1362

Meier RA, Hartnell GG (1994) MRI of right atrial pseudo masses. Is it really a diagnostic problem? J Comput Assist Tomogr 18:398–402

Menegus MA, Greenberg MA, Spindola-Franco H, et al. (1992) Magnetic resonance imaging of suspected atrial tumors. Am Heart J 123:1260–1268

Mirowitz SA, Gutierrez FR (1992) Fibromuscular elements of the right atrium: pseudomass at MR imaging. Radiology 182:231–233

Mohiaddin RH, Longmore DB (1993) Functional aspects of cardiovascular nuclear magnetic resonance imaging. Techniques and application. Circulation 88:264–281

Mohiaddin RH, Amanuma M, Kilner PJ, Pennell DJ, Manzara C, Longmore DB (1991) MR phase-shift velocity mapping of mitral and pulmonary venous flow. J Comput Assisted Tomogr 15:237–243

Murray TI, Boxt LM, Katz J, Reagan K, Barst RJ (1994) Estimation of pulmonary artery pressure in patients with primary pulmonary hypertension by quantitative analysis of magnetic resonance images. J Thorac Imaging 9:198–203

Paz R, Mohiaddin RH, Longmore DB (1993) Magnetic resonance assessment of the pulmonary arterial trunk anatomy, flow, pulsatility and distensibility. Eur Heart J 14:1524–1530

Pennell DJ, Keegan J, Firmin DN, Gatehouse PD, Underwood SR, Longmore DB (1993) Magnetic resonance imaging of the coronary arteries: techniques and preliminary results. Br Heart J 70:315–326

Protopapas Z, Westcott J (1995) Left pulmonic recess of the pericardium: findings at CT and MR imaging. Radiology 196:85–86

Rogers WJ, Shapiro EP, Weiss JL, et al. (1991) Quantification of and correction for left ventricular systolic long-axis shortening by magnetic resonance tissue tagging and slice isolation. Circulation 84:721–731

Sechtem U, Tscholakoff D, Higgins CB (1986) MRI of the abnormal pericardium. Am J Roentgenol 147:245–252

Tardivon A, Mousseaux E, Tasu JP, et al. (1995) Etude morphologique et fonctionnelle des arteres pulmonaires par IRM. Ann Radiol (Paris) 38:98–110

Wang SJ, Nishimura DG, Macovski A (1992) Fast angiography using fast selective inversion recovery. Magn Reson Med 23:109–121

3 Congenital Heart Disease

W.A. Helbing, R.A. Niezen, and A. De Roos

CONTENTS

3.1 Introduction

With an incidence of approximately 5–8 per 1000 live-born children, congenital heart disease is an important cause of morbidity and mortality worldwide (CLARK 1995). As a result of important improvements in diagnostics and surgical procedures,

W.A. HELBING, MD, PhD, Department of Pediatrics (Division of Pediatric Cardiology), Leiden University Medical Center, Albinusdreef 2, P.O. Box 9600, 2300 RC Leiden, The Netherlands
R.A. NIEZEN, MD, Department of Diagnostic Radiology, Leiden University Medical Center, Albinusdreef 2, P.O. Box 9600, 2300 RC Leiden, The Netherlands
A. DE ROOS, MD, PhD, Professor of Radiology, Department of Diagnostic Radiology, Leiden University Medical Center, Albinusdreef 2, P.O. Box 9600, 2300 RC Leiden, The Netherlands

survival of patients with congenital heart disease has significantly increased in recent decades. Presently, it is estimated that in the United States each year 10 000 children who have been operated on for congenital heart disease reach adulthood (ALLEN et al. 1992). Several diagnostic modalities are available for assessment of cardiac and large vessel anatomy and function. For initial anatomical diagnosis, echocardiography is the most widely used technique in infants and children (CHUNG et al. 1988; LUNDSTROM 1995). If specific hemodynamic information is required, for instance on pulmonary vascular resistance, heart catherization is still the gold standard and method of choice. In recent years magnetic resonance imaging (MRI) techniques have become a well-established diagnostic modality in patients with congenital heart disease. As a result of continuing technical developments, the role of MRI in cardiovascular examinations is expanding rapidly. Currently, cardiovascular MRI has been demonstrated to be an adequate technique to evaluate several important aspects of ventricular function, intracardiac flow dynamics, including valve regurgitation and stenosis, and large vessel flow. Furthermore, MRI has been shown to be an important technique in the anatomical characterization of complex congenital abnormalities, particularly of the venous connections, atrial arrangement, and ventricular/large vessel relationships (BANK 1993; PERLOFF 1994; WEXLER and HIGGINS 1995; GEVA et al. 1994).

Because of residual lesions many of the patients operated on for congenital heart disease require close follow-up. In these patients, transthoracic echocardiography may result in poor image quality as a result of scars, sternal wires, and lung interposition. With MRI, access to the chest is unlimited, as is the choice of imaging planes. A stack of MR sections is commonly acquired, encompassing the entire heart in contiguous imaging slices with a section thickness of 1 cm or less. This allows complete evaluation of the anatomical relationships and, with multiphase techniques, of the function of both ventricles and atria. Eventually, MRI may help to reduce the number of invasive procedures required in pre- and postoperative evaluation of patients with congenital heart disease (PARSONS and BAKER 1990; HIRSCH et al. 1994; Ho et al. 1996). In this chapter the role of different MRI techniques for the evaluation of various types of congenital heart disease will be discussed.

3.2
Technical Considerations Regarding Use of MRI in Congenital Heart Disease

The MRI techniques used in the evaluation of congenital heart defects are similar to those used in other types of heart disease. For technical details on these techniques the reader is referred to other chapters of this book. In the following section, the MRI techniques that are commonly used in the assessment of anatomy and function in patients with congenital heart disease will be discussed briefly.

3.2.1
Spin-Echo MRI

For assessment of cardiac and large vessel anatomy, ECG-triggered, multislice spin-echo (SE) MRI is the most commonly applied MR pulse sequence (REES 1989). This MRI sequence displays flowing blood as dark signal or a signal void, providing a natural contrast between flowing blood and surrounding structures. Images with high spatial resolution are usually obtained in several, usually orthogonal, planes with a slice thickness of 8–10 mm (Fig. 3.1). A range of oblique imaging planes can be used, tailored to the anatomical areas of interest. Depending on the patient's size and the structures under investigation, slice thickness can be reduced to several millimeters, improving anatomical detail and reducing partial volume effects. SE MR images are acquired with relatively short repetition times (TR, dependent on the heart rate when using ECG triggering) and short echo times (TE 20–30 ms) with two to four averages to optimize the signal-to-noise ratio.

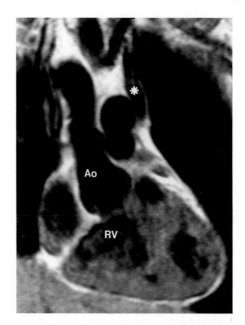

Fig. 3.1. Example of a coronal SE image of the chest of a patient who has undergone corrective surgery for tetralogy of Fallot. Note right ventricular (*RV*) hypertrophy, a right-sided aortic (*Ao*) arch, and a persistent left superior vena cava (*asterisk*)

a high temporal resolution by using a short TR, a short TE, and small flip angles. Images are not acquired real time but in 128–256 heart beats and then reconstructed to be displayed in a cine (movie) loop, representing one cardiac cycle. Of this cardiac cycle, multiple phases (time frames) are displayed, usually of multiple slices of the heart (CHUNG et al. 1988; DIDIER et al. 1993). GE cine loops reveal turbulent flow as areas of signal void contrasting with the high signal intensity of normal, organized flow. This feature of the GE technique can be used to visualize shunt flow and flow across stenosed or regurgitant valves. The visualization of these flow voids is heavily dependent on a number of technical parameters, most notably the TE. Assessment of the functional aspects of the contraction phase of the heart requires multiphase imaging with temporal resolution adequate to isolate the end-diastolic and end-systolic time points. For this purpose multiphase GE MRI of multiple slices of the heart can be used.

3.2.2
Gradient-Echo MRI

Gradient-echo (GE) MRI displays flowing blood with a bright signal intensity. GE images are acquired with

3.2.3
MR Angiography

Magnetic resonance angiography comprises a number of GE-based MR techniques that allow the

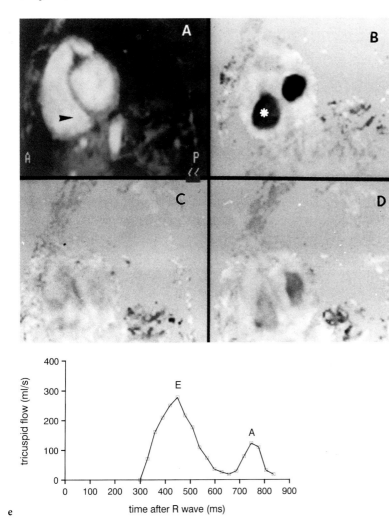

Fig. 3.2. A magnitude image perpendicular to the tricuspid orifice (*arrowhead*) obtained after double oblique angulation with the flow-adjusted gradient. Velocity maps in a section corresponding to **A** are given in **B–D**. Dark signal indicates flow out of the image plane (ventricular filling). Proportional to change in the flow velocity across the imaged plane, gray values vary during diastole, with an early filling peak (dark signal intensity) (**B**), mid-diastolic stationary flow (midgray signal intensity) (**C**), and a second minor filling peak following atrial contraction, in late ventricular diastole (**D**). The tricuspid valve plane is indicated (*asterisk*). After manual outlining of the tricuspid valve area, spatial velocities may be used to calculate tricuspid flow throughout the cardiac cycle. **E** Tricuspid flow volume plotted against time after the R wave in a healthy child. *E*, Early filling peak (ml/s); *A*, atrial filling peak (ml/s)

noninvasive visualization of flowing blood. MR flow visualization may be accomplished using time-of-flight (TOF) or phase-contrast (PC) techniques, which rely on different MR principles for the visualization of flowing blood (HARTNELL and MEIER 1995; EDELMAN 1992).

With TOF MR angiography, flowing blood and stationary tissue acquire different signal intensities as a result of the continuous wash-in of unsaturated blood and wash-out of saturated blood within an imaging section. The resulting image displays bright vessels on a dark background (BRADLEY 1988). In the PC method, a modified GE sequence is used that applies a velocity-encoding magnetic field gradient in the direction of flow (MOHIADDIN and LONGMORE 1993). When magnetic spins of intravascular protons flow along the magnetic field gradient, they acquire a phase shift proportional to their velocity. A velocity-encoded phase image can be reconstructed in addition to the conventional GE image. MR velocity mapping thus provides a 2D map of velocity distribution across the imaging plane. PC MR velocity mapping has been validated both in vitro and in vivo as an accurate technique for the performance of flow measurements (REBERGEN et al. 1993; FIRMIN et al. 1987). The clinical usefulness and accuracy of MR velocity mapping for measuring flow in the heart and great arteries has been demonstrated extensively (REBERGEN et al. 1993a; UNDERWOOD et al. 1987; MOHIADDIN and LONGMORE 1993). This MR technique has also been used successfully to quantify flow in the superior vena cava, pulmonary veins, coronary circulation, across cardiac valves, and in other vascular structures throughout the body (Fig. 3.2) (BOGREN et al. 1989; MOHIADDIN et al. 1990, 1991a,b).

3.3
Analysis of Cardiovascular Anatomy Using MRI

The value of MRI for the evaluation of morphology of the heart and great vessels has been widely recognized (KERSTING-SOMMERHOFF et al. 1989; BAKER et al. 1989). In patients with congenital heart disease, MRI has been found to allow accurate diagnosis of anatomical anomalies in more than 90% of cases, irrespective of the complexity of the malformations (DIDIER et al. 1986; FELLOWS et al. 1992; NIWA et al. 1994).

3.3.1
Segmental Analysis

Segmental analysis is the basis for a proper diagnosis in any type of congenital heart defect. It requires accurate identification of atrial situs, atrioventricular connections, ventricular morphology, and ventriculoarterial connections (HIGGINS 1992; GUIT 1990; TYNAN et al. 1979). Congenital heart defects are categorized by the connections between these anatomical segments and by the identification of additional defects. This approach has been particularly useful for accurate definition of complex forms of congenital heart disease (TYNAN et al. 1979) (Fig. 3.3).

3.3.2
Atrial Situs

Normally, the morphological right atrium is located on the right side and the morphological left atrium on the left side of the patient. This is called atrial situs solitus. In atrial situs inversus, the mirror image of the normal situation is present. Generally, atrial situs is in accordance with abdominal or visceral situs. In situs solitus, the short main bronchus, the liver, and the inferior vena cava are right-sided structures, whereas the long main bronchus, the stomach, the spleen, and the abdominal aorta are located on the left side of the patient. Morphology of the main bronchi is usually well visualized on coronal SE MR images and is a reliable indicator of atrial situs. Under normal conditions, the right pulmonary artery is located entirely ventral to the right main bronchus, whereas the left pulmonary artery crosses over the left main bronchus. In situs ambiguus the atrial and/or visceral position is uncertain or cannot

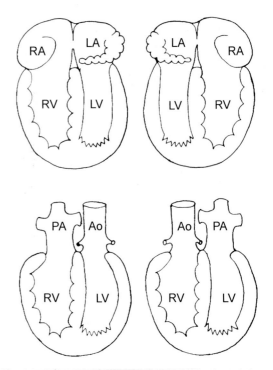

Fig. 3.3. Schematic drawings of some examples of the use of segmental analysis. *Upper left*: situs solitus of the atria, atrioventricular concordance. *Upper right*: situs inversus of the atria, atrioventricular concordance. Ventriculoarterial connections are not given in the upper panels. *Lower left*: ventriculoarterial concordance. *Lower right*: ventriculoarterial discordance. Atrioventricular connections are not given in lower panels. *Ao*, Aorta; *LA*, left atrium; *LV*, left ventricle; *PA*, pulmonary artery; *RA*, right atrium; *RV*, right ventricle. (Courtesy of Margot. M. Bartelings, Laboratory of Anatomy and Embryology, Leiden University, The Netherlands)

be determined. Situs ambiguus is diagnosed when symmetry of the main bronchi and pulmonary arteries is present, and it may occur as bilateral left-sidedness (left isomerism) or bilateral right-sidedness (right isomerism). When right isomerism exists, the spleen is usually absent (asplenia syndrome). Left isomerism is usually associated with multiple spleens (polysplenia syndrome). Situs ambiguus is usually associated with complex cardiovascular malformations. In asplenia syndrome, bilateral short main bronchi, a large symmetrical liver, absence of the spleen, and location of the inferior vena cava and abdominal aorta on the same side of the spine are encountered in conjunction with complex cardiac abnormalities. In polysplenia syndrome, bilateral long main bronchi, multiple spleens, and interruption of the hepatic segment of the inferior vena cava with azygos or hemiazygos vein continuation are characteristic (HAGLER and O'LEARY 1995).

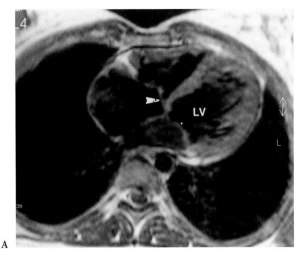

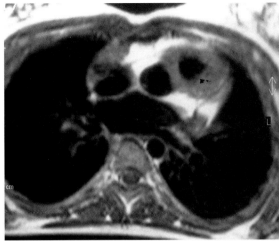

A   B

Fig. 3.4. A transverse SE image of a patient who underwent surgical closure of a perimembranous VSD. All four cardiac chambers are shown. The more apical attachment of the septal part of the tricuspid valve, indicating RV morphology, is clearly demonstrated (*arrowhead*). Note RV hypertrophy, caused in this patient by peripheral pulmonary stenosis. *LV,* Left ventricle. **B** Transverse SE image of the same patient as in **A**. Image at the level of the base of the heart. The muscular infundibulum (*arrowhead*), characteristic for a morphological right ventricle, is demonstrated

Using MRI, atrial morphology can usually be determined from the configuration of the atrial appendages. The morphological right atrium has a triangular-shaped appendage with a wide-based connection to the atrial chamber. The morphological left atrium has a tubular-shaped appendage with a narrow ostium connecting it to the main chamber. In most patients, the atrium connected to the inferior vena cava is the morphological right atrium. Sometimes the atrial appendages are difficult to identify on transverse images, and the bronchial anatomy may be more easily seen on coronal SE images, allowing reliable determination of atrial situs in most patients.

3.3.3
Ventricular Morphology

Since the location of the ventricle may be abnormal in complex cardiac malformations and the wall thickness will vary depending on the loading conditions of the ventricle, the position of a ventricular compartment or its wall thickness cannot be used by itself as a marker of morphology (HUGGON et al. 1992). Morphology of the ventricles can be determined in most patients by studying specific anatomical characteristics. Transverse SE MR images at a midventricular level will usually reveal the presence of the trabecula septomarginalis (moderator band) as a landmark for a morphological right ventricle.

This muscular structure, part of the supraventricular crest, traverses the right ventricle from the anterior wall to the septum. The trabecular pattern of the right ventricle is coarse, whereas the left ventricle displays a finer trabeculation. Usually, this is most evident at the septal surface of either ventricle. Furthermore, the septal attachment of the atrioventricular valve of a morphological right ventricle is closer to the cardiac apex than that for a morphological left ventricle, as seen to best advantage on transverse SE images (Fig. 3.4A). In addition, the presence of a muscular infundibulum is a reliable anatomical marker of a morphological right ventricle in most instances (Fig. 3.4B) (KERSTING-SOMMERHOF and HIGGINS 1990). When morphology cannot be identified reliably, the ventricle is diagnosed as being of indeterminate type. After evaluation of atrial situs and ventricular morphology, the atrioventricular connections are defined.

3.3.4
Ventriculoarterial Connections

The aorta and pulmonary artery are characterized by their usual branching pattern. The vessels and their branches are well visualized on transverse and coronal SE MR images (REES et al. 1987; VICK et al. 1990). After identification of the vessels their positions relative to each other are described, as are ventriculoarterial connections.

3.3.5
Associated Defects and Postsurgical Findings

The final step is to identify any associated defect and/
or postoperative abnormalities. Thoracic arteries
and veins can be depicted using SE, GE, or MR
angiography techniques and any concomitant vascular abnormality can be readily visualized (CHOE et al.
1994). Among the important advantages of MRI are
the depiction of extracardiac vascular malformations and the full visualization of surgical grafts
which connect the heart with the pulmonary arteries
(HOPPE et al. 1996).

3.4
MR Evaluation of Cardiovascular Function

For assessment of the volume and ejection fraction
of both ventricles with MRI, GE cine series are commonly obtained. Tailored to the clinical situation,
these GE cine series may be combined with velocity
maps of large vessel or atrioventricular valve flow to
provide additional information on systolic or diastolic ventricular function.

3.4.1
Systolic Ventricular Function

In patients with congenital heart disease, prognosis
often depends on right ventricular (RV) function
or the function of a single ventricle (GRAHAM 1991).
Evaluation of ventricular function is dependent
on accurate measurement of ventricular volumes.
Transthoracic echocardiography, the most widely
applied technique for this purpose, may be hampered by the absence of appropriate acoustic
windows and the requirement of geometrical
assumptions for ventricular volume measurements.
Various echocardiographic approaches have been
used to assess RV function but none has found general acceptance, since all assumptions of the complex
shape of the right ventricle are intrinsically inaccurate, particularly with abnormal loading conditions
(LANGE et al. 1985; JIANG et al. 1994; HELBING et al.
1995a). The semi-invasive nature of the alternative
echo method, transesophageal echocardiography,
limits the value and clinical applicability of this potentially more accurate approach (JIANG et al. 1994).
  Contrast ventriculography has been considered
the best method for in vivo calculation of RV volumes and function (GRAHAM et al. 1973; REDINGTON

et al. 1988). In addition, the combination of
angiographic volume data with invasive pressure recordings enables calculation of indices of cardiac
performance that are less load dependent than measurements of ejection fraction (REDINGTON et al.
1988). However, the invasive character and the use
of ionizing radiation preclude repetitive use of
angiographic studies in the follow-up of patients
with congenital heart disease. Furthermore, geometric assumptions are used that may lead to overestimation of true RV volume (GRAHAM et al. 1973).
In contrast, GE MRI does not require geometric
assumptions. Consequently multislice, multiphase
GE MRI has important advantages for accurate
imaging and measurement of ventricular volumes
(PATTYNAMA et al. 1993; MARKIEWICZ et al. 1987).
The clinical utility and accuracy of GE MRI of left
ventricular (LV) volumes have been validated extensively. Several studies have also validated the use of
MRI for measurement of RV function (MARKIEWICZ
et al. 1987; PATTYNAMA et al. 1995).
  HELBING et al. (1995b) studied RV volumes with
MRI in 20 children with different types of congenital
heart disease affecting the right ventricle and 22
healthy children between 5 and 16 years of age (Fig.
3.5). Biventricular volumetrics were obtained using
GE imaging, and MR flow mapping was performed to
determine great vessel and tricuspid flow volumes.
In this study a success rate of 97% (42 of 43 children)
was obtained for the use of cardiac multisection GE
MR imaging in the group of nonsedated children, 21
of whom were less than 10 years of age. This clearly
demonstrates the clinical utility of this technique,
not only in adults but also in children.
  Given the lack of a generally accepted in vivo
reference method, assessment of the accuracy of
tomographic MR RV volume measurements has
depended on comparison of RV volumes to MR
measurements with validated accuracy, such as
tomographic LV volume measurements and stroke
volume measurements obtained with velocity mapping. The accuracy of RV volume measurements in
healthy children as well as in patients was demonstrated in a similar way in the above-mentioned
study. Furthermore, intra- and interobserver variability in that study was small and similar to results
of comparable studies performed in adults
(HELBING et al. 1995b). Similar results were reported
by NIWA et al. (1996) in a study of 45 children with
congenital heart disease, with a mean age of 2.6 years
(range 4 months to 8 years). This study included
patients with a variety of complex congenital heart
disease, and used contrast ventriculography as the

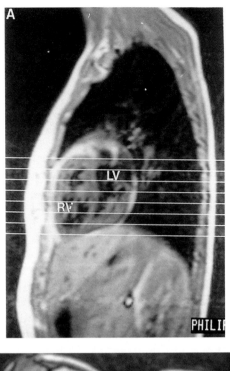

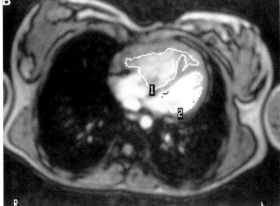

Fig. 3.5. A SE localizing view in the sagittal plane in a patient with atrial-level correction (Senning operation) of transposition of the great arteries. Coronal and sagittal images of this type are used to plan the location and orientation of subsequent GE multislice examinations. *Solid lines* indicate the orientation of transverse sections, encompassing the ventricles. Eight sections with 8 mm slice thickness were planned in this patient. *LV*, Left ventricle; *RV*, right ventricle. **B** Transverse GE MR image at end diastole, in a patient with atrial-level correction of transposition of the great arteries. The endocardial border of the right ventricle (*1*) and left ventricle (*2*) are outlined. Ventricular volumes were calculated by summation of ventricular cavity areas manually outlined on the multisection, multiphase tomographic GE image set of a specific time frame and multiplied by section thickness. In a similar manner, epicardial borders may be outlined and used for calculation of ventricular wall mass (see text). [Reprinted with permission from HELBING et al. Am Heart J (1995b) 130:828–837]

reference method. Correlation for ventricular volumes between the imaging methods was generally good ($r = 0.89$ to 0.94 for RV end-systolic volume and LV end-diastolic volume respectively) (NIWA et al. 1996).

The clinical importance of MRI for assessment of RV function was demonstrated in another study, comparing several echocardiographic methods with results of MRI for assessment of RV function in 17 children with congenital heart disease and 16 age-matched healthy children (HELBING et al. 1995a). The authors concluded that results of echocardiographic measurements of RV function in the follow-up of patients with congenital heart disease should only be compared if RV shape remains constant. If RV shape changes, MRI should be used to obtain accurate measurements of biventricular function (HELBING et al. 1995a).

The MR evaluation of systolic LV function can be further refined by combining MR-derived volumetrics with blood pressure recordings (AUFFERMANN et al. 1991). This allows the assessment of wall stress, which is regarded as one of the primary determinants of cardiac function and oxygen demand at the myocardial level. Wall stress, defined as the force acting on the cross-sectional surface of the myocardial wall divided by its surface area, can be calculated using mathematical models that take into account ventricular cavity dimensions, wall dimensions, and intracavity blood pressure. Combining measurement of ventricular volumes with blood pressure recordings also allows evaluation of myocardial contractility with the use of pressure-volume relations (PATTYNAMA et al. 1994).

3.4.2
Diastolic Ventricular Function

It has become increasingly clear that the filling phase (diastole) of the ventricles plays an important role in various cardiac disease states, including congenital heart disease (GATZOULIS et al. 1995; VANOVERSCHELDE et al. 1990; VERMILION et al. 1990). Usually, ventricular filling occurs in a triphasic pattern: an initial rapid filling phase is followed by a second phase of diastasis with very slow diastolic filling and finally by a third phase of filling as a consequence of atrial contraction (Fig. 3.2E) (MOSTBECK et al. 1993). After closure of the semilunar valve and before opening of the atrioventricular valve the ventricle relaxes while the ventricular volume remains constant. This is the isovolumetric relaxation period. Relaxation, which is in part an active process, continues into the following rapid filling phase. After the completion of relaxation, filling is primarily influenced by compliance of the ventricle and its surroundings, including the pericardium. The rapid filling phase can be characterized by parameters such as peak filling rate, time-to-peak filling rate, acceleration and deceleration slope of the early filling peak, deceleration time, and duration of the rapid filling period (NISHIMURA et al. 1989). The atrial filling peak is usually quantified by the peak filling rate. The ratio of early and atrial peak filling rate (E/A ratio) is another parameter of diastolic function.

Diastolic function of both ventricles is generally derived from time-velocity curves obtained with Doppler echocardiography, which has been proven to be a practical and fairly accurate method, validated against invasive measurements (NISHIMURA et al. 1989). With echo-Doppler it is assumed that the flow velocity as measured in the sample volume is representative of velocity across the valve area and that the valve area does not change during diastole. Transmitral or transtricuspid time-volume curves obtained with GE MRI may also be used to evaluate diastolic function (SUZUKI et al. 1991; HARTIALA et al. 1993; HELBING et al. 1996; REBERGEN et al. 1995). The main advantage of this method is that the actual volume of flow into the ventricle may be quantified (HARTIALA et al. 1993). Furthermore, MRI may be applied when Doppler echocardiography is difficult because of limitations to the acoustic window. These limitations to the acoustic window particularly impair evaluation of tricuspid valve flow in adults with congenital heart disease (HARTIALA et al. 1993; HELBING et al. 1996; REBERGEN et al. 1995). The transtricuspid volume flow measured by MR velocity mapping agrees closely with tomographically measured RV stroke volumes (REBERGEN et al. 1995). Agreement with Doppler echocardiography is such that MRI time-volume curves may be interpreted in a way similar to Doppler echocardiographic data (SUZUKI et al. 1991; HELBING et al. 1996). If inflow into a ventricle occurs from more than one source, interpretation of Doppler echocardiographic data becomes a problem (GATZOULIS et al. 1995; NISHIMURA et al. 1989). In this situation addition of MR time-volume curves from both inflow sources may provide time-volume curves that represent filling of the entire ventricle, as has been demonstrated for the right ventricle in patients with pulmonary regurgitation (HELBING et al. 1996). This is an important option that is not available when using other diagnostic tools. Other possible applications of combining velocity maps include the analysis of LV diastolic function in patients with aortic insufficiency.

3.4.3
Measurement of Ventricular Wall Mass

Alterations in ventricular wall mass may influence ventricular performance, both systolic and diastolic. MRI has been validated for measurements of LV and RV wall mass (DOHERTY et al. 1992; PATTYNAMA et al. 1993, 1995). At present, MRI is the only available method to assess RV wall mass in patients. Ventricular wall mass is calculated by outlining endo- and epicardial contours on a stack of image sections of a specific time frame encompassing the ventricles (Fig. 3.5B). Ventricular wall volume is then calculated as myocardial area (epicardial minus endocardial area) multiplied by the sum of slice and interslice gap thickness. A specific gravity of 1.05 g/ml is assumed.

3.4.4
Assessment of Intracardiac Left-to-Right Shunts

Accurate assessment of the ratio of pulmonary (Q_p) to systemic flow (Q_s) is mandatory for adequate management of patients with intracardiac left to right shunts. Shunts of this type most commonly occur in patients with atrial septal defects or ventricular septal defects. The decision to close these defects is generally made if the Q_p/Q_s ratio exceeds 1.5, since chronic left-to-right shunting with increased blood flow to the lungs may lead to an irreversible elevation of pulmonary resistance, the so-called Eisenmenger physiology.

The Q_p/Q_s ratio is usually derived from oximetric data from heart catheterization. Other methods to calculate shunt size are Doppler echocardiography and radionuclide angiography. The accuracy of all these measurements has been questioned (BOEHRER et al. 1992; RITTOO et al. 1993; BRENNER et al. 1992; HUNDLEY et al. 1995). The most widely used technique, heart catheterization, requires invasive studies, generally entailing the use of ionizing radiation. Using MRI, from a multislice GE image set encompassing both ventricles, LV and RV stroke volumes can be determined, also allowing calculation of the Q_p/Q_s ratio (BRENNER et al. 1992; SIEVERDING et al. 1992). However, this method is rather time-consuming. With velocity mapping MRI, accurate flow quantification in both great arteries may be used to quantify Q_p/Q_s (BRENNER et al. 1992; HUNDLEY et al. 1995; SIEVERDING et al. 1992; REES et al. 1989; MOHIADDIN et al. 1995). Agreement between MRI and other methods for calculation of shunt size has been demonstrated to be good (BRENNER et al. 1992; HUNDLEY et al. 1995). Importantly, this technique was shown to allow accurate differentiation between patients with a Q_p/Q_s ratio of <1.5 and those with a Q_p/Q_s ratio of >1.5 (HUNDLEY et al. 1995).

3.5
MR Evaluation of Specific Cardiovascular Abnormalities

3.5.1
Atrial Septal Defects

Atrial septal defect (ASD) is the most common type of congenital heart disease found in adult patients. The ostium secundum type ASD is located in the region of the fossa ovalis; the sinus venosus type is often associated with anomalous return of the right upper pulmonary vein into the superior vena cava or right atrium; the ostium primum type ASD is part of the spectrum of atrioventricular septal defects.

Although most ASDs are diagnosed during infancy or childhood, all types of ASD may go undetected until adult life despite hemodynamically significant left-to-right shunting (EICHHORN et al. 1995). Definite diagnosis is usually established with 2D echocardiography demonstrating the septal defect itself and concomitant signs of right heart volume overload. Additional Doppler color flow techniques can be used to visualize the shunt flow across the defect. Transesophageal echocardiography has further improved the diagnostic accuracy of echocardiographic examinations, but even with this technique a definite diagnosis of ASD may be difficult to establish (MORIMOTO et al. 1990). SE MR techniques have been used for the anatomical evaluation of the interatrial septum, with a sensitivity and specificity exceeding 90% for the diagnosis of ASD (KERSTING-SOMMERHOFF et al. 1989; LOWELL et al. 1986; DINSMORE et al. 1985). An ostium secundum type ASD may be diagnosed when a sharp and thickened edge is identified. Sometimes differentiation between a true defect and a thin fossa ovalis is difficult (KERSTING-SOMMERHOFF et al. 1989). In this situation, analysis of adjacent imaging sections and the use of additional imaging planes may help to make the correct diagnosis. Sometimes,

identification with GE images of the jet of shunt flow can be helpful in diagnosing an ASD. Shunt size can be calculated as discussed in Sect. 3.4.4.

3.5.2
Coarctation of the Aorta

Coarctation of the aorta is the third most common congenital malformation of the cardiovascular system (incidence: approximately 4 per 10 000 newborns) STEFFENS et al. 1994). Aortic coarctation consists in a narrowing of the proximal descending thoracic aorta, most often located just distal to the left subclavian artery, opposite the insertion of the ductus arteriosus. Associated lesions include hypoplasia of the aortic arch and/or stenosis of the aortic valve. Coarctation of the aorta results in decreased blood flow to the descending aorta. This will lead to the development of a collateral blood supply via the subclavian and intercostal arteries, the extent of which depends on the severity of the aortic coarctation.

Coarctation is classified according to the anatomical location, the narrowing of the stenosed area compared with the upstream diameter, and the severity of the pressure gradient across the stenosed area. A coarctation is considered moderate to severe when a pressure gradient of more than 20–25 mmHg is found.

The utility of MRI for evaluating coarctation of the aorta has been well established (VON SCHULTHESS et al. 1986; BANK et al. 1987). Thin-section SE imaging in oblique sagittal or straight sagittal orientations can be used to determine the exact site and degree of narrowing and also allows visualization of the extent of coarctation and the presence of collateral vessels (GLAZER et al. 1985) (Fig. 3.6). Measurement of the aortic diameter at the coarctation site relative to the diameter of the ascending and descending aorta allows assessment of stenosis severity. In addition, GE MRI and MR velocity mapping can be used to gain insight into the functional significance of the aortic coarctation. GE MRI may reveal abnormal flow patterns caused by the aortic coarctation as a signal void originating from the site of narrowing (SIMPSON et al. 1988). MR velocity mapping can be applied to measure the highest velocity across the stenosed vessel. The pressure gradient across the coarctation can be estimated with the aid of the modified Bernouilli equation: Pressure gradient = $K \times (V_{max})^2$ (19), where K is the loss coefficient, generally taken to be 4. However,

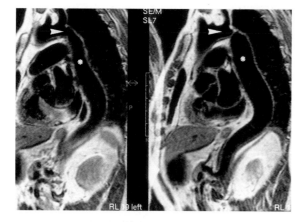

Fig. 3.6. Two adjacent oblique sagittal SE images at the level of the aortic arch in a patient with recoarctation. Note the stenosis in the descending aorta distal to the subclavian artery (*arrowhead*) and the poststenotic dilation (*asterisk*)

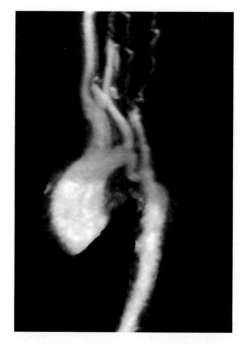

Fig. 3.7. Gadolinium-enhanced MR angiogram in a patient with a bicuspid aortic valve and a hypoplastic segment of the aortic arch. Note the narrowing of the ascending aorta in this patient suffering from Turner's syndrome

recently OSHINSKI et al. (1996), using MRI and velocity mapping, demonstrated that the loss coefficient actually depends on the severity of the stenosis, and is less than 4 in mild stenoses and more than 4 in severe stenosis. Therefore, for accurate noninvasive assessment of pressure gradients across the coarctation, stenosis severity should be taken into account. MRI is an excellent technique for this purpose (OSHINSKI et al. 1996). It should be noted that MR velocity mapping may be a problem in patients with long and tortuous coarctation segments (SECHTEM 1995).

Treatment is aimed at relieving the stenosis, preferably by resection and end-to-end anastomosis, and may in rare surgical cases require the use of prosthetic material. Since aortic cross-clamping may result in spinal cord ischemic injury with insufficient collateral circulation, information on the amount of collateral circulation is crucial in surgical planning. A method to calculate the amount of collateral flow was described recently by STEFFENS et al. (1994). In their study volume flow was calculated at the coarctation site and above the diaphragm using velocity mapping MRI, and collateral flow was expressed as the percentage of flow increase from the coarctation site to the distal descending thoracic aorta.

An important late complication of coarctation repair is systemic hypertension, which may develop years after repair. This may result from several factors, including aortic wall abnormalities or neurohormonal effects, but also from recoarctation. Recoarctation and aneurysms that may develop after repair are common reasons for further evaluation

during follow-up of patients who have undergone coarctation treatment (KAPPETEIN et al. 1994). In this situation, both conventional 2D imaging and MR angiography have been advocated as adequate techniques (Fig. 3.7) (GREENBERG et al. 1995; PARKS et al. 1995; BOGAERT et al. 1995).

At present, MRI is not an adequate technique for studies of coarctation in infants and young children, as a result of mismatch between the size of the region of interest and feasible slice thickness in this age group. The contribution of new techniques such as ultrafast 3D contrast-enhanced MR angiography in the diagnosis of aortic coarctation is currently being evaluated.

3.5.3
Transposition of the Great Arteries

In patients with transposition of the great arteries the ascending aorta arises from the morphological right ventricle, whereas the pulmonary artery originates from the morphological left ventricle. The aorta is located anterior to the main pulmonary artery, as can be clearly depicted with SE MRI (GLAZER et al. 1985). The arterial switch operation, during which ventriculoarterial concordance is restored, is

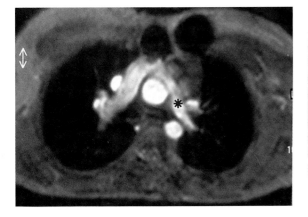

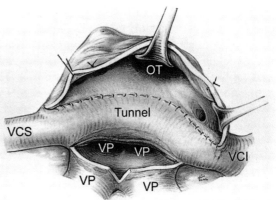

Fig. 3.8. Transverse GE image at the level of the pulmonary bifurcation in a patient after an arterial switch procedure for transposition of the great arteries. Note the narrowing of the left pulmonary artery (*asterisk*). After the arterial switch procedure the pulmonary trunk and right pulmonary artery are located anterior to the aorta

Fig. 3.9. Drawing of the intracardiac situation after the Senning operation for transposition of the great arteries. An intra-atrial "tunnel," consisting of right atrial wall and atrial septum, connects they systemic veins with the mitral valve orifice. The pulmonary veins drain into the right ventricle through the tricuspid valve. *OT*, Tricuspid valve orifice; *VCI*, inferior vena cava; *VCS*, superior vena cava; *VP*, pulmonary vein

the preferred surgical procedure in patients with transposition of the great arteries. This procedure is feasible in almost all forms of transposition of the great arteries in neonates and has excellent results (KIRKLIN et al. 1992; SERRAF et al. 1993). Postoperative complications include supravalvular stenosis, particularly of the pulmonary artery. MRI was found to be superior to echocardiography in detecting postoperative complications of the pulmonary arteries (Fig. 3.8) (BLANKENBERG et al. 1994).

Before the introduction of the arterial switch operation in the late 1970s, atrial redirection, with either the Mustard or the Senning technique, was the surgical procedure used in most patients with transposition of the great arteries. These procedures were designed to redirect the pulmonary venous return to the anatomical right ventricle and the systemic venous return to the anatomical left ventricle, thus creating a "physiologically correct" circulation. (Fig. 3.9). In this situation the right ventricle remains subjected to the loading conditions of a systemic ventricle. Since this ventricle is not ideally suited for systemic performance, RV failure may become evident in these patients (REES et al. 1988). Other postoperative complications in these patients include obstruction of both systemic and pulmonary venous pathways and baffle leakage. MRI, particularly a combination of multisection GE tomography and velocity mapping, can be used to demonstrate these clinically important problems (Fig. 3.10) (SAMPSON et al. 1994). In the case of symptomatic obstruction of the pulmonary vein, inferior vena cava, or superior vena cava, or an obstructed atrial baffle, inter-

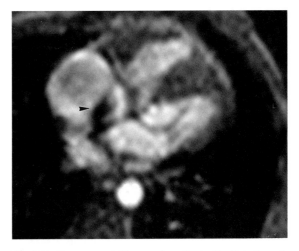

Fig. 3.10. Transverse GE image of a patient with clinical suspicion of pulmonary venous obstruction after a Mustard procedure for transposition of the great arteries. The image, obtained in diastole at the level of the pulmonary venous conduit, reveals an area of signal loss (*arrowhead*) representing turbulent flow across the stenosis. At surgery, a pinpoint stenosis of the pulmonary venous conduit was found

vention is recommended. This may consist in balloon dilation, stenting, or surgical intervention (LOCK et al. 1984; WARD et al. 1995).

Although for the majority of patients the long-term results of the atrial redirection procedures are good, it is essential to monitor RV function in these patients, preferably with a noninvasive technique (HELBING et al. 1995b). As has been discussed previously, MRI is an excellent tool to measure RV systolic as well as diastolic function in this patient group (REBERGEN et al. 1995). LORENZ et al. (1995) used MR techniques to evaluate ventricular function and wall mass after atrial redirection operations in 22 patients with transposition of the great arteries. In comparison with 24 controls, a significant increase in RV wall mass and a significant decrease in interventricular septal and LV wall mass were noted. Furthermore RV size in the patients was normal, and RV ejection fraction mildly reduced (LORENZ et al. 1995). As diastolic filling abnormalities may precede systolic dysfunction, the assessment of diastolic function may provide early information on the development of RV dysfunction after Mustard and Senning operations. In patients who have undergone Mustard or Senning repair, abnormal tricuspid flow patterns as demonstrated by Doppler echocardiography have been attributed to reduced compliance and impaired relaxation of the hypertrophied right ventricle. REBERGEN et al. (1995) have demonstrated abnormal tricuspid flow profiles in patients after Mustard or Senning repair using MR velocity mapping. Thus, MRI allows comprehensive assessment of anatomy and function after Mustard or Senning repair.

3.5.4
Pulmonary Atresia

In many forms of congenital heart disease, significant abnormalities of pulmonary arterial supply may exist, with a profound impact on treatment options. Significant abnormalities of the pulmonary artery are most frequently encountered in patients with pulmonary atresia and ventricular septal defect. In these patients, the size and distribution of the pulmonary arterial system are often highly abnormal, and frequently large portions of the lung are supplied by systemic collaterals. The anatomy of the pulmonary arterial system and of the systemic collaterals shows immense variation between patients. Prior to treatment, detailed knowledge of pulmonary vascular supply is crucial for planning of subsequent surgical or interventional procedures. Many of the various developmental abnormalities of the pulmonary circulation that may occur require repeated evaluation during follow-up. For the purpose of evaluating aortopulmonary collaterals and pulmonary artery branches, transthoracic echocardiography cannot be used (VICK et al. 1994). Hypoplastic central pulmonary arteries may be diffi-

cult to catheterize and angiography depends on adequate flow, which is sometimes absent (KERSTING-SOMMERHOFF et al. 1988; REES et al. 1987).

With MRI, the size and course of the central pulmonary vessels and the collateral supply may be adequately imaged, provided slice thickness can be tailored to the size of the patients (KERSTING-SOMMERHOFF et al. 1988). This may be problematic in neonates and infants, in whom a slice thickness of less than 4 mm is required. For distal aortopulmonary collateral anatomy, GE MRI is superior to SE MRI (VICK et al. 1994). Another advantage of MR is its potential to assess the size and patency of systemic-to-pulmonary artery shunts in these patients (KERSTING-SOMMERHOFF et al. 1988).

3.5.5
Conduits

Multiple surgical approaches have been designed to increase pulmonary blood flow in patients with congenital heart defects characterized by cyanosis and decreased pulmonary blood flow. Many of these approaches include the use of conduits, which may be installed with or without valves (Fig. 3.11). The materials used for these conduits may be human, animal, or artificial (HAAS et al. 1991). These conduits all have a significant inherent risk for obstruction. Obstruction may or may not include the formation of calcifications (AGARWAL 1981), and may lead to dysfunction of the ventricle supporting flow through the conduit. For these reasons, conduits require serial follow-up.

In a study of 52 patients, MARTINEZ et al. (1992) showed the usefulness of SE MRI in the assessment of extracardiac ventriculopulmonary conduits. In this study the success rate of imaging the conduits was significantly higher (90%) for MRI than for echocardiography (17%) (MARTINEZ et al. 1992). Calcifications cannot be visualized with SE MR techniques, and provide aspecific dark images with GE techniques. As well as for anatomical depiction of the conduits, MR velocity mapping can be used to calculate the pressure gradient across the obstructed conduit using the modified Bernouilli equation, as was discussed in the section on coarctation of the aorta (MARTINEZ et al. 1992). Furthermore, this technique may provide information on valve function if a valved conduit has been used. 3D reconstruction of MR images of extracardiac conduits may provide additional information, which may be important for surgical planning (BORNEMEIER et al. 1996).

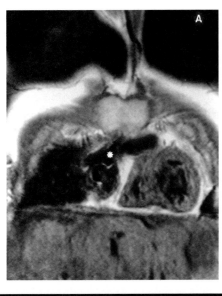

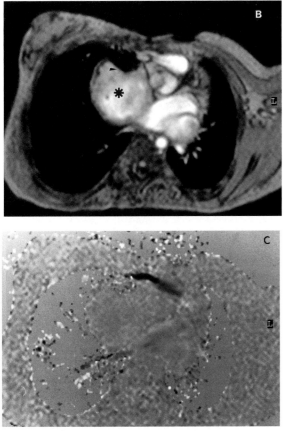

Fig. 3.11. A Coronal SE image at the level of a valved atriopulmonary conduit (*asterisk*) in a patient after Fontan surgery for pulmonary atresia. B Transverse GE image shows enlargement of the right atrium (*asterisk*) and an area of signal loss (*arrowhead*) in the proximal part of the conduit caused by metal components of the artificial valve. C A velocity map obtained at the same level reveals a jet of high velocity distal in the conduit, indicating an obstruction of the valve. [Reprinted with permission from REBERGEN et al. (1996) Radiographics 16:467–481]

3.5.6
Fontan Circulation

The Fontan procedure was designed to separate pulmonary and systemic circulation in patients with obligatory intracardiac mixing of saturated and desaturated blood in the presence of a congenital heart defect with a (functional) single ventricle. The Fontan procedure is used in patients with tricuspid atresia and in those with various other complex cardiac malformations, and redirects total systemic venous return directly into the pulmonary artery (FONTAN and BAUDET 1971). Several modifications of the original Fontan procedure have been used. Therefore a "Fontan circulation" may consist of a connection between the right atrium and right ventricle (if judged of adequate size) or of a direct atriopulmonary connection between the right atrium and pulmonary artery (Fig. 3.11). Currently, the most frequently used type of Fontan operation includes total cavopulmonary connection by means of a tunnel of baffle across the atria, connecting the inferior vena cava and pulmonary artery, and thus excluding the right ventricle. In many centers, a Fontan circulation is established in several stages, in which creation of a bidirectional cavopulmonary connection (between the superior vena cava and pulmonary artery) precedes total cavopulmonary connection.

Preoperatively, MRI can be used to depict the exact course and connection of the pulmonary and systemic veins as well as any associated defects, thus providing a valuable contribution to the planning of surgery (MICHIELON et al. 1993). Pulmonary artery size is one of the factors affecting the outcome of these procedures. Therefore, repeated evaluation of pulmonary artery size is required in these patients. FOGEL et al. (1994), in a study of 36 patients, showed that MRI, including 3D reconstruction, may alleviate the need for angiography throughout the Fontan stages in this patient group. MR velocity mapping provides a means to evaluate pulmonary flow patterns, including volume of flow and selective measurements of flow to either lung, in patient groups with different types of Fontan connections (REBERGEN et al. 1993b). In a study by REBERGEN et al. (1993b), patients with an atriopulmonary connection revealed biphasic forward flow in the pulmonary artery, reflecting the expected, normal venous flow. Monophasic systolic pulmonary flow was seen in half of the patients with atrioventricular Fontan connections, indicating a significant contribution of RV contraction to pulmonary blood flow. In the remaining half of the patients with an atrioventricular connection, the forward flow in the pulmonary artery was biphasic, indicating that pulmonary blood flow was not dependent on RV contraction. In addition, it was shown that measurement of flow velocity alone, as with Doppler echocardiography, may give a false impression of forward pulmonary flow and thus of the possible contribution of the right ventricle to the Fontan circulation (REBERGEN et al. 1993b).

Another possible application of MRI in this patient group is the assessment of global ventricular function, wall mass, and wall motion (AKAGI et al. 1992). Abnormalities of wall mass (hypertrophy) and wall motion may have a negative impact on the outcome after Fontan procedures (AKAGI et al. 1993; FOGEL et al. 1996). FOGEL et al. (1996), in a study of 35 functional single ventricle patients, found important changes in ventricular dimensions, wall mass, and wall motion and a reduced ejection fraction after complete Fontan operation, compared with preoperative data. The results of FOGEL et al. were obtained with cine GE MRI in the large majority of patients, and showed acceptable agreement with ventriculographic data from their and other patient groups (FOGEL et al. 1996; AKAGI et al. 1993). This again suggests that MRI is an attractive technique for repeated measurements during follow-up.

3.5.7
Tetralogy of Fallot

Tetralogy of Fallot is characterized by a ventricular septal defect, overriding of the aorta, RV outflow obstruction, and RV hypertrophy. The most frequent associated anomalies are a right-sided aortic arch, a persistent left superior vena cava, and anomalies of the coronary arteries. Tetralogy can be complicated by a stenosis at the level of the pulmonary valve or by peripheral pulmonary artery hypoplasia and/or stenosis. Cyanosis is the hallmark of the clinical picture of these patients.

Surgical repair aims at relief of the RV outflow obstruction and closure of the ventricular septal defect. Nowadays, most Fallot patients undergo total surgical correction in infancy (SOUSA UVA et al. 1995; BRICKER 1995). Before total correction a palliative shunt procedure may be performed, in which the subclavian artery is connected with the pulmonary artery (Blalock shunt). This is meant to improve pulmonary blood flow, thus decreasing cyanosis and stimulating growth of the often small pulmonary arteries. Pulmonary stenosis and pulmonary regurgita-

tion are common postoperative lesions after repair of tetralogy of Fallot. Pulmonary regurgitation results from relief of RV outflow obstruction, which is achieved by pulmonary valvotomy or the application of patches in the right ventricular outflow and/or common pulmonary artery. Sometimes transannular patches are required. These procedures may destroy pulmonary valve competence. Chronic pulmonary regurgitation in Fallot patients has been associated with RV dilation and impaired RV systolic and diastolic function as well as with impaired LV function (Fig. 3.12) (BOVE et al. 1983; KAVEY et al. 1984; REBERGEN et al. 1993c; SANDOR et al. 1987; WAIEN et al. 1992). This has resulted in diminished exercise tolerance in postoperative Fallot patients with pulmonary regurgitation (WESSEL et al. 1980).

Tetralogy of Fallot and associated cardiovascular abnormalities can be readily demonstrated using SE imaging. The defect in the ventricular septum and the pulmonary stenosis are best demonstrated on transverse tomograms. In addition, 3- to 5-mm slices through pulmonary arteries can be acquired to assess their size. Multislice, multiphase GE imaging can be used to perform measurements of ventricular volumetrics and to calculate ejection fraction, as an indicator of global ventricular performance. Since RV hypertrophy may impair the function of the right ventricle and is a risk factor for sudden death, MRI may be used to monitor ventricular wall mass (Fig. 3.13) (BRICKER 1995; NIEZEN et al. 1996).

Currently, MR velocity mapping is the only practical method for actual quantification of pulmonary regurgitation (REBERGEN et al. 1993c). This technique has been used in a recent study on the effects

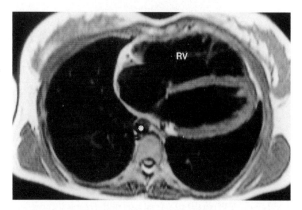

Fig. 3.12. Transverse SE image of a patient who has undergone corrective surgery for tetralogy of Fallot. Enlargement of the right ventricle (*RV*) caused by severe pulmonary regurgitation is clearly demonstrated. Note the right-sided descending aorta (*asterisk*)

of pulmonary regurgitation on biventricular systolic function in young Fallot patients (NIEZEN et al. 1996). In 19 Fallot patients, aged 12 ± 3 years, operated on at the age of 1.5 ± 1 years, and 12 age-matched controls, biventricular volumes, ejection fraction and mass, and pulmonary flow volumes were measured using transverse GE images covering both ventricles and velocity maps of the pulmonary artery. In patients, RV ejection fraction was significantly lower and RV mass was higher than in con-

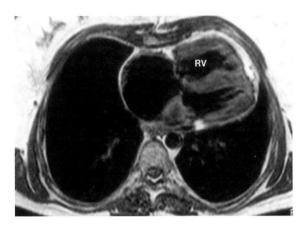

Fig. 3.13. Transverse SE image of patient with residual pulmonary stenosis after correction of tetralogy of Fallot. Hypertrophy of the RV wall is clearly demonstrated

trols; LV ejection fraction was significantly lower and correlated directly with the amount of pulmonary regurgitation. Exercise performance correlated inversely with the amount of pulmonary regurgitation, as had been reported previously (WESSEL et al. 1980; HORNEFFER et al. 1990; ROWE et al. 1991). Also in accordance with previous reports was the marked RV hypertrophy, despite the absence of residual pulmonary stenosis in this patient group (MITSUNO et al. 1993). Furthermore, the MRI study by NIEZEN et al. (1996) confirmed previous reports that there is an effect of pulmonary regurgitation on LV function (KONDO et al. 1995). The relation between pulmonary regurgitation and LV dysfunction has been attributed to RV dilatation and alterations in the function of the interventricular septum. Other proposed causes for LV dysfunction after correction of tetralogy of Fallot have included an older age at surgery, repeated episodes of acute hypoxia, and long operative procedures (WAIEN et al. 1992; BOROW et al. 1980; DE LORGERIL et al. 1984).

Recently it was shown that restriction to late diastolic filling of the right ventricle, indicated by diastolic forward flow in the pulmonary artery following atrial contraction, may reduce pulmonary regurgitation and increase exercise capacity in adult Fallot patients (GATZOULIS et al. 1995). This observation underlines the need for adequate assessment of dias-

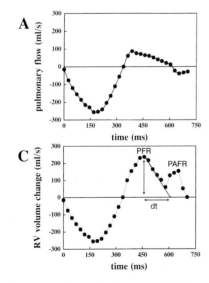

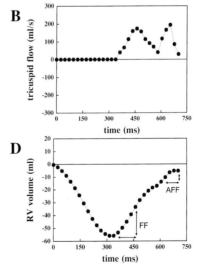

Fig. 3.14. Time-volume curve flow velocity curves of pulmonary artery flow (**A**) and tricuspid flow (**B**), RV time-volume change curve (**C**) and RV time-volume curve (**D**) of a Fallot patient with residual pulmonary regurgitation after surgical correction. Negative values indicate flow out of the right ventricle (**A–C**) or decrease in RV volume (**D**). Notice pulmonary regurgitation (**A**) and late diastolic forward flow, a marker of restrictive RV diastolic function (**A** and **C**). The curve in **C** was obtained by summation of curves **A** and **B**, and the curve in **D** by integration of curve **C**. *AFF*, Atrial filling fraction; *dt*, deceleration time; *FF*, filling fraction in first third of diastole; *PFR*, peak filling rate; *PAFR*, atrial filling fraction; *RV*, right ventricle. [Reprinted with permission from HELBING et al. (1996) J Am Coll Cardiol 28:1827–1835]

tolic RV function in these patients. With conventional methods, such as Doppler echocardiography, RV early diastolic filling cannot be quantified adequately with pulmonary regurgitation. Assuming that changes in RV volume are equal to the sum of the volume of flow entering or leaving through the tricuspid valve and pulmonary artery, RV time-volume change curves can be reconstructed by summation of the respective MR velocity mapping volume flow data (Fig. 3.14). From these curves the usual parameters of diastolic ventricular function may be derived (HELBING et al. 1996). In addition, MR flow mapping can be used to identify patients with or without late diastolic forward flow in the pulmonary artery, as a possible marker of restrictive physiology. Using this approach, we demonstrated abnormalities in RV diastolic function in young patients with residual pulmonary regurgitation after surgical "correction" of tetralogy of Fallot. Two different filling patterns could be recognized in this group: (a) prolonged early filling (as indicated by longer deceleration times) and low early filling rates; (b) increased early filling rates and decreased deceleration time. Pattern (a) is consistent with impaired relaxation, while pattern (b) is present when restriction to filling occurs. Patients with pattern (b) also had late diastolic forward pulmonary flow, confirming restrictive RV physiology. In patients with predominantly restrictive RV physiology, exercise performance was clearly diminished. This could only be explained in this study by differences in diastolic function, not by differences in ventricular size, ejection fraction, or the amount of pulmonary regurgitation. This study nicely demonstrated the potential of combined MRI techniques to increase the understanding of cardiovascular dynamics in congenital heart disease.

Acknowledgements. Large parts of this chapter are based on studies performed at the Departments of Radiology, Paediatric Cardiology and Cardiology of Leiden University Hospital, Leiden, The Netherlands. The contributions of S.A. Rebergen, J. Ottenkamp, E.E. van der Wall, J. Doornbos, and R. van der Geest to these studies and this chapter are gratefully acknowledged.

References

Agarwal KC (1981) Clinicopathological correlates of obstructed right-sided porcine valved extracardiac conduits. J Thorac Cardiovasc Surg 81:591

Akagi T, Benson LN, Green M, et al. (1992) Ventricular performance before and after Fontan repair for univentricular atrioventricular connection: angiographic and radionuclide assessment. J Am Coll Cardiol 20:920–926

Akagi T, Benson LN, Williams W, Freedom RM (1993) Regional ventricular wall motion abnormalities in tricuspid atresia after the Fontan procedure. J Am Coll Cardiol 22:1182–1188

Allen HD, Gersony WM, Taubert KA (1992) Insurability of the adolescent and young adult with heart disease: report from the fifth conference on insurability, October 3–4, 1991. Circulation 86:703–710

Auffermann W, Wagner S, Holt WW, et al. (1991) Noninvasive determination of left ventricular output and wall stress in volume overload and in myocardial disease by cine magnetic resonance imaging. Am Heart J 121:1750–1758

Baker EJ, Ayton V, Smith MA, et al. (1989) Magnetic resonance imaging of coarctation of the aorta in infants: use of a high field strength. Br Heart J 62:97–101

Bank ER (1993) Magnetic resonance of congenital cardiovascular disease. An update [review]. Radiol Clin North Am 31:553–572

Bank ER, Aisen AM, Rocchini AP, Hernandez RJ (1987) Coarctation of the aorta in children undergoing angioplasty: pretreatment and posttreatment MR imaging. Radiology 162:235–240

Blankenberg F, Rhee J, Hardy C, Helton G, Higgins SS, Higgins CB (1994) MRI vs echocardiography in the evaluation of the Jatene procedure. J Comput Assisst Tomogr 18:749–754

Boehrer JD, Lange RA, Willard JE, Grayburn PA, Hillis LD (1992) Advantages and limitations of methods to detect, localize, and quantitate intracardiac left-to-right shunting [review]. Am Heart J 124:448–455

Bogaert J, Gewillig M, Rademakers F, et al. (1995) Transverse arch hypoplasia predisposes to aneurysm formation at the repair site after patch angioplasty for coarctation of the aorta. J Am Coll Cardiol 26:521–527

Bogren HG, Klipstein RH, Firmin DN, et al. (1989) Quantitation of antegrade and retrograde blood flow in the human aorta by magnetic resonance velocity mapping. Am Heart J 117:1214–1222

Bornemeier RA, Weinberg PM, Fogel MA (1996) Angiographic, echocardiographic, and three-dimensional magnetic resonance imaging of extra-cardiac conduits in congenital heart disease. Am J Cardiol 78:713–717

Borow KM, Green LH, Castaneda AR, Keane JF (1980) Left ventricular function after repair of tetralogy of Fallot and its relationship to age at surgery. Circulation 61:1150–1158

Bove EL, Byrum CJ, Thomas FD, et al. (1983) The influence of pulmonary insufficiency on ventricular function following repair of tetralogy of Fallot. J Thorac Cardiovasc Surg 85:691–696

Bradley WG (1988) Flow phenomena in MR imaging. AJR 150:983–994

Brenner LD, Caputo GR, Mostbeck G, et al. (1992) Quantification of left to right atrial shunts with velocity-encoded cine nuclear magnetic resonance imaging. J Am Coll Cardiol 20:1246–1250

Bricker JT (1995) Sudden death and tetralogy of Fallot. Circulation 92:162–163

Choe YH, Lee HJ, Kim HS, Ko JK, Kim JE, Han JJ (1994) MRI of total anomalous pulmonary venous connections. J Comput Assist Tomogr 18:243–249

Chung KJ, Simpson IA, Newman R, Sahn DJ, Sherman FS, Hesselink JR (1988) Cine magnetic resonance imaging for evaluation of congenital heart disease: role in pediatric cardiology compared with echocardiography and angiography. J Pediatr 113:1028–1035

Clark EB (1995) Epidemiology of congenital cardiovascular malformations. In: Emmanouilides GC, Allen HD,

Riemenschneider TA, Gutgesell HP (eds) Moss and Adams heart disease in infants, children and adolescents. Williams and Wilkins, Baltimore, pp 60-70

de Lorgeril M, Friedli B, Assimacopoulos A (1984) Factors affecting left ventricular function after correction of tetralogy of Fallot. Br Heart J 1984;52:536-541

Didier D, Higgins CB, Fisher MR, Osaki L, Silverman NH, Cheitlin MD (1986) Congenital heart disease: gated MR imaging in 72 patients. Radiology 158:227-235

Didier D, Ratib O, Friedli B, et al. (1993) Cine gradient-echo MR imaging in the evaluation of cardiovascular diseases. Radiographics 13:561-573

Dinsmore RE, Wismer GL, Guyer D, et al. (1985) Magnetic resonance imaging of the interatrial septum and atrial septal defects. AJR 145:697-703

Doherty NE III, Fujita N, Caputo GR, Higgins CB (1992) Measurement of right ventricular mass in normal and dilated cardiomyopathic ventricles using cine magnetic resonance imaging. Am J Cardiol 69:1223-1228

Edelman RR (1992) Basic principles of magnetic resonance angiography. Cardiovasc Intervent Radiol 15:3-13

Eichhorn P, Vogt P, Ritter M, Widmer V, Jenni R (1995) Abnormalities of the atrial septum in adults: kind, prevalence and clinical relevance. Schweiz Med Wochenschr 125:1336-1341

Fellows KE, Weinberg PM, Baffa JM, Hoffman EA (1992) Evaluation of congenital heart disease with MR imaging: current and coming attractions [review]. AJR Am J Roentgenol 159:925-931

Firmin DN, Nayler GL, Klipstein RH, Underwood SR, Rees RSO, Longmore DB (1987) In vivo validation of MR velocity imaging. J Comput Assist Tomogr 11:751-756

Fogel MA, Donofrio MT, Ramaciotti C, Hubbard AM, Weinberg PM (1994) Magnetic resonance and echocardiographic imaging of pulmonary artery size throughout stages of Fontan reconstruction. Circulation 90:2927-2936

Fogel MA, Weinberg PM, Chin AJ, Fellows KE, Hoffmann EA (1996) Late ventricular geometry and performance changes of functional single ventricle throughout staged Fontan reconstruction assessed by magnetic resonance imaging. J Am Coll Cardiol 28:212-221

Fontan F, Baudet E (1971) Surgical repair of tricuspid atresia. Thorax 26:240-248

Gatzoulis MA, Clark AL, Cullen S, Newman CGH, Redington AN (1995) Right ventricular diastolic function 15 to 35 years after repair of tetralogy of Fallot. Restrictive physiology predicts superior exercise performance. Circulation 91:1775-1781

Geva T, Vick W, Wendt RE, Rokey R (1994) Role of spin echo and cine magnetic resonance imaging in presurgical planning of heterotaxy syndrome. Circulation 90:348-356

Glazer HS, Gutierrez FR, Levitt RG, Lee JT, Murphy WA (1985) The thoracic aorta studied by MR imaging. Radiology 157:149-155

Graham TP Jr. (1991) Ventricular performance in congenital heart disease. Circulation 84:2259-2274

Graham TP, Jarmakani JM, Atwood GF, Canent RV (1973) Right ventricular volume determinations in children. Circulation 47:144-153

Greenberg SB, Balsara RK, Faerber EN (1995) Coarctation of the aorta: diagnostic imaging after corrective surgery. J Thorac Imaging 10:36-42

Guit G (1990) Situs, atrioventricular and ventriculoarterial connection by magnetic resonance imaging. In: Higgins CB, Kersting-Sommerhoff BA, Silverman NH, Schmidt K (eds) Congenital heart disease. Echocardiography and

magnetic resonance imaging. Raven Press, New York, pp 89-98

Haas G, Laks H, Perloff JK (1991) The selection, use, and long-term effects of prosthetic materials. In: Perloff JK, Childs JS (eds) Congenital heart disease in adults, 1st edn W.B. Saunder, Philadelphia, pp 213-223

Hagler DJ, O'Leary PW (1995) Cardiac malpositions and abnormalities of atrial and visceral situs. In: Emmanouilides GC, Allen HD, Riemenschneider TA, Gutgesell HP (eds) Moss and Adams' heart disease in infants, children and adolescents. Williams and Wilkins, Baltimore, pp 1307-1336

Hartiala JJ, Mostbeck GH, Foster E, et al. (1993) Velocity-encoded cine MRI in the evaluation of left ventricular diastolic function: measurement of mitral valve and pulmonary vein flow velocities and flow volume across the mitral valve. Am Heart J 125:1054-1066

Hartnell GG, Meier RA (1995) MR angiography of congenital heart disease in adults. Radiographics 15:781-794

Helbing WA, Bosch H, Maliepaard C, et al. (1995a) Comparison of echocardiographic methods with magnetic resonance imaging for assessment of right ventricular function in children. Am J Cardiol 76:589-594

Helbing WA, Rebergen SA, Maliepaard CM, et al. (1995b) Quantitation of right ventricular function with magnetic resonance imaging in children with normal hearts and with congenital heart disease. Am Heart J 130:828-837

Helbing WA, Niezen RA, LeCessie S, van der Geest RJ, Ottenkamp J, de Roos A (1996) Right ventricular diastolic function in children with pulmonary regurgitation after repair of tetralogy of Fallot: volumetric evaluation by magnetic resonance velocity mapping. J Am Coll Cardiol 28:1827-1835

Higgins CB (1992) MRI of congenital heart disease. In: Higgins CB (ed) Essentials of cardiac radiology and imaging. J.B. Lippincott, New York, pp 283-331

Hirsch R, Kilner PJ, Connelly MS, Redington AN, St John Sutton MG, Somerville J (1994) Diagnosis in adolescents and adults with congenital heart disease. Prospective assessment of individual and combined roles of magnetic resonance imaging and transesophageal echocardiography. Circulation 90:2937-2951

Ho VB, Kinney JB, Sahn DJ (1996) Contributions of newer MR imaging strategies for congenital heart disease. Radiographics 16:43-60

Hoppe UC, Dederichs B, Deutsch HJ, Theissen P, Schicha H, Sechtem U (1996) Congenital heart disease in adults and adolescents: comparative value of transthoracic and transesophageal echocardiography and MR imaging. Radiology 199:669-677

Horneffer PJ, Zahka KG, Rowe SA, et al. (1990) Long-term results of total repair of tetralogy of Fallot in childhood. Ann Thorac Surg 50:179-185

Huggon IC, Baker EJ, Maisey MN, et al. (1992) Magnetic resonance imaging of hearts with atrioventricular valve atresia or double inlet ventricle. Br Heart J 68:313-319

Hundley WG, Li HF, Lange RA, et al. (1995) Assessment of left-to-right intracardiac shunting by velocity-encoded, phase difference magnetic resonance imaging. A comparison with oximetric and indicator dilution techniques. Circulation 91:2955-2960

Jiang L, Siu SC, Handschumacher MD, et al. (1994) Three-dimensional echocardiography. In vivo validation for right ventricular volume and function. Circulation 89:2342-2350

Kappetein AP, Zwinderman AH, Bogers AJ, Rohmer J, Huysmans HA (1994) More than thirty-five years of coarctation repair. An unexpected high relapse rate. J Thorac Cardiovasc Surg 107:87–95

Kavey REW, Thomas FD, Byrum CJ, Blackman MS, Sondheimer HM, Bove EL (1984) Ventricular arrhythmias and biventricular dysfunction after repair of tetralogy of Fallot. J Am Coll Cardiol 4:126–131

Kersting-Sommerhoff B, Higgins CB (1990) Magnetic resonance imaging of congenital heart disease. In: Brundage BH (ed) Comparative cardiac imaging. Aspen, Rockville, pp 493–503

Kersting-Sommerhoff BA, Sechtem U, Higgins CB (1988) Evaluation of pulmonary blood supply by nuclear magnetic resonance imaging in patients with pulmonary atresia. J Am Coll Cardiol 11:166–171

Kersting-Sommerhoff BA, Diethelm L, Teitel DF, et al. (1989) Magnetic resonance imaging of congenital heart disease: sensitivity and specificity using receiver operating characteristic curve analysis. Am Heart J 118:155–161

Kirklin JW, Blackstone EG, Tchervenkov CI, Castaneda AR (1992) Clinical outcomes after the arterial switch operation for transposition. Circulation 86:1501–1515

Kondo C, Nakazawa M, Kusakabe K, Momma K (1995) Left ventricular dysfunction on exercise long term after total repair of tetralogy of Fallot. Circulation 92 [Suppl II](9):250–255

Lange PE, Seiffert PA, Pices F, Wersel A, Onnasch DGW, Heintzen PH (1985) Value of image enhancement and injection of contrast medium for right ventricular volume determination by two-dimensional echocardiography in congenital heart disease. Am J Cardiol 55:152–157

Lock JE, Bass JL, Castaneda-Zuniga W, Fuhrman BP, Rashkind WJ, Lucas RV (1984) Dilation angioplasty of congenital or operative narrowings of venous channels. Circulation 70:457–464

Lorenz CH, Walker ES, Graham TP Jr, Powers TA (1995) Right ventricular performance and mass by use of cine MRI late after atrial repair of transpostion of the great arteries. Circulation 92(Suppl II):II-233–II-239

Lowell DG, Turner DA, Smith SM, et al. (1986) The detection of atrial and ventricular septal defects with electrocardiographically synchronized magnetic resonance imaging. Circulation 73:89–94

Lundstrom NR (1995) Non-invasive imaging techniques in pediatric cardiology: impact on clinical decision making. Acta Paediatr Suppl 410:5–7

Markiewicz W, Sechtem U, Higgins CB (1987) Evaluation of the right ventricle by magnetic resonance imaging. Am Heart J 113:8–15

Martinez JE, Mohiaddin RH, Kilner PJ, et al. (1992) Obstruction in extracardiac ventriculopulmonary conduits: value of nuclear magnetic resonance imaging with velocity mapping and Doppler echocardiography. J Am Coll Cardiol 20:338–344

Michielon G, Gharagozloo F, Lulsrud PR, Danielson GK, Puga FJ (1993) Modified Fontan operation in the presence of anomalies of systemic and pulmonary venous connection. Circulation 88 (part 2):141–148

Mitsuno M, Nakano S, Shimazaki Y, et al. (1993) Fate of right ventricular hypertrophy in tetralogy of Fallot after corrective surgery. Am J Cardiol 72:694–698

Mohiaddin RH, Longmore DB (1993) Functional aspects of cardiovascular nuclear magnetic resonance imaging. Techniques and application [review]. Circulation 88:264–281

Mohiaddin RH, Wann SL, Underwood R, Firmin DN, Rees S, Longmore DB (1990) Vena caval flow: assessment with cine MR velocity mapping. Radiology 177:537–541

Mohiaddin RH, Amanuma M, Kilner PJ, Pennell DJ, Manzara C, Longmore DB (1991a) MR phase-shift velocity mapping of mitral and pulmonary venous flow. J Comput Assist Tomogr 15:237–243

Mohiaddin RH, Paz R, Theodoropoulos S, Firmin DN, Longmore DB, Yacoub MH (1991b) Magnetic resonance characterization of pulmonary arterial blood flow after single lung transplantation. J Thorac Cardiovasc Surg 101:1016–1023

Mohiaddin RH, Underwood R, Romeira L, et al. (1995) Comparison between cine magnetic resonance velocity mapping and first-pass radionuclide angiocardiography for quantitating intracardiac shunts. Am J Cardiol 75:529–532

Morimoto K, Matzusaki M, Tohma Y, et al. (1990) Diagnosis and quantitative evaluation of secundum type atrial septal defect by transesophageal Doppler echocardiography. Am J Cardiol 66:85–91

Mostbeck GH, Hartiala JJ, Foster E, Fujita N, Dulce M, Higgins CB (1993) Right ventricular diastolic filling: evaluation with velocity-encoded cine MRI. J Comput Assist Tomogr 17:245–252

Niezen RA, Helbing WA, van der Wall EE, van der Geest RJ, Rebergen SA, de Roos A (1996) Biventricular systolic function and mass studied with MR imaging in children with pulmonary regurgitation after Fallot repair. Radiology 201:135–140

Nishimura RA, Abel MD, Hatle LK, Tajik AJ (1989) Assessment of diastolic function of the heart: background and current applications of Doppler echocardiography. Part II. Clinical studies. Mayo Clin Proc 64:181–204

Niwa K, Uchishiba M, Aotsuka H, et al. (1994) Magnetic resonance imaging of heterotaxia in infants. J Am Coll Cardiol 23:177–183

Niwa K, Uchishiba M, Aotsuka H, et al. (1996) Measurement of ventricular volumes by cine magnetic resonance imaging in complex congenital heart diasease with morphologically abnormal ventricles. Am Heart J 131:567–575

Oshinski JN, Parks WJ, Markou CP, et al. (1996) Improved measurements of pressure gradients in aortic coarctation by magnetic resonance imaging. J Am Coll Cardiol 28:1818–1826

Parks WJ, Ngo TD, Plauth WH, et al. (1995) Incidence of aneurysm formation after dacron patch aortoplasty repair for coarctation of the aorta: long-term results and assessment utilizing magnetic resonance angiography with three-dimensional surface rendering. J Am Coll Cardiol 26:266–271

Parsons JM, Baker EJ (1990) The use of magnetic resonance imaging in the investigation of infants and children with congenital heart disease: current status and future prospects. Int J Cardiol 1990:263–275

Pattynama PMT, Lamb HJ, van der Veldo EA, van der Wall EE, de Roos A (1993) Left ventricular measurements by cine and spin-echo MR imaging: a study of reproducibility with variance component analysis. Radiology 187:261–268

Pattynama PM, de Roos A, van der Wall EE, van Voorthuisen AE (1994) Functional magnetic resonance imaging of the heart. Am Heart J 128:595–607

Pattynama PMT, Lamb HJ, van der Geest RJ, van der Velde EA, van der Wall EE, de Ross A (1995) Reproducibility of measurements of right ventricular volumes and myocardial mass with MR imaging. Magn Res Imaging 13:53–63

Perloff JK (1994) Congenital heart disease in the adult: clinical approach. J Thorac Imaging 9:260–268

Rebergen SA, van der Wall EE, Doornbos J, De Roos A (1993a) Magnetic resonance measurement of velocity and flow:

technique, validation and clinical application. Am Heart J 126:1439–1456

Rebergen SA, Ottenkamp J, Doornbos J, van der Wall EE, Chin JG, de Roos A (1993b) Postoperative pulmonary flow dynamics after Fontan surgery: assessment with nuclear magnetic resonance velocity mapping. J Am Coll Cardiol 21:123–131

Rebergen SA, Chin JG, Ottenkamp J, van der Wall EE, de Roos A (1993c) Pulmonary regurgitation in the late postoperative follow-up of tetralogy of Fallot. Volumetric quantitation by nuclear magnetic resonance velocity mapping. Circulation 88:2257–2266

Rebergen SA, Helbing WA, van der Wall EE, Maliepaard C, Chin JGJ, de Roos A (1995) MR velocity mapping of tricuspid flow in healthy children and in patients who have undergone Mustard or Senning repair. Radiology 194:505–512

Rebergen SA, Niezen RA, Helbing WA, van der Wall EE, de Roos A (1996) Cine gradient-echo MR imaging and MR velocity mapping in the evaluation of congenital heart disease. Radiographics 16:467–481

Redington AN, Oldershaw PJ, Shinebourne EA, Rigby ML (1988) A new technique for the assessment of pulmonary regurgitation and its application to the assessment of right ventricular function before and after repair of tetralogy of Fallot. Br Heart J 60:57–65

Rees S (1989) Cardiac magnetic resonance imaging: anatomical display using spin echo images. Br Med Bull 45:933–947

Rees RSO, Somerville J, Underwood SR, et al. (1987) Magnetic resonance imaging of the pulmonary arteries and their systemic connections in pulmonary atresia: comparison with angiographic and surgical findings. Br Heart J 58:621–626

Rees S, Somerville J, Warnes C, et al. (1988) Comparison of magnetic resonance imaging with echocardiography and radionuclide angiography in assessing cardiac function and anatomy following Mustard's operation for transposition of the great arteries. Am J Cardiol 61:1316–1322

Rees S, Firmin D, Mohiaddin R, Underwood R, Longmore D (1989) Application of flow measurements by magnetic resonance velocity mapping to congenital heart disease. Am J Cardiol 64:953–956

Rittoo D, Sutherland GR, Shaw TRD (1993) Quantification of left-to-right shunting and defect size after balloon mitral commissurotomy using biplane transesophageal echocardiography, color flow Doppler mapping, and the principle of proximal flow convergence. Circulation 87:1591–1603

Rowe SA, Zahka KG, Manolio TA, Horneffer PJ, Kidd L (1991) Lung function and pulmonary regurgitation limit exercise capacity in postoperative tetralogy of Fallot. J Am Coll Cardiol 17:461–466

Sampson C, Kilner PJ, Hirsch R, Rees RSO, Somerville J, Underwood SR (1994) Venoatrial pathways after the Mustard operation for transposition of the great arteries; anatomic and functional MR imaging. Radiology 193:211–217

Sandor GGS, Patterson MWH, Tipple M, Ashmore PG, Popov R (1987) Left ventricular systolic and diastolic function after total correction of tetralogy of Fallot. AM J Cardiol 60:1148–1151

Sechtem U (1995) Imaging of the aortic coarctation – difficult choices. Eur Heart J 16:1315–1316

Serraf A, Lacour-Gayet F, Bruniaux J, et al. (1993) Anatomic correction of transposition of the great arteries in neonates. J Am Coll Cardiol 22:193–200

Sieverding L, Jung WI, Klose U, Apitz J (1992) Noninvasive blood flow measurement and quantification of shunt volume by cine magnetic resonance in congenital heart disease. Preliminary results. Pediatr Radiol 22:48–54

Simpson IA, Chung KJ, Glass RF, Sahn DJ, Sherman FS, Hesselink J (1988) Cine magnetic resonance imaging for evaluation of anatomy and flow relations in infants and children with coarctation of the aorta. Circulation 78:142–148

Sousa Uva M, Chardigny C, Galetti L, et al. (1995) Surgery for tetralogy of Fallot at less than six months of age. Is palliation "old-fashioned"? Eur J Cardiothorac Surg 9:453–459; discussion 459–460

Steffens JC, Bourne MW, Sakuma H, O'Sullivan M, Higgins CB (1994) Quantification of collateral blood flow in coarctation of the aorta by velocity encoded cine magnetic resonance imaging. Circulation 90:937–943

Suzuki JI, Change JM, Caputo GR, Higgins CB (1991) Evaluation of right ventricular early diastolic filling by cine nuclear magnetic resonance imaging in patients with hypertrophic cardiomyopathy. J Am Coll Cardiol 18:120–126

Tynan MJ, Becker AE, Macartney FJ, Quero Jimenez M, Shinebourne EA, Anderson RH (1979) Nomenclature and classification of congenital heart disease. Br Heart J 41:544–553

Underwood SR, Firmin DN, Klipstein RH, Rees RSO, Longmore DB (1987) Magnetic resonance velocity mapping: clinical application of a new technique. Br Heart J 57:404–412

Vanoverschelde JLJ, Raphael DA, Robert AR, Cosyns JR (1990) Left ventricular filling in dilated cardiomyopathy: relation to functional class and hemodynamics. J Am Coll Cardiol 15:1288–1295

Vermilion RP, Snider AR, Meliones JN, Peters J, Merida-Asmus L (1990) Pulsed Doppler evaluation of right ventricular diastolic filling in children with pulmonary valve stenosis before and after balloon valvuloplasty. Am J Cardiol 66:79–84

Vick GW III, Rokey R, Huhta JC, Mulvagh SL, Johnston DL (1990) Nuclear magnetic resonance imaging of the pulmonary arteries, subpulmonary region and aorticopulmonary shunts: a comparative study with two-dimensional echocardiography and angiography. Am Heart J 119:1103–1110

Vick GW III, Wendt RE, Rokey R (1994) Comparison of gradient echo with spin echo magnetic resonance imaging and echocardiography in the evaluation of major aortopulmonary collateral arteries. Am Heart J 127:1341–1347

Von Schulthess GK, Higashino SM, Higgins SS, Didier D, Fisher MR, Higgins CB (1986) Coarctation of the aorta: MR imaging. Radiology 158:469–474

Waien SA, Liu PP, Ross BL, Williams WG, Webb GD, McLaughlin PR (1992) Serial follow-up of adults with repaired tetralogy of Fallot. J Am Coll Cardiol 20:295–300

Ward CJ, Mullins CE, Nihill MR, Grifka RG, Vick GW III (1995) Use of intravascular stents in systemic venous and systemic venous baffle obstructions. Short-term follow-up results. Circulation 91:2948–2954

Wessel HU, Cunningham WJ, Paul MH, Bastanier CK, Muster AJ, Idriss FS (1980) Exercise performance in tetralogy of Fallot after intracardiac repair. J Thorac Cardiovasc Surg 80:582–593

Wexler L, Higgins CB (1995) The use of magnetic resonance imaging in adult congenital heart disease. Am J Card Imaging 9:15–28

4 Pericardial Diseases

P. Croisille and D. Revel

4.1
Introduction

The evaluation of pericardial diseases has been radically modified by modern imaging techniques, particularly by the development of echocardiography. Echocardiography is still the first-line modality to explore the pericardium, especially for the diagnosis of pericardial effusion. Computed tomography (CT) and magnetic resonance imaging (MRI) are second-line imaging modalities that have the ability to overcome, in large part, the limitations of echocardiography. MRI has the ability to provide unique information on the pericardium because of its excellent spatial resolution and the inherent contrast between anatomical structures.

P. Croisille, MD, Departement de Radiologie, Hôpital Cardiovasculaire et Pneumologique L. Pradel, BP Lyon Montchat, F-69394 Lyon Cedex 03, France
D. Revel, MD, Departement de Radiologie, Hôpital Cardiovasculaire et Pneumologique L. Pradel, BP Lyon Montchat, F-69394 Lyon Cedex 03, France

4.2
Anatomy

The pericardium is a flask-shaped sac that envelops the heart, extends to the origin of the great vessels, and is attached to the sternum, the dorsal spine, and the diaphragm (Hoit 1990). It is composed of two layers, an inner serous membrane consisting of a monolayer of mesothelial cells and an outer fibro-collagenous layer. The inner serosal layer, termed the *visceral* pericardium, is closely attached to the epicardial surface of the heart and covers a subepicardial layer of conjunctive tissue containing fat and coronary vessels. The serosal layer reflects back on itself to become the inner lining of the outer fibrous layer. Together, these layers form the *parietal* pericardium.

The pericardium contains two major pericardial recesses. The oblique sinus lies behind the left atrium so that the posterior wall of the left atrium is actually separated from the pericardial space. This explains why a posterior pericardial effusion behind the left ventricle is seen behind the left atrium only when it is very large. The transverse sinus is the connection between two tubes of pericardium that envelop the great vessels. The aorta and pulmonary artery are enclosed in one anterosuperior tube, and the vena cava and pulmonary veins are enclosed in a more posterior tube. Pericardial effusion located in the superior recess should not be mistaken for an intimal flap of an aortic dissection.

The pericardial virtual cavity normally contains between 10 and 50 ml of an ultrafiltrate of plasma (Roberts and Spray 1976). The fluid is produced by the visceral pericardium and drainage of the cavity is toward both the thoracic duct and the right lymphatic duct.

4.3
Imaging Technique

Imaging of the pericardium is usually performed using ECG-triggered multislice spin-echo (SE) sequences that provide between five and ten anatomical levels in the same imaging time (LANZER et al. 1984). Image quality will depend, among other factors, on cardiac gating, which can be difficult to obtain in patients with low ECG voltages due to pericardial disease. Respiratory artifacts can be reduced using single slice breath-hold turbo-SE sequences. Images with a higher spatial resolution can be obtained by combining breath-hold acquisition with the use of phased array coils. T2-weighted sequences can be used to provide additional information in an attempt to characterize the lesion, whereas gradient-echo (GE) cine sequences will demonstrate fluid movement during cardiac contraction and will be helpful in studying ventricular function, particularly right ventricular (RV) function in cases of constrictive pericarditis.

4.4
Normal Pericardium in MRI

On MR images, the normal pericardium appears as a low-intensity line that is underlined by the high-intensity mediastinal and subepicardial fat or medium-intensity myocardium (SECHTEM et al. 1986b; STARCK et al. 1984) (Fig. 4.1). In areas adjacent to the lung, the pericardium is more difficult to visualize due to the low intensity of the lung parenchyma. The sensitivity for visualization of the pericardium as determined by SECHTEM et al. (1986b) varies

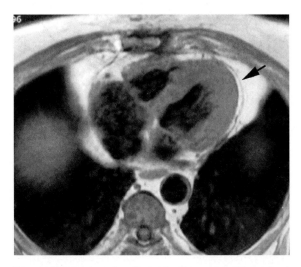

Fig. 4.1. Normal pericardium. Cardiac gated T1-weighted axial scan demonstrating the normal appearance of pericardium as a low signal intensity line (*arrowhead*) surrounded by the subepicardial and pericardial fat in a patient with a hypertrophic cardiomyopathy

from 100% over the region of the right ventricle (because of the presence of fat) to only 61% for the posterolateral portion of the left ventricle because of the lack of fat and the low signal of the pleura and lung parenchyma.

The transverse sinus of the pericardium is much more readily visualized on MR images than on CT images. It can be identified in 80% of cases in the transverse or sagittal plane, and in 70% of cases in the coronal plane (IM et al. 1988). Preaortic and retroaortic recesses of the pericardium can be identified in 67%–100% of the cases. Familiarity with the normal anatomy of the superior pericardial recesses is important in order to avoid misdiagnosis of aortic dissection or confusion with lymph nodes or mediastinal vessels (McMURDO et al. 1985; SOLOMON et al. 1990).

The average thickness of normal pericardium varies from 1.2 mm in diastole to 1.7 mm in systole. Pericardial thickness is also a function of the anatomical level and considerably increases in caudal sections (up to 7 mm), due essentially to the tangential direction of the pericardium with the imaging plane, and the diaphragmatic ligamentous insertions of the pericardium at caudal levels (SECHTEM et al. 1986b). Therefore, measurements of the pericardium should be performed on midventricular slices.

Visualization of the pericardium is improved in systole because the heart can maintain a more consistent shape during the acquisition of successive phase-encoding steps and preserve luminal flow void (CHAKO et al. 1995). It can also be explained by the greater width of the pericardial line, which increases during cardiac contraction (SECHTEM et al. 1986b).

Average pericardial thickness measured on MRI is slightly greater than that determined from anatomical studies (average of 1.4 mm on MRI versus 0.8–1 mm anatomically). The apparent pericardial line thickness actually results from the combination of the low-intensity fibrous parietal pericardium with motion-induced signal loss of the pericardial fluid surrounding the heart .

4.5
Congenital Anomalies

4.5.1
Agenesis of the Pericardium

Agenesis of the pericardium is a rare entity, and results from an abnormal embryonic development that may be secondary to abnormalities in the vascular supply of the pericardium. Agenesis is more common on the left side (70%) than on the right side (4%) or the inferior side (17%) (SECHTEM et al. 1986a). It is more often partial than total (9%) and may be associated, in at least one-third of cases, with other malformations, particularly malformations of the heart (tetralogy of Fallot, atrial septal defect, patent ductus arteriosus) or other types of abnormalities (bronchogenic cyst or hiatus hernia) (LORELL and BRAUNWALD 1988; LETANCHE 1988).

Since the pericardial defect is generally asymptomatic, it will be suggested on the chest X-ray by an abnormal left cardiac contour with better definition and separation of the segments that comprise the cardiac border (GLOVER et al. 1969). A left pericardial defect will be diagnosed on MRI in the absence of the pericardial line over the left cavities, which may lead to direct contact between the lung and the cardiac chambers; a leftward shift of the heart can be associated with this finding (GUTIERREZ et al. 1985). Herniation of the left ventricle through the pericardial window can occur, as can herniation within the pericardium of lung, left hemidiaphragm, or inferior vena cava.

4.5.2
Pericardial Cysts

Pericardial cysts correspond to congenital encapsulated cysts that are essentially anterior mediastinal lesions in the cardiophrenic sulcus (90%), more frequently located on the right side (70%) (Fig. 4.2).

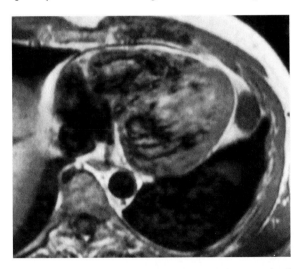

Fig. 4.2. Pericardial cyst. Axial cardiac gated T1-weighted scan shows a sharply demarcated mass lying on the pericardium and contained within pericardial fat. The signal intensity of this mass is equal to that of the muscle

They should not communicate with the pericardial cavity. MRI shows an aspect of paracardial liquid mass, which may be surrounded by a line of low intensity consistent with pericardium (SECHTEM et al. 1986a) (see also 10.4.4.8).

4.5.3
Pericardial Diverticula

Pericardial diverticula can be congenital or acquired, and corresponds to a herniation through a defect in the parietal pericardium that communicates with the pericardial cavity (SECHTEM et al. 1986a).

4.6
Effusive Pericardial Disease

The diagnosis of pericardial effusion is usually accomplished by echocardiography, given its high sensitivity. However, the accuracy of echocardiography can be limited in some circumstances: (1) false-positive cases may occur in the presence of atelectasis, or pleural effusion of mediastinal lesions that mimics pericardial effusion; (2) false-negative cases may occur in the presence of loculated fluid collections, such as in cases of inflammatory adhesions or hemopericardium; (3) there may be difficulties in differentiating fluid from epicardial fat in the anterior or posterior recesses or from pericardial thickening (WALINSKY 1978). MRI is of value compared with echocardiography because of its ability to better identify anatomical structures and interfaces, which reduces the false-positive rate. MRI will provide valuable information regarding the distribution of pericardial fluid, which may vary considerably, even if, in 70% of the cases, fluid collection is observed posterolateral to the left ventricle due to the gravitational dependency of the fluid (SECHTEM et al. 1986a). Another common location of fluid collection is the superior recess, as witnessed in cases of abundant pericardial effusion (Fig. 4.3).

Although MRI can detect pericardial effusion as small as 30 ml, a relationship between the measured width of the pericardial space and total fluid volume cannot be established because of the focal fluid accumulations. Regions in which pericardial width is greater than 4 mm can be regarded as abnormal. Moderate effusions (between 100 and 500 ml of fluid) are associated with a greater than 5 mm pericardial space anterior to the right ventricle (SECHTEM et al. 1986a).

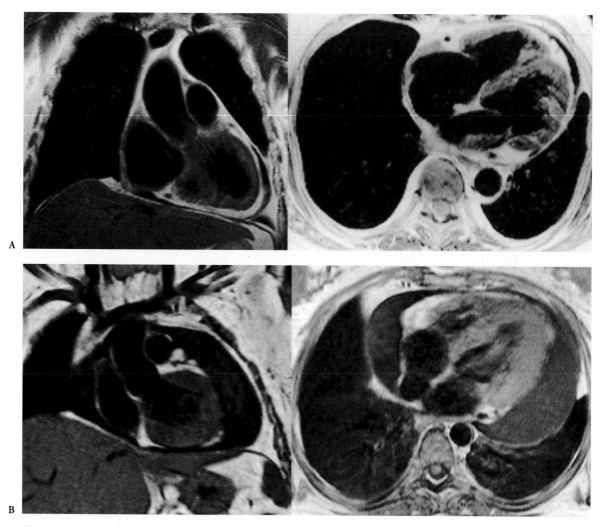

Fig. 4.3 A,B. Pericardial effusion. Cardiac gated T1-weighted coronal and axial images. **A** Localized pericardial effusion with fluid accumulation limited to the anteroapical regions. **B** Large pericardial effusion around the heart and extending up to the superior recesses of the pericardium. Note the changes in signal intensity of the fluid on T1-weighted images, essentially related to fluid motion during the cardiac cycle that prevents accurate characterization

MULVAGH et al. (1989) have shown that MRI is more sensitive that echocardiography for the detection of small pericardial effusions; this improved sensitivity is even more pronounced in the presence of loculated effusions when adhesions occur between the visceral and parietal pericardium. In a such case, it is common to observe a heterogeneous and high signal intensity that can be attributed to a reduction of fluid motion and cellular content.

Attempts to characterize the nature of the effusion based on the signal intensity have been disappointing. While pericardial effusions do vary in signal intensity, they characteristically display a low signal intensity on T1-weighted images. Because of fluid movement during cardiac contraction, flow void effects are apparent which in most cases prevent accurate characterization of pericardial fluid as either transudative or exudative (Fig. 4.4). However, effusions with a high proteinaceous or hemorrhagic content can be recognized by their high signal intensity on T1-weighted images, as well as by the presence of associated signs, such as an irregular pericardial surface suggestive of metastatic or inflammatory disease (Fig. 4.5).

4.7
Pericardial Thickening

Thickening of the pericardium is defined as an increase in the width of the pericardium to greater

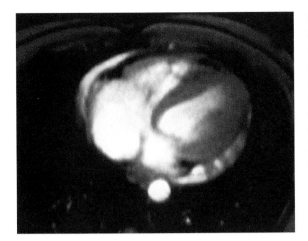

Fig. 4.4. Pericardial fluid motion. Cardiac GE T2-weighted axial image illustrating pericardial fluid motion artifacts in the posterolateral regions

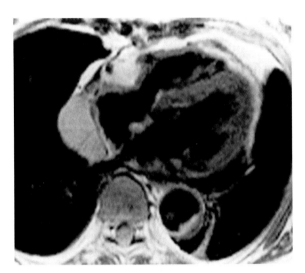

Fig. 4.5. Post-CABG localized hemorrhagic pericardial effusion. Hemorrhagic content appears as a fluid collection of intermediate signal intensity posterior to the right atrium

than 4 mm that can be focal or diffuse and may be associated with pericardial effusion or calcifications (SECHTEM et al. 1986a). It usually corresponds morphologically to a fibrous pericarditis that can be a manifestation of various systemic diseases, such as rheumatoid arthritis, lupus erythematosus, renal disease, scleroderma, infection, irradiation, or hemopericardium.

On MRI, pericardial thickening appears on the first echo of SE images as a widened pericardial line of low signal intensity that is similar in signal to the pericardial effusion. The following criteria are useful to help differentiate pericardial thickening from pericardial effusion: (1) the distribution of a focal or diffuse thickening is different from that of the fluid, which tends to accumulate posterolateral to the left ventricle; (2) an enlargement of the anterosuperior recess is highly suggestive of pericardial effusion; (3) a thickened fibrotic pericardium will maintain a constant thickness during the cardiac cycle whereas distribution of fluid in a nonloculated pericardial effusion will vary because of cardiac contraction. In the presence of inflammatory pericardial thickening, signal will increase on second echo images (MULVAGH et al. 1989; STARCK et al. 1984).

Pericardial calcifications, which may be associated with fibrous pericarditis, will appear as focal regions of decreased signal intensity with irregular shapes (SOULEN et al. 1985), but are much better demonstrated by CT.

4.8
Constrictive Pericarditis

An especially important clinical indication for MRI in pericardial disease is to differentiate constrictive pericarditis from restrictive cardiomyopathy (SOULEN et al. 1985) (see also Chap. 5). In contrast to its ability to demonstrate pericardial effusions, echocardiography is inadequate for the diagnosis of constrictive pericarditis because thickening due to fibrosis or calcification of the pericardium is difficult to characterize.

Today most cases of constrictive pericarditis are late sequelae of viral pericarditis, whereas formerly tuberculous pericarditis accounted for most cases. Other etiologies include infectious pericarditis, connective tissue disease, neoplasm, and trauma. Constriction is also a recognized complication of long-term renal dialysis, cardiac surgery, and radiation therapy (Fig. 4.6). Constrictive pericardial disease results from progressive pericardial fibrosis leading to constriction of the cardiac ventricles during diastole. Pathological findings include calcium deposition in a scarred and fibrotic pericardium that is adherent to the myocardium.

The major dilemma lies in distinguishing constrictive pericarditis from restrictive cardiomyopathy, which is critical since the treatment for constriction is surgery. Clinically, patients with constrictive pericarditis present with evidence of depressed ventricular function and with elevated diastolic filling pressures due to the constraining effect on diastolic filling of the scarred pericardium, while in restrictive myocardial disease the heart muscle is thickened and exhibits decreased compliance.

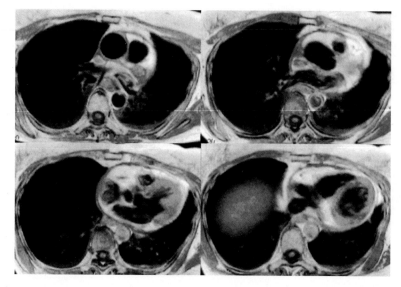

Fig. 4.6. Postradiotherapy constrictive pericarditis. A diffuse thickened pericardium is visible around the right cavities, as well as in the superior recesses of the pericardium

The presence of an abnormally thickened pericardium (exceeding 5 mm) in a patient with a suspected constriction is highly suggestive of the diagnosis (SOULEN et al. 1985) (Fig. 4.6). In chronic constriction, the thickened pericardium appears low in signal intensity because of the fibrous content, whereas in subacute cases (cardiac surgery, irradiation) it can be of high signal intensity (SECHTEM et al. 1986a). Associated calcifications will be identified by the presence of signal voids in conjunction with the thickened pericardium. Other imaging findings associated with this condition include: (1) narrowing (tubular-shaped) of the ventricles (especially the RV); (2) enlargement of one or both atria; (3) narrowing of one or both atrioventricular grooves; (4) dilatation of the vena cava and hepatic vein; and (5) abnormal ventricular contraction and septal wall motion.

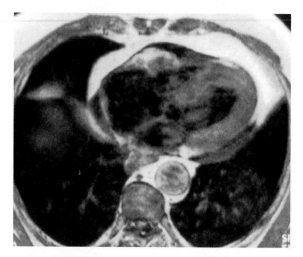

Fig. 4.7. Pericardial tumor which developed in the right atrioventricular sulcus from the visceral pericardium, associated with a reactive pericardial effusion

4.9
Pericardial Tumors

Primary tumors of the pericardium are rare entities, occurring much less frequently than pericardial metastasis. The most common malignant tumor of the pericardium is the mesothelioma, which is often associated with hemorrhagic pericardial effusion (Fig. 4.7). Other primary tumors include malignant fibrosarcoma, angiosarcoma, and benign and malignant teratoma (GOMES et al. 1987).

Pericardial metastases are very common (having a frequency of up to 22% in autopsy series comprising cancer patients) and are, in most cases, secondary to lung or breast carcinoma, leukemia, and lymphoma (HANOCK 1982). They are frequently associated with a large and hemorrhagic effusion that is disproportionate to the amount of tumor present.

Magnetic resonance imaging has advantages over other techniques for the assessment of pericardial tumors because it better delineates the implantation

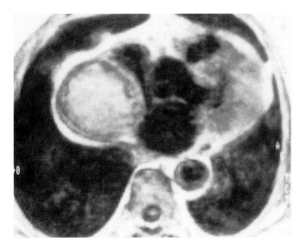

Fig. 4.8. Postsurgical mass with a compressive effect on the right atrium: pericardial foreign body granuloma

of the tumor outlined by either the pericardial fat or the pericardial effusion, and provides additional information on the contiguous anatomical structures (myocardial wall or great vessels). In the assessment of mediastinal tumors, MRI is also the imaging modality of choice to detect tumorous invasion of the pericardium, which can be inferred when there is focal absence of the pericardial line. In cases where malignancy is adjacent to cardiac structures, visualization of the pericardial line indicates that pericardial invasion has not occurred (LUND et al. 1989). Characterization of the pericardial tumor is usually not possible, exceptions being lipoma and liposarcoma, which appear with a high signal intensity due to their fatty content, and pericardial cyst (Fig. 4.8) .

4.10
Conclusion

Despite the unique ability of MRI to evaluate pericardial disease, MRI is not indicated for the primary evaluation of the pericardium, especially because of cost-effectiveness considerations. When further characterization is required after initial screening by echocardiography, such as when combined cardiac and pericardial involvement is suspected or when echocardiography proves inadequate owing to technical limitations, MRI is the imaging modality of choice. MRI will provide a more precise approach to pericardial effusions, especially in cases of loculated pericardial effusion. MRI is the imaging modality of

choice to differentiate constrictive pericarditis from restrictive cardiomyopathy, as well as to explore cardiac and pericardiac tumors, even if tissue characterization on the basis of signal intensity is limited (SECHTEM et al. (1998).

References

Chako AC, Tempany CM, Zerhouni EA (1995) Effect of slice acquisition direction on image quality in thoracic MRI. J Comput Assist Tomogr 19:936–940

Glover LB, Barcia A, Reeves TJ (1969) Congenital absence of the pericardium. Am J Radiol 106:542–548

Gomes AS, Lois JF, Child JS, et al. (1987) Cardiac tumors and thrombus: evaluation with MR imaging. AJR Am J Roentgenol 149:895–899

Gutierrez FR, Shackelford GD, McKnight RC, Levitt RG, Hartmann A (1985) Diagnosis of congenital absence of left pericardium by MR imaging. J Comput Assist Tomogr 9:551–553

Hanock EW (1982) Pericardial disease in patients with neoplasm. In: Reddy PS, Leon DF, Shaver JA (eds) Pericardial disease. Raven Press, New York, p 325

Hoit BD (1990) Imaging the pericardium. Cardiol Clin 8:587–600

Im JG, Rosen A, Webb WR, Gamsu G (1988) MR imaging of the transverse sinus of the pericardium. AJR Am J Roentgenol 150:79–84

Lanzer BH, Botvinick EH, Schiller NB, et al. (1984) Cardiac imaging using gated magnetic resonance. Radiology 150:121–127

Letanche G, Gayer C, Souquet PJ, et al. (1988) Agenesis of the pericardium: clinical, echocardiographic and MRI aspects. Rev Pneumol Clin 44:105–109

Lorell BH, Braunwald E (1988) Pericardial disease. In: Braunwald E (ed) Heart disease, a textbook of cardiovascular medicine. W.B. Saunders, Philadelphia, pp 1484–1485

Lund JT, Ehman RL, Julsrud PR, Sinak LJ, Tajik AJ (1989) Cardiac masses: assessment by MR imaging. AJR Am J Roentgenol 152:469–473

McMurdo KK, Webb WR, von Schulthess GK, Gamsu G (1985) Magnetic resonance imaging of the superior pericardial recesses. AJR Am J Roentgenol 145:985–988

Mulvagh SL, Rokey R, Vick GWD, Johnston DL (1989) Usefulness of nuclear magnetic resonance imaging for evaluation of pericardial effusions, and comparison with two-dimensional echocardiography. Am J Cardiol 64:1002–1009

Roberts WC, Spray TL (1976) Pericardial heart disease: a study of its causes, consequences, and morphologic features. Cardiovasc Clin 7:11–65

Sechtem U, Tscholakoff D, Higgins CB (1986a) MRI of the abnormal pericardium. AJR Am J Roentgenol 147:245–252

Sechtem U, Tscholakoff D, Higgins CB (1986b) MRI of the normal pericardium. AJR Am J Roentgenol 147:239–244

Sechtem U, Neubauer S, Revel D, et al. (1998) The clinical role of magnetic resonance in cardiovascular disease. Report of a Task Force of the European Society of Cardiology in collaboration with the Association of European Pediatric Cardiologists. Eur Heart J 19;19–39

Solomon SL, Brown JJ, Glazer HS, Mirowitz SA, Lee JKT (1990) Thoracic aortic dissection: pitfalls and artifacts in MR imaging. Radiology 177:223–228

Soulen RL, Stark DD, Higgins CB (1985) Magnetic resonance imaging of constrictive pericardial disease. Am J Cardiol 55:480–484

Starck DD, Higgins CB, Lanzer P, et al. (1984) Magnetic resonance imaging of the pericardium: normal and pathologic findings. Radiology 150:469–474

Walinsky P (1978) Pitfalls in the diagnosis of pericardial effusion. Cardiovasc Clin: 9:111–116

5 Myocardial Diseases

J. Bogaert

CONTENTS

5.1 Introduction

The heart is the central circulatory pump of the cardiovascular system. The driving force is generated by a repetitive contraction of the myocardium, which is a thick-walled layer of myocytes lying around a cavity. The myocardium may be involved in a variety of disorders in which the heart muscle is exclusively or preferentially affected (e.g., myocardial ischemia, hypertrophic cardiomyopathy) or in which the myocardial involvement is part of a multiorgan disorder (e.g., hemochromatosis). Not infrequently no underlying etiology can be found for the myocardial disorder, i.e., it is idiopathic. Important causes of myocardial diseases are shown in Table 5.1. Myocardial disorders present clinically in a variety of manners ranging from asymptomatic to fulminant cardiac failure. Assessment of the underlying etiol-

ogy of myocardial disorders is often difficult, and usually based on patients' symptoms, physical examination, and a series of technical investigations (e.g., cardiac imaging, laboratory investigations, endomyocardial biopsy). Since MRI is an excellent technique for assessment of human anatomy, this chapter will focus on the role of MRI in the morphological assessment of myocardial diseases. The repercussions of myocardial diseases for ventricular function are discussed in Chap. 6. MRI also permits evaluation of the effects of coronary artery disease on myocardial perfusion (see Chap. 8) and myocardial viability (see Chap. 7), and study of the metabolic spectra of myocardial diseases (see Chap. 9). The role of MRI in congenital heart diseases is discussed in Chap. 3.

5.2 Signal Characteristics of the Myocardium on MRI

On spin-echo (SE) MRI the myocardium has an intermediate signal intensity or a "gray" appearance similar to that of skeletal muscles, and is clearly distinguishable from the surrounding bright subepicardial fat and the adjacent dark endocavitary blood. The T1 relaxation time of myocardial tissue is about 800 ms (on a 1.5-T MR unit) (Zerhouni et al. 1988), and the T2 relaxation time approximately 45 ms (on a 1.0 T-MR unit) (Lund et al. 1989). Similar to diseases in other parts of the body, myocardial disorders are not infrequently characterized by changes in proton relaxation times. These changes may be helpful since they can be used at least to a certain degree for tissue characterization. For instance, fatty infiltration of the free wall of the right ventricle will be visible as hyperintense intramyocardial spot(s) on T1-weighted SE images and these abnormalities are highly suggestive for arrhythmogenic right ventricular dysplasia. Mature myocardial fibrosis or calcification, on the other hand, appears hypointense on both T1- and T2-

J. Bogaert, MD, PhD, Department of Radiology, University Hospitals Casthuisberg, Catholic University of Leuven, Herestraat 49, B-3000 Leuven, Belgium

Table 5.1. Etiology and patterns of myocardial diseases (cardiomyopathies and myocarditis)

Etiology	Condition	Pattern
Idiopathic	DCM	Dilated
	HCM	Hypertrophic
	Restrictive cardiomyopathy	Restrictive
	AVRD	RV dysfunction/dilation
Genetic	HCM	Hypertrophic
	ARVD	RV dysfunction
	Neuromuscular disorders	
Ischemic		Dilated
Inflammatory	Infective/noninfective	Asymptomatic to fulminant cardiac failure
		Dilated (end-stage)
Infiltrative	Amyloidosis	Restrictive
		Dilated
		May simulate HCM
	Hemochromatosis	Restrictive
		Dilated (end-stage)
	Other storage diseases (e.g., glycogen)	Restrictive
		May simulate HCM
	Neoplastic	Restrictive
	Sarcoidosis	Restrictive/dilated
Fibroplastic	Endomyocardial fibrosis	Restrictive
	Endocardial fibroelastosis	
	Löffler's fibroplastic endocarditis	
	Carcinoid	
Other	Metabolic/toxic (e.g., alcohol)	Dilated
	Hypersensitivity	
	Physical agents (e.g., radiation)	Restrictive
	Hematological	

ARVD, Arrhythmogenic right ventricular dysplasia; DCM, dilated cardiomyopathy; HCM, hypertrophic cardiomyopathy; RV, right ventricular.

weighted sequences and can be found in patients with endomyocardial fibrosis. A hyperintense myocardial area on T2-weighted images in a patient with a recent myocardial infarction is suggestive for increased free water content due to myocardial edema and/or necrosis. The latter finding can thus be used for noninvasive localisation of the myocardial infarction. However, the changes are nonspecific since other conditions, such as acute rejection of a cardiac allograft or myocarditis, are equally characterized by an increased water content and a subsequent rise in T2 relaxation values. In conclusion, changes in relaxation times reflect gross morphological changes but unfortunately are often nonspecific.

5.3
Ischemic Heart Disease

Coronary artery disease is one of the most common causes of morbidity and mortality in the industrialized countries. Since Chap. 7 is entirely focused on the assessment of myocardial viability with MRI, myocardial ischemia is discussed only briefly in this chapter.

The impact of a coronary artery occlusion on myocardial viability is highly variable, and influenced by many factors such as the rapidity and duration of the occlusion, the relation between myocardial oxygen consumption and supply, and the presence of collateral circulation. In the last two decades several therapeutic strategies to salvage the myocardium distal to the occlusion have been developed. Therapeutic approaches such as a mechanical or pharmacological revascularization of the occluded artery and reduction of the myocardial oxygen consumption are now routinely used clinically, while newer strategies such as angiogenesis of collateral vessels by gene therapy are still under investigation (The TIMI Study Group 1985; TAKAHASHI et al. 1997).

Acute occlusion of the coronary artery leads to a cessation of the myocardial contraction within seconds in the area deprived of oxygen. If the occlusion

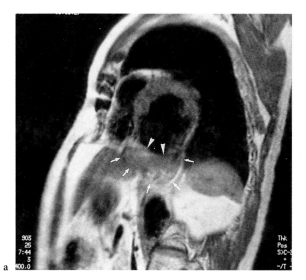 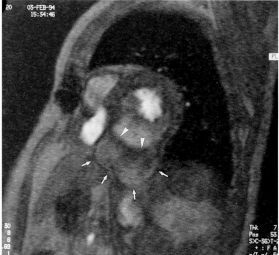

a   b

Fig. 5.1 a,b. Left ventricular aneurysm with thrombus formation in a patient with a previous inferior myocardial infarction. **a** Short-axis T1-weighted SE image; **b** short-axis GE image. There is extreme thinning of the inferior LV wall with aneurysmal wall bulging (*small arrows*). A large thrombus is present in the aneurysmal sac, clearly distinguishable from the LV blood pool (*arrowheads*)

is short-term, no necrosis occurs and this condition is recognized by a reversible postischemic contractile dysfunction after reperfusion has been achieved, i.e., stunned myocardium (TREVI and SHEIBAN 1991). The length of the contractile dysfunction, however, is out of proportion to the duration of coronary artery occlusion, but the longer the ischemia time, the longer will be the contractile dysfunction (LAWRENCE et al. 1992). Prolonged ischemia leads to tissue necrosis which first occurs in the subendocardium after approximately 15 min of ischemia. The subendocardial infarct boundaries are established within the first 40 min and closely correspond to the vascular territory. The infarct progresses towards the subepicardium over a period of 3–6 h. This transmural wave front is much more heterogeneous (REIMER and JENNINGS 1979; REIMER et al. 1977). Extensive transmural infarcts may lead to rupture of the myocardium with subsequent hemopericardium and cardiac tamponade or ventricular septum defect, and to rupture of the papillary muscles with acute valvular regurgitation and pulmonary edema. Chronic complications of acute myocardial infarctions include aneurysmal wall thinning in the infarcted region with thrombus formation, and ischemic cardiomyopathy (Fig. 5.1).

Chronic myocardial ischemia, as a result of severely reduced myocardial blood flow, leads to a series of morphological (e.g., dedifferentiation of the myocytes, progressive loss of myocytes and replacement fibrosis), functional (wall dyssynergia), and metabolic (increased glucose metabolism) changes (MAES et al. 1994). This condition is better known as hibernating myocardium and can be considered as a protective functional downregulation of the myocardium (RAHIMTOOLA 1993). In other words, hibernating myocardium represents a "last defence mechanism" in response to profound and chronic ischemia. However, it does not occur in all patients with chronic myocardial ischemia. In some circumstances the myocardium may undergo ischemic necrosis instead of hibernation, with irreversible structural and functional damage. The mechanism leading to one or other response to chronic ischemia is unclear and may depend on the degree and duration of myocardial ischemia. Since the myocardium at least partially survives, some improvement in the myocardial function can be expected after revascularization (BRAUNWALD and RUTHERFORD 1986). Thus, the detection of hibernating myocardium is clinically important because it indicates that the myocardium is potentially salvageable.

Clinically, the myocardium distal to the coronary artery occlusion often presents a mixture of necrosis, ischemia, and stunned and hibernating myocardium. Reperfusion therapy by means of thrombolytic therapy or angioplastic procedures, intended to salvage myocardial tissue, will further contribute to this inhomogeneity. One of the most important and certainly one of the most difficult aims of cardiac imaging is to detect and differentiate the several forms of myocardial viability (e.g., differentiation between dysfunctional but viable myocardium and irreversible damaged myocardium).

Several strategies have been proposed to assess myocardial viability with MRI in patients with an acute myocardial infarction or a history of such infarction. First, viable but dysfunctional myocardial tissue can be differentiated from infarcted myocardium by means of low-dose dobutamine infusion, because wall thickening will improve in the viable but dysfunctional segments under inotropic stimulation but remains unchanged or may even worsen in infarcted myocardium (PIÉRARD et al. 1990). In chronic infarcts, quantification of myocardial thickness and systolic wall thickening with and without positive inotropic stimulation can be applied to detect dysfunctional but viable myocardium (BAER et al. 1994). Second, acute and subacute myocardial infarctions may be depicted by changes in proton-density relaxation times, especially T2 relaxation times (CAPUTO et al. 1987). These changes however, reflect the ischemic area more than they do the true infarcted myocardium. Third, the use of paramag-

netic contrast media, especially infarct-avid contrast agents, may be appealing for the localization and quantification of infarcted myocardium (DE ROOS et al. 1989a; MARCHAL et al. 1996). Finally, measurement of metabolite concentrations within the infarct area using MR spectroscopy is another approach to assess myocardial viability (WEISS et al. 1990; NEUBAUER et al. 1992) (see Sect. 9.4.5).

5.4
Myocardial Hypertrophy

Increase in myocardial mass may occur as a consequence of physical training ("athlete's heart") (Fig. 5.2), is found in a variety of diseases including cardiomyopathies (see Sect. 5.5), increased afterload (e.g., aortic or pulmonary stenosis, systemic or pulmonary arterial hypertension), and increased preload (e.g., volume overload), and may occur as a compensatory mechanism following myocardial infarction. This ventricular remodeling represents an adaptive process and very likely consists in a combination of myocardial hyperplasia and hypertrophy. Tradition-

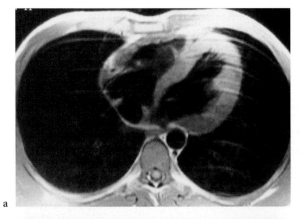

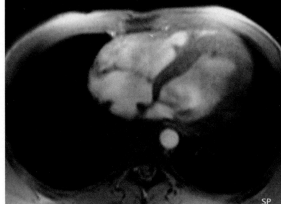

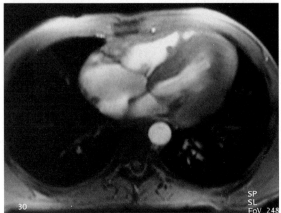

Fig. 5.2 a–c. Left ventricular hypertrophy in a professional cyclist (athlete's heart). **a** Axial turbo SE image; **b, c** axial breath-hold GE images at end-diastole (**b**) and end-systole (**c**). There is global thickening of the LV wall (end-diastolic wall thickness 18 mm), expressing a normal systolic wall motion. Since the end-diastolic wall thickness exceeds 16 mm, differentiation between physiological (athlete's heart) and pathological wall thickening (e.g., HCM) is difficult

ally, two types of ventricular hypertrophy are described which differ not only in presentation but also in underlying physiopathology. First, concentric left ventricular (LV) hypertrophy occurs as a consequence of pressure overload and is characterized by an increase in wall thickness and little or no change in cavity size (Fig. 5.3).

Second, eccentric hypertrophy is due to a volume overload with primarily an increase in cavity size and only a moderate increase in wall thickness (Fig. 5.4). The wall thickness-to-chamber radius ratio is a good parameter to express the changes in ventricular morphology. As discussed in Sect. 5.5.2, dilated cardiomyopathy represents an extreme (or "decompensated") form of eccentric LV hypertrophy, in which the increase in cavity volume is out of proportion to the increase in wall thickness.

Assessment of the extent and location of the myocardial hypertrophy is important not only as a prognostic indicator but also to permit follow-up of the effects of treatment. MRI is an excellent technique for quantitation of ventricular volumes and masses and regional and global ventricular function (see Chap. 6). Normal LV end-diastolic wall thickness is less than 12 mm; it may increase up to 16 mm in highly trained athletes, while in patients with severe arterial hypertension it may exceed 20 mm (BELENKOV et al. 1992; MARON et al. 1995).

5.5 Cardiomyopathies

Cardiomyopathies are diseases of the myocardium. The term cardiomyopathy was introduced by Harvey and Brigden four decades ago (BRIGDEN et al. 1957; HARVEY et al. 1964). In the classification of the World Health Organization (WHO), the term "cardiomyopathy" is reserved for myocardial diseases of unknown etiology, while other diseases that affect the myocardium but are of known cause or are part of a generalized systemic disorder are termed specific heart muscle diseases. However, since the clinical presentation of a given cardiomyopathy and a specific heart muscle disease is often similar, it is preferable to use the term *secondary* cardiomyopathy to identify those patients with a specific heart muscle disease that clinically closely simulates an idiopathic or *primary* cardiomyopathy. The etiology and pattern of the most frequent myocardial diseases causing cardiomyopathies are shown in Table 5.1. Three basic types of cardiomyopathies have been described by the WHO: *hypertrophic* cardiomyopathies (HCM), *dilated* cardiomyopathies (DCM) (formerly called congestive), and *restrictive* cardiomyopathies (FEJFAR 1968). Each type of cardiomyopathy corresponds with a basic type of functional impairment. However, overlap between the different types may exist. Hypertrophic cardiomyopathies are

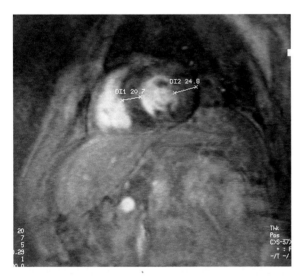

Fig. 5.3. Concentric LV hypertrophy in a patient with severe arterial hypertension. Short-axis GE image obtained at end-diastole. Excessive thickening of the LV wall (septum: 20.7 mm, lateral wall 24.8 mm) and a normal-sized LV cavity

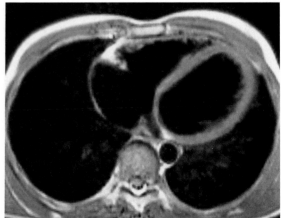

Fig. 5.4. Eccentric ventricular hypertrophy in a 12-year-old patient with chronic hemodialysis. There is enlargement of the cardiac chambers, especially the left ventricle, due to volume overload as a consequence of the arteriovenous fistula in the left arm. Little or no thickening of the LV wall.

Table 5.2. Morphological and functional abnormalities in cardiomyopathy

	Dilated	Hypertrophic	Restrictive
Morphology			
LV ± RV enlargement	+++	–	–
Myocardial hypertrophy	+	+++	–/+
Atrial dilation	++	+	++
Pleural effusion	+		+
Pericardial effusion	(+)	–	+
Ventricular thrombi (apex)	+	–	–
Dilation of IVC/SVC	+	–	+++
Myocardial function			
Global dysfunction	+++	+	(+)
Segmental variation	+	+++	(+)
Diastolic dysfunction	+	+(+)	+++
Valvular function			
Mitral regurgitation	++	++	+
Tricuspid regurgitation	+	–	+

IVC, Inferior vena cava; LV, left ventricular; RV, right ventricular; SVC, superior vena cava.

characterized by an inappropriate LV hypertrophy, usually with a preserved contractile function; dilated cardiomyopathies are characterized by ventricular dilatation and a contractile dysfunction, while in restrictive forms, impaired diastolic filling is the most prominent finding. The findings of the different cardiomyopathies on cardiac imaging are shown in Table 5.2. Most forms of secondary cardiomyopathy are characterized by the dilated cardiomyopathy pattern; less frequently the restrictive pattern is present. Other conditions such as arrhythmogenic right ventricular dysplasia are difficult to fit into this traditional classification scheme and are therefore discussed in separate sections. The changes in metabolic spectra in patients with DCM and in patients with HCM and other forms of myocardial hypertrophy are discussed in Sects. 9.4.3 and 9.4.4.

5.5.1
Hypertrophic Cardiomyopathy

The characteristic finding of HCM is an inappropriate myocardial hypertrophy in the absence of an obvious cause for the hypertrophy, such as systemic hypertension or aortic stenosis. Familial clustering is often observed, and the disease is genetically transmitted in about half of the cases. The disease has a variable natural history and may cause sudden death due to arrhythmia (SARDANELLI et al. 1993). Histologically, HCM is characterized by a disorganization and malalignment of the myofibrils, i.e., myofibrillar disarray, which is not unique to HCM but is clearly

more extensive in this disorder than in secondary myocardial hypertrophy from pressure overload or congenital heart disorders (MARON et al. 1981). This entity predominantly involves the upper portion of the interventricular septum of a nondilated left ventricle. Atypical locations of myocardial hypertrophy are the midportion of the ventricular septum, the apex, and the lower portion of the septum; severe concentric hypertrophy may also occur.

Asymmetric septal HCM, previously also called "idiopathic hypertrophic subaortic stenosis" and "muscular subaortic stenosis," is the most frequent subtype of HCM. It is characterized by a disproportionately thickened interventricular septum in comparison to the posterolateral wall of the left ventricle (Fig. 5.5). Asymmetric septal HCM may be responsible for an obstruction of the left ventricular outflow tract as demonstrated by a pressure gradient across the outflow tract of the left ventricle (BRAUNWALD et al. 1960; WIGLE et al. 1962). The anterior movement and apposition of the anterior mitral valve leaflet to the septum during systole contribute to the outflow obstruction. However, it is clearly recognized that not all patients have severe outflow tract pressure gradients while abnormalities in diastolic function are common (STEWARD et al. 1968). The less common apical form of HCM has a high prevalence in Japan. These patients have no outflow obstruction but present with a severe apical LV hypertrophy, giant negative T waves on their ECG, and a typical spade-shaped LV cavity (ABELMANN and LORELL 1989). In a recent study by SOLER et al. (1997) using MRI, three types of apical HCM were described: (a)

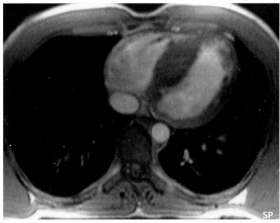

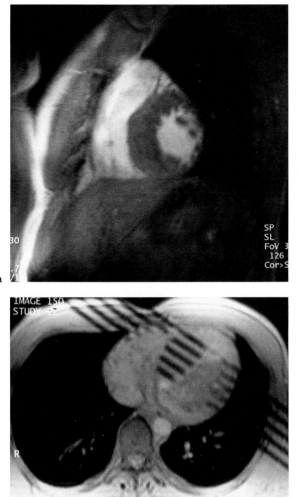

Fig. 5.5 a–c. Asymmetric septal HCM. **a** Short-axis GE image; **b, c** axial GE images without (**b**) and with (**c**) tag lines. There is excessive thickening of the basal two-thirds of the interventricular septum. Cine MRI and MR myocardial tagging depict not only a reduced wall thickening but also a profoundly impaired longitudinal shortening of the hypertrophic part of the interventricular septum

the true apical form, (b) involvement of the apex and symmetric hypertrophy of the four ventricular wall segments, and (c) involvement of the apex with asymmetric involvement of the wall segments. Another form of HCM is midventricular hypertrophy. These patients present with a gradient between the LV apical region and the remainder of the chamber. This may progress to a noncontractile apical aneurysm with apical thrombus formation (ABELMANN and LORELL 1989).

Although the role of MRI in the diagnosis of HCM is not yet established, MRI allows evaluation of the presence, distribution, and severity of the hypertrophic process (BEEN et al. 1985; HIGGINS et al. 1985; GAUDIO et al. 1992). A good correlation between the MRI findings and ECG abnormalities has been demonstrated. MRI permits differentiation between obstructive and nonobstructive forms of sep-

tal HCM, because obstructive forms will lead to a flow acceleration in the narrowed LV outflow tract, resulting in an area of signal void on cine MRI (DI CESARE et al. 1994) (Fig. 5.6). Accurate assessment of the LV obstruction is important as treatment modalities differ according to whether HCM is obstructive or nonobstructive and according to the severity of obstruction (MARON et al. 1987). The impact of the myocardial hypertrophy on the global and regional ventricular function can be precisely assessed. An advantage of MRI over other cardiac imaging modalities is the use of angled planes, which allows accurate measurement of the myocardial wall thickness (ARRIVE et al. 1994). In patients with HCM the end-diastolic wall thickness is increased. In the asymmetric septal form of HCM, the mean ratio of septal-to-free wall thickness is higher than 1.5 ± 0.8, compared with 0.9 ± 0.3 in normal volunteers and 0.8

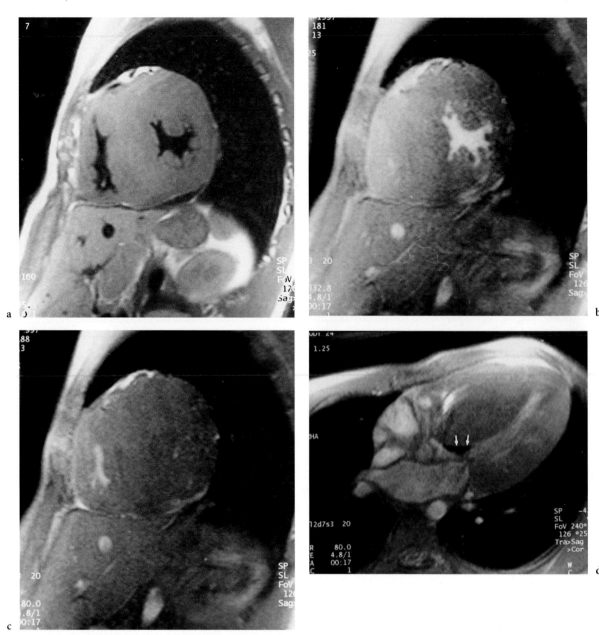

Fig. 5.6 a–d. Extreme case of obstructive HCM in an 11-year-old patient. **a** Short-axis turbo SE image; **b, c** short-axis GE images at end-diastole (**b**) and end-systole (**c**); **d** horizontal long-axis GE image obtained at mid-systole. There is excessive fusiform thickening of the interventricular septum (exceeding 50 mm), and to a lesser degree the anterior and posterior LV wall and the papillary muscles. Concomitant thickening of the RV free wall is present, very likely secondary to obstruction of the RV outflow tract by the hypertrophic interventricular septum. During cardiac systole there is a complete obliteration of the LV cavity (**c**). Narrowing of the LV outflow tract is causing a pressure gradient across the outflow tract. The flow acceleration in the narrowed outflow tract is visible as a hypointense jet on cine MR (*small arrows*) (**d**)

± 0.2 in patients with LV hypertrophy (BEEN et al. 1985). On the other hand, thickening of the septal wall during systole is markedly reduced, which is related to muscle disorganization (MARON et al. 1987; ARRIVE et al. 1994). Diastolic dysfunction of the right ventricle has been assessed by means of cine MRI in patients with HCM (SUZUKI et al. 1991a).

Another major advantage of MRI is the possibility of noninvasive study of the myocardial strain, i.e., myocardial deformation (see Chap. 6). By means of selective presaturation pulses, tag lines or a grid pattern can be imprinted on the myocardium, a technique called MRI myocardial tagging. This technique has not only been used to analyze the myocardial strain in normal circumstances but also been applied in patients with HCM. Using a two-dimensional SPAMM, i.e., spatial modulation of magnetization technique, tagging method, MAIER et al. (1992) demonstrated a reduction in the cardiac rotation in the posterior region and a reduced radial displacement in the inferior septal region. However, in a study by YOUNG et al. (1994) using a 3D SPAMM technique, significantly increased ventricular torsion was demonstrated in patients with HCM. These authors showed a significant reduction in the longitudinal ventricular shortening and to a lesser extent in the radial motion. In a study by KRAMER et al. (1994) using a similar technique, in HCM circumferential shortening was depressed in the septum and the inferior and anterior regions while longitudinal shortening was reduced in the basal septum. DONG et al. (1994), using the radial myocardial tagging technique, demonstrated a heterogeneously thickened myocardium. The fractional wall thickening and circumferential shortening were reduced compared with healthy volunteers, and inversely related to the local thickness. In summary, these studies show a profound and diffuse alteration of the myocardial contraction pattern in patients with HCM.

Gadolinium (Gd)-DTPA administration may be useful to differentiate normal from disorganized myocardial tissue (TSUKIHASHI et al. 1994). After Gd-DTPA administration, the hypertrophic myocardium in patients with HCM shows a higher signal intensity ratio than nonhypertrophic regions and than myocardium in normal subjects, and a delayed decay of the signal intensity is present. The areas of abnormally high signal intensity in LV myocardium seem to reflect myocardial ischemia and fibrosis due to small-vessel disease, or myocardial degeneration and necrosis (KOITO et al. 1995).

5.5.2
Dilated Cardiomyopathy

Dilated cardiomyopathy (DCM) is a syndrome characterized by LV or biventricular enlargement, cardiac hypertrophy, and severely depressed systolic function (DEC and FUSTER 1994). A series of morphological changes are found in the myocardial wall. At the cellular level, a combination of atrophy and hypertrophy of the myocytes is demonstrated. The myocardial hypertrophy consists in myocyte elongation with an in-series addition of newly formed sarcomeres, which is the major factor responsible for the increase in chamber size (BELTRAMI et al. 1995). The myocyte diameter also increases, although the lateral expansion of myocytes is modest and inadequate to preserve the ratio of the wall thickness to the chamber diameter at normal values (BELTRAMI et al. 1995). The structural correlate in the extracellular matrix is an excessive deposition of collagen in the ventricular wall (SCHAPER et al. 1991). The combination of ventricular dilatation and an inadequate increase in myocardial wall thickness leads to a decompensated eccentric hypertrophy, and a consequent increase in ventricular wall stress (FUJITA et al. 1993).

Although the cause of DCM is often not definable (idiopathic DCM), a variety of cytotoxic, metabolic, immunological, familial, and infectious mechanisms can produce the clinical manifestations of DCM (DEC and FUSTER 1994). It is likely that DCM represents the final common pathway that is the end result of myocardial damage.

The clinical presentation of DCM is variable. The most common symptom is left heart failure. Many patients, however, have minimal or no symptoms and the progression of the disease in these patients is unclear (REDFIELD et al. 1994). Right heart failure is rather uncommon and is found only in severe cases. On chest x-ray, DCM usually reveals generalized cardiomegaly and pulmonary vascular redistribution; interstitial and alveolar edema is less common on initial presentation (DEC and FUSTER 1994). However, a normal cardiac silhouette may be present in patients with DCM and can be explained on the basis of a counterclockwise transverse rotation of the heart within the thorax (KONO et al. 1992). Pleural effusions may be present, and the azygos vein and superior vena cava may be dilated when right heart failure supervenes.

Cardiac imaging techniques are used to evaluate the size of the ventricular cavity and the thickness of the ventricular walls, to exclude concomitant valvular and pericardial disease, and to detect the repercussions of the LV dilatation for valvular function (Fig. 5.7). They are also useful to detect LV thrombi, which are usually located in the apex (see Fig. 10.4). Functional studies reveal increased end-diastolic and end-systolic LV volumes, reduced ejection fractions in one or both ventricles, and wall motion abnormalities. Although segmental wall motion abnormalities are not uncommon in DCM, they are still more characteristic of ischemic heart disease, whereas diffuse global dysfunction is more typical of DCM.

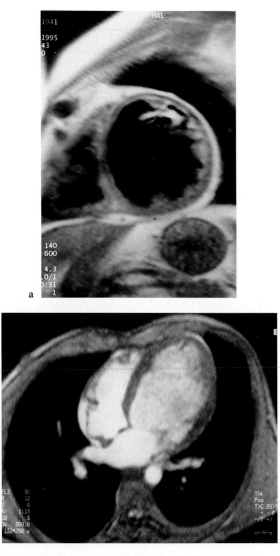

Fig. 5.7 a,b. Extreme case of dilated cardiomyopathy. **a** Short-axis HASTE image; **b** horizontal long-axis GE image. Huge dilation of the LV cavity (EDV: 250 ml), with a global thinning of the LV wall

disappeared in patients with DCM (BUSER et al. 1990). Calculations showed that the RV mass in patients with DCM was not significantly different from that in normals, whereas the LV mass was significantly greater (DOHERTY et al. 1992a). IMAI et al. (1992) demonstrated an enlargement of the LV trabeculae in patients with DCM. In normal subjects, LV trabeculae are seen at the free walls of the left ventricle, but not at the septal wall. These trabeculae were larger in patients with DCM than in normals, while in patients with old myocardial infarction the trabeculae were scarce and the inner sides of the myocardium became very smooth. KOITO et al. (1996) demonstrated an abnormally high signal intensity on Gd-DTPA enhanced MR images in patients with DCM. These regions may reflect areas of myocardial degeneration, necrosis, and fibrosis, and the high signal intensity may predict the severity of LV dysfunction in DCM.

Cine MRI is able to depict global and/or segmental wall motion abnormalities in patients with DCM (Fig. 5.8). FUJITA et al. (1993), using cine MRI, showed an inverse relation between the regional end-systolic wall stress and the regional ejection fraction in the left ventricle in patients with DCM. Diastolic abnormalities, i.e., increase in the time-to-peak filling rate and impaired filling fraction, were detected in the right ventricle showing a normal volume and normal systolic function in patients with DCM (SUZUKI et al. 1991b). It is likely that changes in LV morphology and function in patients with DCM will influence the behavior even of a normal-appearing right ventricle (DONG et al. 1995). Cine MRI has also been used to evaluate the potential beneficial effects of ACE inhibitor therapy on the ejection fraction in patients with DCM (DOHERTY et al. 1992b). MACGOWAN et al. (1997) used myocardial tagging to study the impact of the structural abnormalities on the fiber and cross-fiber shortening in patients with DCM.

Magnetic resonance imaging is able to accurately describe the morphological and functional abnormalities of DCM. At present, MRI is very likely the preferred imaging technique to quantify ventricular volumes and functional parameters, to measure the ventricular wall thickness, to calculate the right ventricular (RV) and LV mass, and to evaluate the presence of RV enlargement in patients with DCM (SEMELKA et al. 1990; BUSER et al. 1990; GAUDIO et al. 1991; DOHERTY et al. 1992a). Buser et al. showed a significantly more heterogeneous end-diastolic LV wall thickness in patients with DCM compared with normals (Fig. 5.8). Furthermore, the normal gradient in systolic wall thickening between LV base and apex

5.5.3
Restrictive Cardiomyopathy

The hallmark of restrictive cardiomyopathy is abnormal diastolic function. Restrictive cardiomyopathy is characterized hemodynamically by increased RV and LV filling pressures as a consequence of increased myocardial stiffness. The influence of restrictive cardiomyopathy on LV output is variable. The contractile function is often unimpaired. Thus, functionally restrictive cardiomyo-

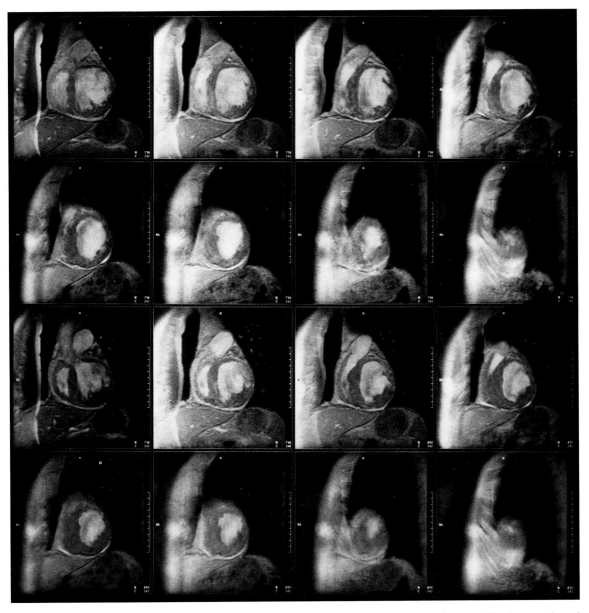

Fig. 5.8. Short-axis cine MRI study in a patient with DCM. The *upper two rows* demonstrate the left ventricle at end-diastole (LV base: *top left*; LV apex: *bottom right*). The *lower two rows* demonstrate the corresponding images at end-systole. Note the irregularities in wall thickness and systolic wall thickening of a mildly dilated left ventricle. Especially the anterolateral wall appears very thin and exhibits little or no wall thickening. Global LV parameters: end-diastolic volume, 119 ml; end-systolic volume, 87 ml; stroke volume, 32 ml; ejection fraction, 27%

pathy resembles constrictive pericarditis, which is also characterized by normal or nearly normal systolic function but abnormal ventricular filling. Differentiation between the two can be difficult on clinical grounds, but is critical for decisions regarding the therapeutic approach, since constrictive pericarditis requires surgical resection or stripping of the pericardium whereas nonsurgical management is used for restrictive cardiomyopathy (SHABETAI 1986; WENGER et al. 1986) (see also Sect. 4.8). In both conditions right atrial and inferior vena caval enlargement is observed, while the ventricles have a small or normal size (Fig. 5.9). Differentiation of the two diseases is dependent on the demonstration of a thickened pericardium. The pericardium, and any thickening thereof, can be very nicely demonstrated by means of SE MRI. MASUI et al. (1992) demonstrated that the identification of pericardial thicken-

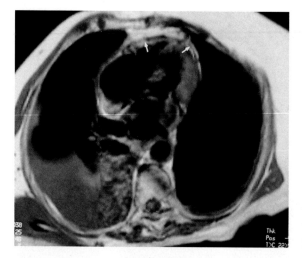

Fig. 5.9. Restrictive cardiomyopathy. Horizontal long-axis T1-weighted SE image. Small ventricles are present and there is dilation of both atria and the inferior vena cava. The thickness of the pericardium is within normal limits (*small arrows*). Note the presence of a right-sided pleural effusion

ing, i.e., pericardial thickness greater than 4 mm, on MRI has a diagnostic accuracy of 93% in patients with symptoms and signs suggestive of constrictive pericarditis.

A variety of specific pathological processes may result in restrictive cardiomyopathy, although the cause often remains unknown. Restrictive cardiomyopathy may result from myocardial fibrosis, infiltration, myocardial storage, or endomyocardial scarring (see Sect. 5.5.4). Furthermore, patients with HCM, for instance, may also demonstrate a restrictive pattern due to the increased stiffness of the myocardium.

5.5.4
Secondary Cardiomyopathies or Specific Heart Muscle Diseases

Table 5.1 shows the most common causes of secondary cardiomyopathies. The role of MRI in the diagnosis of some entities will be discussed in the following subsections.

5.5.4.1
Amyloidosis

Cardiac amyloidosis is a common cause of secondary restrictive cardiomyopathy. Cardiac amyloidosis is characterized by myocardial wall thickening as a consequence of intramyocardial accumulation of amyloid fibrils. The cardiac amyloid deposits generally cause severe cardiac dysfunction with a poor prognosis (SIVARAM et al. 1985). Although the therapeutic means are limited and treatment is generally unsatisfactory, the diagnosis is important to exclude the potentially curable conditions which it may mimic.

Cardiac amyloidosis has no specific patterns on MRI (VON KEMP et al. 1989). It is unknown whether intramyocardial amyloid deposits cause changes in myocardial relaxation times on MRI. However, severe concentric hypertrophy of both normal sized ventricles in the absence of arterial hypertension or valvular heart disease and in conjunction with positive extramyocardial biopsy is highly suspicious of cardiac amyloidosis (SHIREY et al. 1980) (Fig. 5.10). Other findings include thickening of the papillary muscles, valve leaflets, and the interatrial septum. Pleural and pericardial effusions are not infrequently recognized. Systolic wall thickening and global LV function are impaired and the left atrium is enlarged. Another hallmark of cardiac amyloidosis is diastolic dysfunction, with an abnormal relaxation pattern and a restrictive pattern of transmitral valve flow in the advanced stage. However, differentiation from other restrictive cardiomyopathies is not feasible. The increase in myocardial wall thickness in cardiac amyloidosis may mimic HCM (SIQUEIRA-FILHO et al. 1981). Asymmetric septal hypertrophy is found in 15%–55% of cases of cardiac amyloidosis in combination with a systolic anterior motion of the mitral valve and early systolic closure of the aortic valve.

5.5.4.2
Sarcoidosis

Cardiac involvement is diagnosed clinically in only 5% of patients with sarcoidosis, although it is present in the myocardium at autopsy in 20%–30% of patients. Patients with myocardial sarcoidosis usually have minimal or no clinical evidence of extracardiac organ involvement and the illness is rarely diagnosed before death (VIRMANI et al. 1980). Because sudden death is a common initial manifestation, occurring in as many as 60% of these patients, a noninvasive method to diagnose myocardial sarcoidosis would be valuable.

Sarcoidosis can invade the myocardium in multiple regional sites, leading to postinflammatory scarring. Sarcoid infiltrates present as zones of increased intramyocardial signal intensity that are

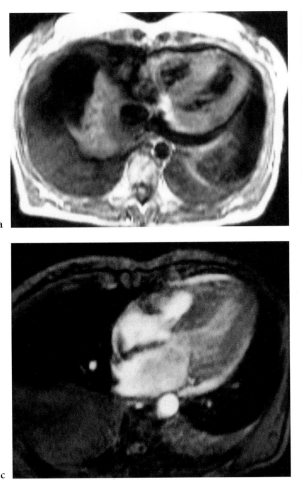

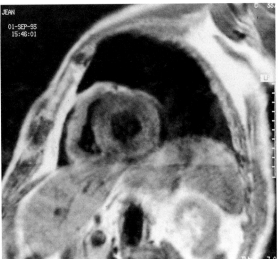

Fig. 5.10 a–c. Cardiac amyloidosis in a patient presenting with restrictive heart failure. **a** Axial and **b** short-axis T1-weighted SE images; **c** horizontal long-axis GE image. Concentric thickening of the RV and LV walls is seen. There is moderate pericardial and pleural effusion

more pronounced on T2-weighted images than on T1-weighted images. Moreover, it is possible to follow up the response of these lesions to steroid therapy and observe their partial regression (DUPUIS et al. 1994). These nonspecific appearances may be observed in all inflammatory conditions but, in the context of systemic sarcoidosis, are very suggestive of cardiac involvement. MRI is helpful in locating the site and extent of sarcoid lesions and in guiding an endomyocardial biopsy (DUPUIS et al. 1994). Regional scarring, even when limited to the subendocardium, may be detected by means of MRI as a focal area of diminished or absent systolic wall thickening or even systolic wall thinning (CHANDRA et al. 1996a). In addition, regional and global ventricular function can be simultaneously quantified and extracardiac signs of sarcoidosis, e.g., mediastinal adenopathy, can be imaged. Thus, one should consider performing MRI when cardiac sarcoidosis is suspected.

5.5.4.3
Iron Overload Cardiomyopathy

Iron overload cardiomyopathy is defined as the presence of systolic or diastolic cardiac dysfunction secondary to increased deposition of iron in the heart. This cardiac dysfunction is independent from other concomitant processes, such as atherosclerosis, ischemia, or valvular disease (LIU and OLIVIERI 1994). It can result from primary or secondary hemochromatosis, which is classically defined as iron overload in the parenchymal cells in tissues, e.g., iron deposition in the liver cells leading to cirrhosis or in the cardiac myocytes leading to heart failure. Primary hemochromatosis is an autosomal recessive disease affecting one in 220 persons, and usually presents late in life. Secondary hemochromatosis is a common cause of mortality in the young adult population in the developed world. This is the result of the large population with hereditary anemias, such as thalassemia or sickle cell anemia. These patients require chronic red cell transfusion starting at a young

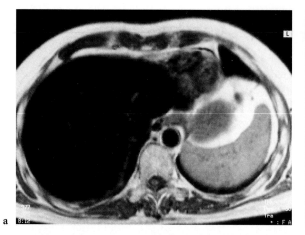

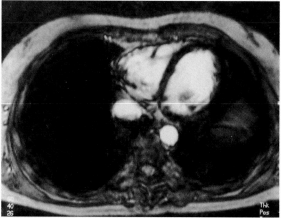

a

b

Fig. 5.11 a,b. Iron overload cardiomyopathy. a Axial T1-weighted SE image through the liver; b T2-weighted GE image. Extremely low signal intensity of the liver is caused by iron deposition (a). Iron overload in the myocardium leads to a low myocardial signal intensity, as shown in b, with mild dilation of the left ventricle

age. However, one of the complications of this transfusion therapy is iron overload. Chelation therapy may delay or prevent the occurrence of iron-induced heart failure. Other conditions in which iron overload may occur in body organs include chronic alcoholic disease and chronic hemodialysis.

Initially, myocardial iron overload is totally asymptomatic. There is a mild increase in LV wall thickness and end-diastolic chamber diameter. Diastolic function abnormalities usually precede systolic function abnormalities and are characterized by a restrictive filling pattern (BENSON et al. 1989; LIU et al. 1993a). Systolic function abnormalities usually do not appear until the iron concentration reaches a critical level, but then there is often a rapid deterioration in cardiac function.

Magnetic resonance imaging can be used to identify the presence of iron in the heart and potentially to quantitate the iron levels from the image signal intensity or the calculated T2 relaxation time (CHAN et al. 1992). Imaging with MR is based on the differences in signal intensity among tissues with intrinsically different relaxation parameters in a homogeneous magnetic field. The presence of iron disturbs the magnetic field homogeneity and enhances tissue T2 relaxation. MRI techniques that are sensitive to tissue T2 changes will be able to detect a marked decrease in signal intensity on T2-weighted images (STARK et al. 1985; HARDY and HENKELMAN 1989) (Fig. 5.11). The degree of signal attenuation is related to the intrinsic tissue iron levels, but not the serum ferritin concentration (LESNEFSKY et al. 1992). The T2 relaxation time is the best independent parameter to detect the iron content directly in the heart and so predict cardiac complications, and can be used for monitoring therapy (LIU et al. 1993b).

5.5.4.4
Endomyocardial Disease (Löffler Endocarditis and Endomyocardial Fibrosis)

Endomyocardial disease is a common form of secondary restrictive cardiomyopathy, and includes Löffler endocarditis and endomyocardial fibrosis (PARRILLO 1990). Although they were previously thought to be two variants of a single disease, these entities have not only a different geographical distribution but also a different clinical presentation. Löffler endocarditis occurs in temperate countries, has a more aggressive and rapidly progressive course, and is related to hypereosinophilia, while endomyocardial fibrosis occurs most commonly in equatorial Africa and is not related to hypereosinophilia. The restrictive pattern is caused by an intensive endocardial fibrotic wall thickening of the apex and subvalvular regions of one or both ventricles, resulting in an inflow obstruction of blood. The underlying pathogenesis of Löffler endocarditis is complex and probably related to hypereosinophilia, with a toxic effect of eosinophils on the heart causing necrosis, endomyocarditis, and formation of intramyocardial thrombi (WELLER and BUBLEY 1994). In a later phase localized or extensive replacement fibrosis causes thickening of the ventricular wall (Fig. 5.12). Atrioventricular valve regurgitation, as a result of progressive scarring of the chordae tendinae, may occur, with enlargement of the atria.

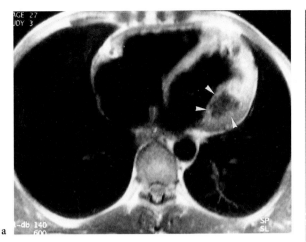

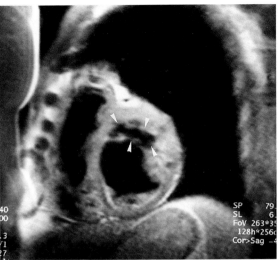

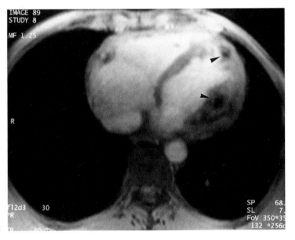

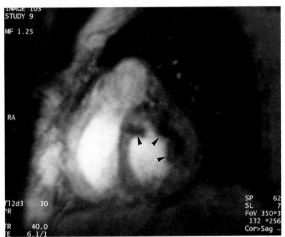

Fig. 5.12 a–d. Endomyocardial fibrosis. **a** Axial and **b** short-axis HASTE images; **c** axial and **d** short-axis GE images. There is inhomogeneous thickening of the anterolateral wall and apex of the left ventricle with several hypointense areas at the inner side of the myocardium (*arrowheads*) representing fibrotic or calcified areas

The increased stiffness of the ventricles and the reduction of the ventricular cavity by organized thrombus causes a restrictive filling pattern. MRI is helpful in the diagnosis of endomyocardial disease and in the evaluation of effects of medical treatment (D'Silva et al. 1992; Lombardi et al. 1995; Chandra et al. 1996b; Pitt et al. 1996; Huong et al. 1997). Areas of myocardial fibrosis appear as areas of low signal intensity. The right, left, or both ventricular walls are grossly thickened, with subsequent narrowing of the ventricular cavities. Ventricular volumes and atrioventricular regurgitation can be accurately quantified.

5.5.4.5
Glycogen and Other Metabolic Storage Diseases

Cardiac involvement in metabolic storage diseases such as type I or II glycogenosis, Gaucher and Neimann-Pick diseases, galactosialidosis, and mucopolysaccharidosis is characterized by LV wall thickening, valvular involvement, and LV diastolic dysfunction while LV systolic function is often normal. The LV wall thickening may even mimic HCM with or without obstruction of the LV outflow (Fig. 5.13). In clinical practice, M-mode, two-dimensional, and Doppler echocardiography are used for the determination of LV wall thickness, systolic function, anatomical derangement, valvular dysfunction, and LV diastolic function; the role of MRI remains to be established (Senocak et al. 1994).

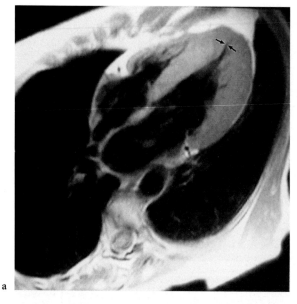 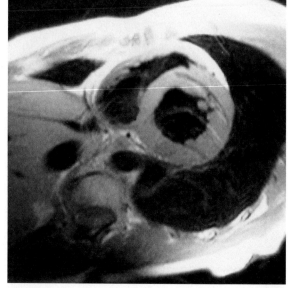

a   b

Fig. 5.13 a,b. Fabry's disease (metabolic storage disease). **a** Horizontal long-axis and **b** short-axis turbo-SE image. There is diffuse thickening of the myocardial wall. Although the LV apex is relatively less affected, the apposition of the thickened septum and lateral wall may lead to a false impression of LV apical hypertrophy (*small arrows*). Metabolic storage diseases may mimic other causes of myocardial hypertrophy such as HCM

5.5.5
Arrhythmogenic Right Ventricular Dysplasia

Arrhythmogenic right venticular dysplasia (ARVD) or cardiomyopathy (ARVD) is defined as a primary disorder of the right ventricle characterized by partial or total displacement of muscle by fatty or fibrous tissue (BLAKE et al. 1994; FONTAINE et al. 1998). It occurs predominantly in males and may be familial. The mean age of patients when symptoms arise is 30 years, and the symptoms frequently occur during exercise. This entity can result in recurrent ventricular tachyarrhythmias of RV origin and must be distinguished from exercise-induced automatic ventricular tachycardias originating from the RV outflow tract in patients with normal RV anatomy. The risk of sudden death in ARVD is substantial, whereas it appears to be negligible in patients with RV outflow tract tachycardia.

At histological examination, an inflammatory infiltrate with necrosis and fibroadipose replacement is found (BURKE et al. 1998). Although initially regarded as a congenital or complete congenital absence of ventricular myocardium, there is convincing clinical and pathological evidence that it is an acquired disorder with a continuous, chronic process of injury and repair (ANGELINI et al. 1996). In ARVD, the fibrous-fatty replacement almost exclusively involves the RV free wall; involvement of the septum and left ventricle is much less frequent. In a later phase, focal or diffuse thinning is noticed with bulging of the ventricular wall. Functionally, the involved regions demonstrate an a- or dyskinetic wall motion.

The diagnosis of AVRD relies on the demonstration of intramyocardial adipose deposits, wall thinning, and abnormal wall motion. Angiocardiography and echocardiography are able to depict only focal or diffuse ventricular bulging. MRI, however, has the capability also to depict the fatty myocardial degeneration, wall thinning, and abnormal contractility in patients with ARVD (Figs. 5.14, 5.15). Adipose tissue has a high signal intensity on T1-weighted images and stands in clear contrast with the intermediate signal intensity of the myocardium (CASOLO et al. 1987; MENGHETTI et al. 1996) (Figs. 5.16, 5.17). Detailed MR images of the RV wall allow detection of small intramyocardial fatty deposits. The best approach to study the free wall of the right ventricle is to position the subject in the prone position, and to use a surface coil over the precordium (BLAKE et al. 1994) (Fig. 5.18). In order to maximize the spatial resolution of the RV free wall, a small field of view can be used. Flow signal artifact, displayed in the phase-encoding direction, can produce factitious bright signal foci in the free wall of the right ventricle. Therefore, double saturation bands placed

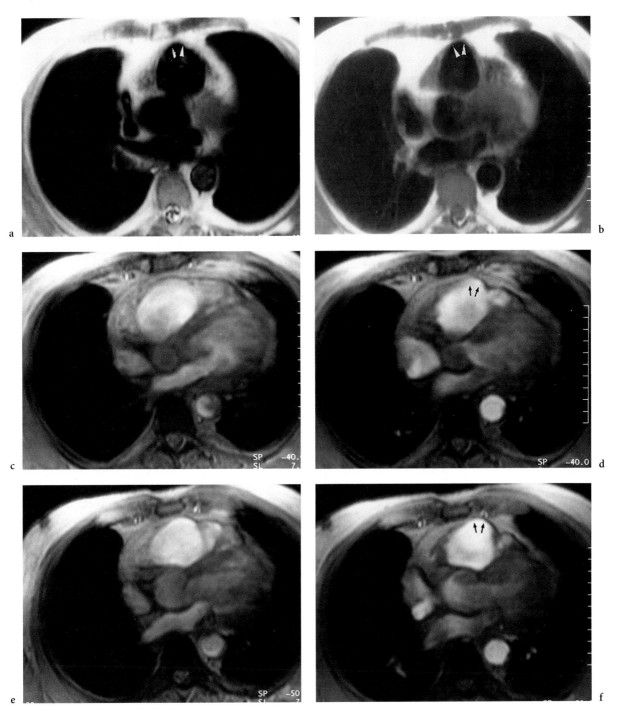

Fig. 5.14 a–f. Arrhythmogenic right venticular dysplasia **a, b** Axial HASTE images; **c–f** axial GE images at end-diastole (**c, e**), and end-systole (**d, f**), obtained at two different cardiac levels. There is focal thinning and bulging of the RV free wall (**a, b**): (*arrowheads*). Dyskinetic wall motion is seen on cine MRI (**c–f**): (*arrows*)

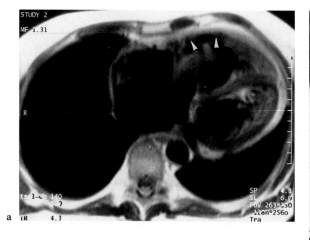

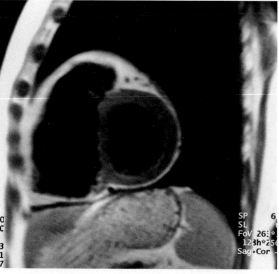

Fig. 5.15 a,b. End-stage arrhythmogenic right ventricular dysplasia. **a** Axial and **b** short-axis HASTE images. There is thinning of the basal portion of the RV free wall (*arrowheads*), showing dyskinesis on cine MRI (not shown) Dilation of the right ventricle and atrium is present

behind the free wall will suppress flow artifacts from the ventricular blood pool. Focal or diffuse abnormalities in myocardial contractility can be studied with cine MRI. Thus, MRI can be used with other procedures in the initial diagnostic evaluation and is a useful alternative tool in the long-term follow-up of patients with ARVD.

Recently, White and colleagues also reported morphologic and functional abnormalities in patients with RV arrhythmia in the absence of ARVD (WHITE et al. 1998). These abnormalities included fixed wall thinning, fatty myocardial infiltration and local bulging, most often located in the lower infundibular part of the RV. Similarities in MR imaging findings with ARVD suggests that these conditions are related, and that MR imaging appears to be an extremely valuable imaging technique, possibly the best, for assessment of the right ventricle for cardiomyopathy predisposing to arrhythmia.

5.6
Myocarditis

Myocarditis is defined as an inflammatory infiltrate of the myocardium with necrosis or degeneration of the adjacent myocytes not typical of ischemic damage associated with coronary artery disease (ARETZ et al. 1986). The clinical presentation and outcome are highly variable (LIEBERMAN et al. 1991). Patients with acute myocarditis usually present with a profound ventricular dysfunction which may progress to DCM, whereas patients with chronic persistent myocarditis usually have no ventricular dysfunction despite foci of myocyte necrosis. Although the etiology is often unknown (i.e., idiopathic), myocarditis can be found in a variety of diseases affecting the myocardium and/or other parts of the heart. Though virtually any infectious agent may cause myocarditis, most cases of acute myocarditis are caused by viruses (e.g., Coxsackie virus) (REMES et al. 1990; RAMAMURTHY et al. 1993) (Fig. 5.19). Myocarditis may also be caused by allergic reactions and pharmacological agents, as well as occurring during the course of some systemic diseases such as vasculitis. Endomyocardial biopsy is required for diagnosis and classification (ARETZ et al. 1986).

Though its role remains to be established, MRI has been proposed as a noninvasive method to detect inflammatory changes within the myocardium. The histological findings in acute myocarditis are similar to those in acute cardiac allograft rejection (see below). The increase in myocardial water content (due to interstitial edema) is characterized by a prolongation of the proton relaxation time (especially T2 relaxation time) and a hyperintense appearance of the myocardium on T2-weighted MRI sequences. In a preliminary study by GAGLIARDI et al. (1991), promising results were reported regarding discrimination of infants and children with from those without

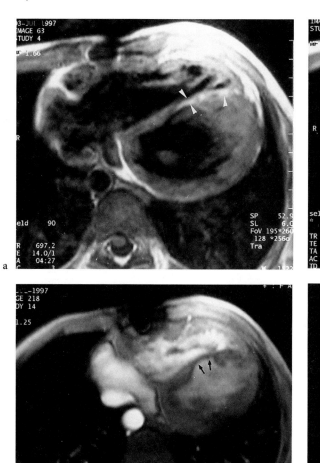

Fig. 5.16 a–d. Arrhythmogenic right venticular dysplasia involving the interventricular septum in a patient with tetralogy of Fallot. (**a, b**) Axial turbo-SE images; **c, d** axial (**c**) and short-axis (**d**) breath-hold GE images. Areas of increased signal intensity in the apical portion of the interventricular septum and moderator band (*arrowheads*) represent fatty infiltration (**a, b**). There is focal thinning of the interventricular septum showing dyskinetic wall motion (**c, d**: *arrows*)

acute myocarditis, based on T2-weighted MRI sequences. Furthermore, administration of paramagnetic contrast agent (Gd-DTPA) can be helpful in identifying the exact region of myocardial damage due to myocarditis and to monitor the myocarditis activity (MATSOUKA et al. 1994 and FRIEDRICH et al. 1998). In addition, a similar enhancement is shown in the pericardium if this part of the heart is involved in the inflammatory process. In the following sections the role of MRI in the diagnosis of Lyme disease, Chagas' heart disease, Wegener's granulomatosis, and systemic lupus erythematosus is highlighted.

5.6.1
Lyme Disease

Lyme disease is caused by the spirochete *Borrelia burgdorferi*, and is characterized by a multisystem disorder primarily affecting the skin, joints, heart,

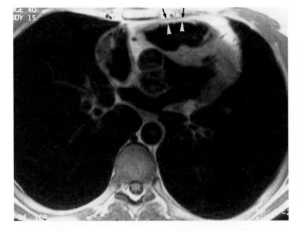

Fig. 5.17. Arrhythmogenic right venticular dysplasia? Axial turbo-SE image obtained with the patient in the prone position. Is there fatty infiltration of the RV free wall? No, the subepicardial fat between the thin RV free wall (*arrowheads*) and the pericardial sac (*black arrows*) gives a false impression of fatty infiltration. In addition, there was no bulging or evidence of abnormal wall motion on cine MRI in this case (not shown)

and central nervous system (NATHWANI et al. 1990). The most common cardiac manifestation of Lyme carditis is affection of the conduction system with transient atrioventricular block. Other manifestations like rhythm disturbances, myopericarditis, and heart failure are less common (VAN DER LINDE et al. 1991). The cardiac manifestations are usually self-limited, though it has been suggested that *Borrelia burgdorferi* may be associated with or even play an etiological role in the development of DCM (STANKE et al. 1991). Abnormalities of Lyme carditis on MRI include myopericarditis with myocardial wall thickening and areas of increased signal intensity within the myocardium, the presence of a subtle to moderate pericardial effusion, and ventricular dysfunction with regional or global hypokinesia (PONSONNAILLE et al. 1986; HANNEBICQUE et al. 1989; BERGLER et al. 1993; GLOBITS et al. 1994) (Fig. 5.20).

5.6.2
Chagas' Heart Disease

American trypanosomiasis (Chagas' disease) is a zoonosis caused by the protozoan parasite *Trypanosoma cruzi*. Chagas' disease is endemic in almost all Latin American countries, where it is one of the leading causes of death (WHO Expert Committee 1984). The disease is characterized by three phases: acute,

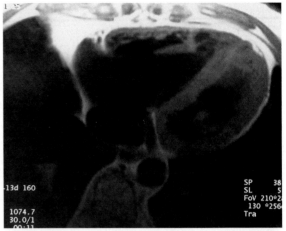

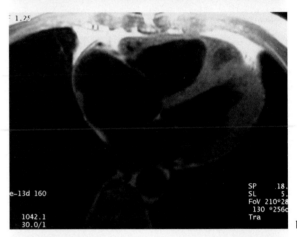

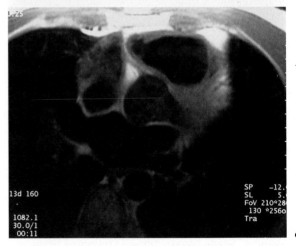

Fig. 5.18 a–c. Preferred evaluation of the RV free wall with the patient in the prone position. Axial turbo-SE images (obtained in breath-hold). Detailed anatomical images are obtained of the RV free wall, which is most frequently affected in arrhythmogenic right ventricular dysplasia. In this patient the myocardium exhibits a normal signal intensity

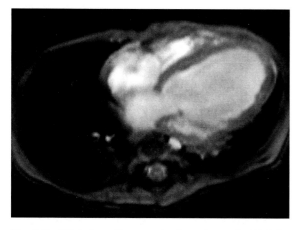

Fig. 5.19. Dilated cardiomyopathy in a 2-month-old baby with a recent history of Coxsackie myocarditis. Axial GE image. Note the huge dilation of the left ventricle, which exhibits a hypocontractile wall motion

Coronary arteritis involving the proximal aorta with dilation and wall thickening is found in another 50% of patients. Myocarditis with granuloma which may produce acute cardiac failure and progress to cardiomyopathy is seen in 25%. It may also present as mass lesions within the ventricles and may result in obstruction (KOSOVSKY et al. 1991). Valve abnormalities secondary to dilation of the aorta or left ventricle and conduction abnormalities are less common findings in Wegener's granulomatosis of the heart. Noninvasive cardiac imaging modalities, such as transthoracic and transesophageal echocardiography and MRI, may be helpful in identifying and delineating cardiac and proximal aortic involvement in Wegener's granulomatosis and also have a potentially important role in following the response to treatment (KOSOVSKY et al. 1991; GOODFIELD et al. 1995).

indeterminate, and chronic. The heart is the most commonly affected organ in chronic Chagas' disease, and lymphocytic myocarditis is often observed. It is associated with diffuse interstitial fibrosis, myocyte hypertrophy, and atrophy. Patients present with severely impaired LV function and refractory heart failure, or have episodes of sustained ventricular tachycardia without severe LV dysfunction (BELLOTTI et al. 1996). MRI after gadolinium infusion may be helpful in detecting areas of intense myocardial inflammation (KALIL-FILHO and DE ALBUQUERQUE 1995). In a recent study by BELLOTTI et al. (1996), seven out of eight patients showed a high signal intensity after gadolinium infusion in the inferolateral free wall of the left ventricle and in the RV septum in one patient. MRI may be helpful in guiding endomyocardial biopsy and seems a promising alternative method for the diagnosis of an inflammatory process in Chagas' heart disease.

5.6.3
Wegener's Granulomatosis

Wegener's granulomatosis is a systemic inflammatory disorder of unknown etiology. Cardiac involvement in Wegener's granulomatosis is not as uncommon as generally thought, occurring in 6%–44% of patients (GRANT et al. 1994). It may take many forms and varies from the principal clinical feature to mild or subclinical disease. Pericarditis and pericardial effusion are found in 50% of patients with cardiac involvement (FORSTOT et al. 1980).

5.6.4
Systemic Lupus Erythematosus

Systemic lupus erythematosus (SLE) is a disease of unknown etiology, thought to be autoimmune in nature (DOHERTY and SIEGEL 1985). The most common cardiac manifestations of this systemic disorder are nonbacterial "verrucous" endocarditis (Libman-Sacks endocarditis) (see Sect. 10.4.4.2), pericardial effusion, pericardial thickening, and myocarditis. Myocarditis is clinically diagnosed in 10% of patients with SLE. However, in autopsy studies the incidence approaches 40%. Myocardial injury is probably caused by immune complex deposition, but the in vivo diagnosis of myocarditis is difficult. MRI may be a valuable technique to detect myocardial involvement in patients with SLE but its clinical role is unclear. In a paper by BEEN et al. (1988) the myocardial signal intensity on T1-weighted images was significantly higher in patients with SLE than in normal volunteers or patients with HCM. Furthermore, patients with active disease, indicated by the lupus activity criteria count, showed significantly higher T1 values than patients with inactive disease. In addition, T1 values showed a negative correlation with serum C3 in the group with SLE. The increase in T1 shows a diffuse pattern and is probably caused by a cellular (lymphocytic) infiltration. Whether SLE causes changes in T2 relaxation is as yet unknown. Myocardial involvement in SLE will also lead to an impairment of LV diastolic function in the absence of systolic abnormalities (SASSON et al. 1992).

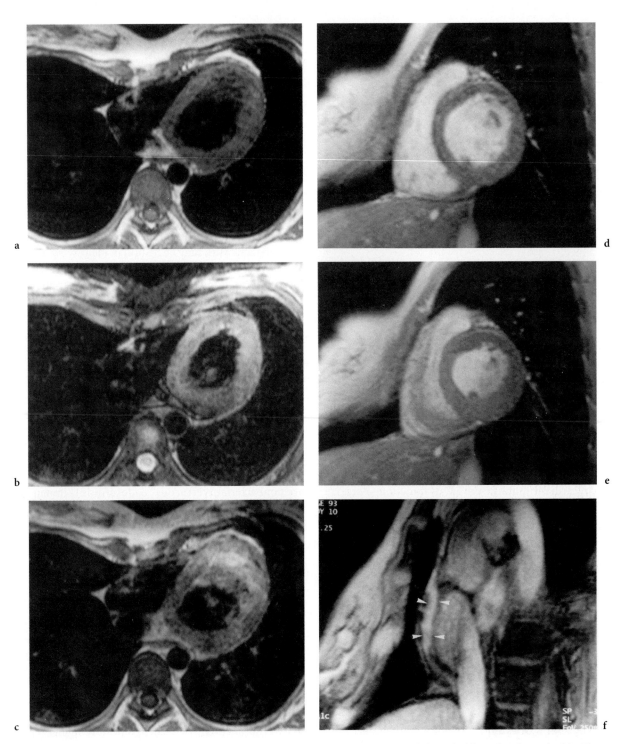

Figure 5.20. Lyme disease in a 20 year old female, with a history of a thick bite three months previously and a positive Lyme antibody titer, presenting with neurological symptoms and congestive heart failure (a-e). (a) Axial T1-weighted turbo-SE (obtained in breath-hold) through the left ventricle. Slightly enlarged left ventricle with a normal thickness of the LV wall. (b) Axial T2-weighted turbo-SE (TIR sequence). Note the slightly inhomogeneous, hyperintense appearance of the myocardium. (c) Axial contrast-enhanced T1-weighted turbo-SE (obtained in breath-hold). Inhomogeneous appearance of the myocardium, especially the LV apex, apical septum and anterior wall are strongly enhancing. (d-e) Short-axis breath-

hold cine MR at end-diastole (**d**) and end-systole (**e**). The anterior wall and anterior septum have an inhomogeneous appearance with a dark subendocardium and midwall and a bright subepicardium. Functionally this part of the LV demonstrates a pronounced reduction in wall thickening and centripetal wall motion during systole. (**f**) Short-axis two-dimensional coronary MR angiography of the right coronary artery. Huge dilatation of the proximal and middle part of the right coronary artery (up to 7 mm) (*arrows*). Coronary artery aneurysm is a late but extremely rare complication of Lyme disease.

5.7
Heart Transplantation

Heart transplantation is being performed with increasing frequency and success, making it an appropriate life-saving procedure in patients with end-stage heart disease. One of the major causes of death during the first year post transplantation is acute allograft rejection. Thus, a crucial factor in improving results is accurate evaluation of the severity and extent of cardiac rejection, with differentiation of rejection from other conditions such as infection (WALPOTH et al. 1995).

In the early phase, myocardial rejection consists in interstitial edema and mononuclear cell infiltration, which progresses towards myocytolysis or myocyte necrosis (SASAKI et al. 1987). Therefore, early diagnosis and adequate treatment before the occurrence of myocardial necrosis are mandatory. However, the clinical presentation of acute cardiac rejection may be silent in patients receiving cyclosporin treatment. Right endomyocardial biopsy and histological grading is the gold standard for the detection of myocardial rejection (CAVES et al. 1973; BILLINGHAM 1982). However, endomyocardial biopsy has several drawbacks: it is invasive and costly, 6–12 h is required before the diagnostic results become available, experienced pathologists are required for the histological diagnosis, and it is prone to sampling error (NISHIMURA et al. 1988; SMART et al. 1993).

Therefore, a noninvasive modality that would guide the timing of endomyocardial biopsy and assess the response to changes in immunosuppressive therapy would be advantageous. With the advent of MRI as a noninvasive cardiovascular imaging modality, one of the great aims was for this technique to become a preferred noninvasive diagnostic method for the assessment of early cardiac rejection and the effects of immunosuppressive therapy. Basically, four pathways have been explored: (a) tissue characterization by means of proton relaxation times, especially T2 relaxation time, (b) administration of paramagnetic contrast agents, (c) changes in myocardial wall thickness, and (d) myocardial MR spectroscopy (see Sect. 9.4.3). Despite the initially very promising results in animals and also in patient studies, at the moment MRI is unable to replace endomyocardial biopsy in human cardiac transplants.

The signal intensity is dependent on several parameters, including proton density, T1 (spin-lattice) and T2 (spin-spin) relaxation times, and flow (PYKETT 1982). Changes in proton relaxation times are related to the water and local chemical environment of tissue and permit the detection of various pathological states in vivo, including ischemia, infarction, and tumors (KOUTCHER et al. 1978; WESBEY et al. 1984). Since one of the early findings in cardiac rejection is an increase in the myocardial water content, principally due to myocardial edema, assessment of relaxation times may provide a sensitive measure of rejection (SCOTT et al. 1983).

Animal studies have shown an increase in relaxation times in cardiac transplants as early as 2 days after transplantation (SASAGURI et al. 1985; HUBER et al. 1985, TSCHOLAKOFF et al. 1985; AHERNE et al. 1986; LECHAT et al. 1986; EUGENE et al. 1986; NISHIMURA et al. 1987, 1988). T2 relaxation time, and to a much lesser extent T1 relaxation time, was found to be a reliable indicator of cardiac rejection, showing a linear relation with the myocardial water content. With progression of the rejection process, an increase in T2 relaxation time was shown, while cyclosporin treatment suppressed T2 relaxation time, except in cases with histological evidence of rejection. Studies in patients, however, were more disappointing. While some investigators showed an increase in T2 relaxation times in patients with cardiac rejection (WISENBERG et al. 1987; SMART et al. 1993), others could not confirm these results (REVEL et al. 1989; DOORNBOS et al. 1990). DOORNBOS and colleagues (1990) showed slightly (but not statistically significant) higher myocardial T2 relaxation times in patients in early stages of cardiac rejection than in nonrejecting patients and normal volunteers. The authors reported a large degree of overlap between the T2 values of normal volunteers, patients without signs of cardiac rejection, and patients with such signs. In other words, the absence of a demarcation value between normal or nonrejected and rejected myocardium precludes the clinical application of T2 relaxation times for assessment of cardiac rejection (KURLAND et al. 1989; DOORNBOS et al. 1990).

The contradictory results between the animal and patient studies can be explained in several ways. First, for technical reasons, e.g., cardiac and respiratory motion and signal from flowing blood, good T2-weighted images and reliable T2 relaxation times are difficult to obtain in humans. Second, animal studies represent optimized conditions while the clinical situation is far more complex. Factors such as variable ischemia time of the donor heart or effects of immunosuppressive therapy may contribute to changes in T2 relaxation time. In conclusion, further improvements in T2 measurements are needed before this technique can be used clinically (KURLAND et al. 1989; DOORNBOS et al. 1990).

Paramagnetic contrast agents, particular gadolinium in the form of Gd-diethylenetriamine penta-acetic acid (DTPA) and Gd-tetra-azacyclododecane tetra-acetic acid (DOTA), shorten the T1 relaxation time and can improve visualization and characterization of myocardial injury during ischemic disease (PESHOCK et al. 1986; REHR et al. 1986; DE ROOS et al. 1988, 1989b). Several investigators have evaluated the role of paramagnetic contrast agents for the assessment of cardiac transplant rejection. Animal studies have shown that in the absence of rejection, Gd-DTPA induced mild homogeneous myocardial enhancement (NISHIMURA et al. 1987; KONSTAM et al. 1988; KURLAND et al. 1989) while moderate and severe allograft rejection were characterized by one or more areas of intense myocardial enhancement. The extent and distribution of intense myocardial enhancement corresponded to the severity and extent of histological rejection. In contrast to T2- relaxation time, Gd-DTPA allowed differentiation between mild and moderate or severe degrees of cardiac rejection. MOUSSEAUX and colleagues (1993) showed a significantly greater myocardial enhancement in patients with histological rejection of the cardiac transplant than in patients without signs of rejection or normal volunteers. However, myocardial enhancement was not significantly different in patients with mild histological rejection compared with those with moderate or severe rejection. Since the pattern of myocardial enhancement was predominantly focal, regional myocardial enhancement seems a better measurement than mean myocardial enhancement for distinguishing focal histological changes when the rejection process is beginning. The visualization of myocardial regions with intense enhancement may furthermore be helpful in guiding endomyocardial biopsy, and thus reducing the sampling error.

An increase in myocardial wall thickness due to myocardial edema or cellular infiltrate was shown in acute allograft rejection in both animals and patients, while normal values were obtained in normal cardiac allografts and in patients during the resolving phase of an acute rejection episode (TSCHOLAKOFF et al. 1985; REVEL et al. 1989). The role of the myocardial wall thickness in predicting myocardial rejection, however, has not been established.

Besides acute allograft rejection, chronic allograft rejection and interstitial fibrosis may interfere with graft survival. However, since the MRI appearance of chronic cardiac rejection is close to normal, there is probably no role for MRI in diagnosing chronic rejection (REVEL et al. 1989). Finally, MRI may be helpful in detecting complications of cardiac transplantation, such as pleural or pericardial effusion or hemorrhage and endocavitary processes (LUND et al. 1987; REVEL et al. 1989; MOUSSEAUX et al. 1993).

5.8
Conclusion

The myocardium may be affected by a large number of diseases. The presentation is often atypical, necessitating invasive procedures such as endomyocardial biopsy for assessment of the underlying etiology, and often no cause can be found. The present role of MRI consists in demonstrating the morphological myocardial abnormalities in addition to other cardiac or extracardiac abnormalities. Changes in myocardial relaxation times may be helpful in depicting and localizing certain myocardial abnormalities, though their role in the detection of rejection of cardiac transplants is limited. The impact of the myocardial disease on the (global and regional) ventricular function and valvular function can be simultaneously and precisely assessed by MRI. This technique is the preferred imaging modality in some myocardial diseases such arrhythmogenic right ventricular dysplasia, and in the differentiation between constrictive pericarditis and restrictive cardiomyopathies. Some authors have stressed the importance of paramagnetic contrast agents in the detection of myocardial abnormalities. In the future, newly developed tissue- or disease-specific contrast agents will certainly increase the role of MRI in the diagnosis of myocardial diseases.

Acknowledgements. The author would like to thank S. DYMARKOWSKI, MD, and B. CLAIKENS, MD, for their help in the preparation of this chapter; Mr. W. DESMEDT for producing illustrations; F. VAN DE WERF, MD, PhD, from the Department of Cardiology, M. GEWILLIG from the Department of Pediatric Cardiology, and other colleagues for their cooperation in the patient MRI studies.

References

Abelmann WH, Lorell BH (1989) The challenge of cardiomyopathy. J Am Coll Cardiol 13:1219–1239

Aherne T, Tscholakoff D, Finkbeiner W, et al. (1986) Magnetic resonance imaging of cardiac transplants: the evaluation of rejection of cardiac allografts with and without immunosuppression. Circulation 74:145–156

Angelini A, Basso C, Nava A, Thiene G (1996) Endomyocardial biopsy in arrhythmogenic right ventricular cardiomyopathy (editorial). Am Heart J 132:203–206

Aretz HT, Billingham ME, Edwards WD, et al. (1986) Myocarditis: a histopathologic definition and classification. Am J Cardiovasc Pathol 1:3–14

Arrive L, Assayag P, Russ G, Najmark D, Brochet E, Nahum H (1994) MRI and cine MRI of asymmetric septal hypertrophic cardiomyopathy. J Comput Assist Tomogr 18:376–382

Baer FM, Theissen P, Schneider CA, Voth E, Schicha H, Sechtem U (1994) Magnetic resonance imaging techniques for the assessment of residual myocardial viability. Herz 19:51–64

Baer FM, Voth E, Deutsch HJ, et al. (1996) Predictive value of low dose dobutamine transesophageal echocardiography and fluorine-18 fluorodeoxyglucose positron emission tomography for recovery of regional left ventricular function after successful revascularization. J Am Coll Cardiol 28:60–69

Been M, Kean D, Smith MA, Douglas RH, Best JJ, Muir AL (1985) Nuclear magnetic resonance in hypertrophic cardiomyopathy. Br Heart J 54:48–52

Been M, Thomson BJ, Smith MA, et al. (1988) Myocardial involvement in systemic lupus erythematosus detected by magnetic resonance imaging. Eur Heart J 9:1250–1256

Belenkov Y, Vikhert OA, Belichenko OI, Arabidze GG (1992) Magnetic resonance imaging of cardiac hypertrophy in malignant arterial hypertension. Am J Hypertens 5:195S–199S

Bellotti G, Bocchi EA, de Moreas A, et al. (1996) In vivo detection of *Trypanosoma cruzi* antigens in hearts of patients with chronic Chagas' heart disease. Am Heart J 131:301–317

Beltrami CA, Finato N, Rocco M, et al. (1995) The cellular basis of dilated cardiomyopathy in humans. J Mol Cell Cardiol 27:291–305

Benson L, Liu P, Olivieri N, Rose V, Freedom R (1989) Left ventricular function in young adults with thalassemia. Circulation 80:274

Bergler KJ, Sochor H, Stanek G, Globits S, Ullrich R, Glogar D (1993) Indium 111-monoclonal antimyosin antibody and magnetic resonance imaging in the diagnosis of acute Lyme myopericarditis. Arch Intern Med 153:2696–2700

Billingham ME (1982) Diagnosis of cardiac rejection by endomyocardial biopsy. Heart Transpl 1:25–30

Billingham ME, Caves PK, Dong EJ, Shumway NE (1973) The diagnosis of canine orthotopic cardiac allograft rejection by transvenous endomyocardial biopsy. Transplant Proc 5:741–743

Blake LM, Scheinman MM, Higgins CB (1994) MR features of arrhythmogenic right ventricular dysplasia. Am J Roentgenol 162:809–812

Braunwald E, Rutherford JD (1986) Reversible ischemic left ventricular dysfunction: evidence for the "hibernating myocardium". J Am Coll Cardiol 8:1467–1470

Braunwald E, Morrow AG, Cornwell WP, Aygen MM, Hillbish TF (1960) Idiopathic hypertrophic subaortic stenosis. Clinical, hemodynamic, and angiographic manifestations. Am J Med 29:924–945

Brigden W (1957) The noncoronary cardiomyopathies. Lancet II:1179–1243

Burke AP, Farb, A, Tashko G, Virmani R (1998) Arrhythmogenic right ventricular cardiomyopathy and fatty replacement of the right ventricular myocardium. Are they different diseases? Circulation 97: 1571-1580

Buser PT, Wagner S, Auffermann W, et al. (1990) Three-dimensional analysis of the regional contractility of the normal and the cardiomyopathic left ventricle using cine-magnetic resonance imaging (in German). Z Kardiol 79:573–579

Caputo GR, Sechtem U, Tscholakoff D, Higgins CB (1987) Measurement of myocardial infarct size at early and late time intervals using MR imaging: an experimental study in dogs. Am J Roentgenol 149:237–244

Casolo GC, Poggesi L, Boddi M, et al. (1987) ECG-gated magnetic resonance imaging in right ventricular dysplasia. Am Heart J 113:1245–1248

Caves PK, Stinson EB, Graham AF, Billingham ME, Grehl TM, Shumway NE (1973) Percutaneous transvenous endomyocardial biopsy. JAMA 225:288–291

Chan PCK, Liu P, Cronin C, Heathcote J, Uldall R (1992) The use of nuclear magnetic resonance imaging in monitoring total body iron in hemodialysis patients with hemosiderosis treated with erythropoietin and phlebotomy. Am J Kidney Dis 19:484–489

Chandra M, Silverman ME, Oshinski J, Pettigrew R (1996a) Diagnosis of cardiac sarcoidosis aided by MRI. Chest 110:562–565

Chandra M, Pettigrew RI, Eley JW, Oshinski JN, Guyton RA (1996b) Cine-MRI-aided endomyocardectomy in idiopathic hypereosinophilic syndrome. Ann Thorac Surg 62:1856–1858

Dec GW, Fuster V (1994) Idiopathic dilated cardiomyopathy. N Engl J Med 331:1564–1574

de Roos A, Doornbos J, van der Wall EE, van Voorthuisen AE (1988) MR imaging of acute myocardial infarction: value of Gd-DTPA. Am J Roentgenol 150:531–534

de Roos A, Doornbos J, Matheijssen N, van der Laarse A, van der Wall E (1989a) Gd-DTPA enhanced MRI in the assessment of myocardial reperfusion. Medicamundi 34:99–102

de Roos A, van Rossum AC, van Der Wall E, et al. (1989b) Reperfused and nonreperfused myocardial infarction: diagnostic potential of Gd-DTPA-enhanced MR imaging. Radiology 172:717–720

Di Cesare E, Marsili L, Chichiarelli A, Di Renzi P, Costanzi A, Lupattelli L (1994) Characterization of hypertrophic cardiomyopathy with magnetic resonance (in Italian). Radiol Med (Torino) 87:614–619

Doherty NE, Siegel RJ (1985) Cardiovascular manifestations of systemic lupus erythematosus. Am Heart J 110:1257–1265

Doherty NIII, Fujita N, Caputo GR, Higgins CB (1992a) Measurement of right ventricular mass in normal and dilated cardiomyopathic ventricles using cine magnetic resonance imaging. Am J Cardiol 69:1223–1228

Doherty NIII, Seelos KC, Suzuki J, et al. (1992b) Application of cine nuclear magnetic resonance imaging for sequential evaluation of response to angiotensin-converting enzyme inhibitor therapy in dilated cardiomyopathy. J Am Coll Cardiol 19:1294–1302

Dong SJ, MacGregor JH, Crawley AP, et al. (1994) Left ventricular wall thickness and regional systolic function in patients with hypertrophic cardiomyopathy. Circulation 90:1200–1209

Dong SJ, Crawley AP, MacGregor JH, et al. (1995) Regional left ventricular systolic function in relation to the cavity geometry in patients with chronic right ventricular pressure overload. A three-dimensional tagged magnetic resonance study. Circulation 91:2359–2370

Doornbos J, Verwey H, Essed CE, Balk AH, de Roos A (1990) MR imaging in assessment of cardiac transplant rejection in humans. J Comput Assist Tomogr 14:77–81

D'Silva SA, Kohli A, Dalvi BV, Kale PA (1992) MRI in right ventricular endomyocardial fibrosis. Am Heart J 123:1390–1392

Dupuis JM, Victor J, Furber A, Pezard P, Lejeune LL, Tadei A (1994) Value of magnetic resonance imaging in cardiac sarcoidosis. Apropos of a case (in French). Arch Mal Coeur Vaiss 87:105–110

Eugene M, Lechat P, Hadjiisky P, Teillac A, Grosgogeat Y, Cabrol C (1986) Nuclear magnetic resonance and proton relaxation times in experimental heterotopic heart transplantation. J Heart Transpl 5:39–45

Fejfar Z (1968) Accounts of international meetings: idiopathic cardiomegaly. Bull WHO 38:979–992

Fontaine G, Fontaliran F, Frank R (1998) Arrhythmogenic right ventricular cardiomyopathies. Clinical forms and main differential diagnoses. Circulation 97:1532-1535

Forstot JZ, Overlie PA, Neufeld GK, Harmon CE, Forstot SL (1980) Cardiac complications of Wegener's granulomatosis: a case report of complete heart block and review of the literature. Semin Arthritis Rheum 10:148–154

Friedrich MG, Strohm O, Schulz-Menger J, Marciniak H, Luft FC, Dietz R (1998). Contrast-enhanced magnetic resonance imaging visualizes changes in the course of viral myocarditis. Circulation 97: 1802-1809

Fujita N, Duerinckx AJ, Higgins CB (1993) Variation in left ventricular regional wall stress with cine magnetic resonance imaging: normal subjects versus dilated cardiomyopathy. Am Heart J 125:1337–1345

Gagliardi MG, Bevilacqua M, Di Renzi P, Picardo S, Passariello R, Marcelletti C (1991) Usefulness of magnetic resonance imaging for diagnosis of acute myocarditis in infants and children, and comparison with endomyocardial biopsy. Am J Cardiol 68:1089–1091

Gaudio C, Tanzilli G, Mazzarotto P, et al. (1991) Comparison of left ventricular ejection fraction by magnetic resonance imaging and radionuclide ventriculography in idiopathic dilated cardiomyopathy. Am J Cardiol 67:411–415

Gaudio C, Pelliccia F, Tanzilli G, Mazzarotto P, Cianfrocca C, Marino B (1992) Magnetic resonance imaging for assessment of apical hypertrophy in hypertrophic cardiomyopathy. Clin Cardiol 15:164–168

Globits S, Bergler KJ, Stanek G, Ullrich R, Glogar D (1994) Magnetic resonance imaging in the diagnosis of acute Lyme carditis. Cardiology 85:415–417

Goodfield NER, Bhandari S, Plant WD, Morley-Davies A, Sutherland GR (1995) Cardiac involvement in Wegener's granulomatosis. Br Heart J 73:110–115

Grant SCD, Levy RD, Venning MC, Ward C, Brooks NH (1994) Wegener's granulomatosis and the heart. Br Heart J 71:82–86

Hannebicque G, Becquart J, Gommeaux A, et al. (1989) Cardiac manifestations of Lyme disease. Apropos of a case (in French). Ann Cardiol Angeiol Paris 38:87–90

Hardy P, Henkelman RM (1989) Transverse relaxation rate enhancement caused by magnetic particles. Magn Reson Imaging 7:265–275

Harvey WP, Segal JP, Gurel T (1964) The spectrum of primary myocardial disease. Prog Cardiovasc Dis 7:17–42

Higgins CB, Byrd B3, Stark D, et al. (1985) Magnetic resonance imaging in hypertrophic cardiomyopathy. Am J Cardiol 55:1121–1126

Huber DJ, Kirkman RL, Kupiec WJ, Araujo JL, Tilney NL, Adams DF (1985) The detection of cardiac allograft rejection by alterations in proton NMR relaxation times. Invest Radiol 20:796–802

Huong DL, Wechsler B, Papo T, et al. (1997) Endomyocardial fibrosis in Behçet's disease. Ann Rheum Dis 56:205–208

Imai H, Kumai T, Sekiya M, et al. (1992) Left ventricular trabeculae evaluated with MRI in dilated cardiomyopathy and old myocardial infarction. J Cardiol 22:83–90

Kalil-Filho R, de Albuquerque CP (1995) Magnetic resonance imaging in Chagas' heart disease. Rev Paul Med 113:880–883

Koito H, Suzuki J, Nakamori H, et al. (1995) Clinical significance of abnormal high signal intensity of left ventricular

myocardium by gadolinium-diethylenetriaminepentaacetic acid enhanced magnetic resonance imaging in hypertrophic cardiomyopathy. J Cardiol 25:163–170

Koito H, Suzuki J, Ohkubo N, Ishiguro Y, Iwasaka T, Inada M (1996) Gadolinium-diethylenetriamine pentaacetic acid enhanced magnetic resonance imaging of dilated cardiomyopathy: clinical significance of abnormally high signal intensity of left ventricular myocardium. J Cardiol 28:41–49

Kono T, Suwa M, Hanada H, Hirota Y, Kawamura K (1992) Clinical significance of normal cardiac silhouette in dilated cardiomyopathy – evaluation based upon echocardiography and magnetic resonance imaging. Jpn Circ J 56:359–365

Konstam MA, Aronovitz MJ, Runge VM, et al. (1988) Magnetic resonance imaging with gadolinium-DTPA for detecting cardiac transplant rejection in rats. Circulation 78:87–94

Kosovsky PA, Ehlers KH, Rafal RB, Williams WM, O'Loughlin JE, Markisz JA (1991) MR imaging of cardiac mass in Wegener granulomatosis. J Comput Assist Tomogr 15:1028–1030

Koutcher JA, Goldsmith M, Damadian R (1978) NMR in cancer. X. A malignancy index to discriminate normal and cancerous tissue. Cancer 41:174–182

Kramer CM, Reichek N, Ferrari VA, Theobald T, Dawson J, Axel L (1994) Regional heterogeneity of function in hypertrophic cardiomyopathy. Circulation 90:186–194

Kurland RJ, West J, Kelley S, et al. (1989) Magnetic resonance imaging to detect heart transplant rejection: sensitivity and specificity. Transplant Proc 21:2537–2543

Lawrence WE, Maughan WL, Kass DA (1992) Mechanism of global functional recovery despite sustained postischemic regional stunning. Circulation 85:816–827

Lechat P, Eugene M, Hadjiisky P, Teillac A, Cabrol C, Grosgogeat Y (1986) Detection of cardiac graft rejection using proton nuclear magnetic resonance (in French). Arch Mal Coeur Vaiss 79:1356–1360

Lesnefsky EJ, Allen KG, Carrea FP, Horwitz LD (1992) Iron-catalyzed reactions cause lipid peroxidation in the intact heart. J Mol Cell Cardiol 24:1031–1038

Lieberman EB, Hutchins GM, Herskowitz A, Rose NR, Baughman KL (1991) Clinicopathologic description of myocarditis. J Am Coll Cardiol 18:1616–1626

Liu P, Olivieri N (1994) Iron overload cardiomyopathies: new insights into an old disease. Cardiovasc Drugs Ther 8:101–110

Liu P, Stone J, Collins A, Olivieri N (1993a) Is there a predictable relationship between ventricular function and myocardial iron levels in patients with hemochromatosis. Circulation 88:183

Liu P, Olivieri N, Sullivan H, Henkelman M (1993b) Magnetic resonance imaging in beta-thalassemia: detection of iron content and association with cardiac complications. J Am Coll Cardiol 21:491

Lombardi C, Rusconi C, Faggiano P, Lanzani G, Campana C, Arbustini E (1995) Successful reduction of endomyocardial fibrosis in a patient with idiopathic hypereosinophilic syndrome. A case report. Angiology 46:345–351

Lund G, Letourneau JG, Day DL, Crass JR (1987) MRI in organ transplantation. Radiol Clin North Am 25:281–288

Lund G, Morin RL, Olivari MT, Ring WS (1988) Serial myocardial T2 relaxation time measurements in normal subjects and heart transplant recipients. J Heart Transpl 7:274–279

MacGowan GA, Shapiro EP, Azhari H, et al. (1997) Shortening in the fiber and cross-fiber directions in the normal human left ventricle and in idiopathic dilated cardiomyopathy. Circulation 96:535–541

Maes A, Flameng W, Nuyts J, et al. (1994) Histological alterations in chronically hypoperfused myocardium: correlation with PET findings. Circulation 90:735–745

Maier SE, Fischer SE, McKinnon GC, Hess OM, Kraeyenbuehl HP, Boesiger P (1992) Evaluation of left ventricular segmental wall motion in hypertrophic cardiomyopathy with myocardial tagging. Circulation 86:1919–1928

Marchal G, Ni Y, Herijgers P, et al. (1996) Paramagnetic metalloporphyrins: infarct avid contrast agents for diagnosis of acute myocardial infarction by MRI. Eur Radiol 6:2–8

Maron BJ, Anan TJ, Roberts WC (1981) Quantitative analysis of the distribution of cardiac muscle cell disorganization in the left ventricular wall of patients with hypertrophic cardiomyopathy. Circulation 63:882–894

Maron BJ, Bonow RO, Cannon ROI, Leon MB (1987) Hypertrophic cardiomyopathy: interrelations of clinical manifestations, pathophysiology, and therapy. N Engl J Med 316:780–789

Maron BJ, Pelliccia A, Spirito P (1995) Cardiac disease in young trained athletes. Insight into methods for distinguishing athlete's heart from structural heart disease, with particular emphasis on hypertrophic cardiomyopathy. Circulation 91:1596–1602

Masui T, Finck S, Higgins CB (1992) Constrictive pericarditis and restrictive cardiomyopathy: evaluation with MR imaging. Radiology 182:369–373

Matsouka H, Hamada M, Honda T, et al. (1994) Evaluation of acute myocarditis and pericarditis by Gd-DTPA enhanced magnetic resonance imaging. Eur Heart J 15:283–284

Menghetti L, Basso C, Nava A, Angelini A, Thiene G (1996) Spin-echo nuclear magnetic resonance for tissue characterisation in arrhythmogenic right ventricular cardiomyopathy. Heart 76:467–470

Mousseaux E, Farge D, Guillemain R, et al. (1993) Assessing human cardiac allograft rejection using MRI with Gd-DOTA. J Comput Assist Tomogr 17:237–244

Nathwani D, Hamlet N, Walker E (1990) Lyme disease: a review (see comments). Br J Gen Pract 40:72–74

Neubauer S, Krahe T, Schindler R, et al. (1992) Direct measurement of spin-lattice relaxation times of phosphorus metabolites in human myocardium. Magn Reson Med 26:300–307

Nishimura T, Sada M, Sasaki H, et al. (1987) Cardiac transplantation in dogs: evaluation with gated MRI and Gd-DTPA contrast enhancement. Heart Vessels 3:141–145

Nishimura T, Sada M, Sasaki H, et al. (1988) Assessment of severity of cardiac rejection in heterotopic heart transplantation using indium-111 antimyosin and magnetic resonance imaging. Cardiovasc Res 22:108–112

Parrillo JE (1990) Heart disease and the eosinophil. N Engl J Med 323:1560–1561

Peshock RM, Malloy CR, Buja LM, Nunnally RL, Parkey RW, Willerson JT (1986) Magnetic resonance imaging of acute myocardial infarction: gadolinium diethylenetriamine pentaacetic acid as a marker of reperfusion. Circulation 74:1434–1440

Piérard LA, De Landsheere CM, Berthe C, Rigo P, Kulbertus HE (1990) Identification of viable myocardium by echocardiography during dobutamine infusion in patients with myocardial infarction after thrombolytic therapy: comparison with positron emission tomography. J Am Coll Cardiol 15:1021–1031

Pitt M, Davies MK, Brady AJ (1996) Hypereosinophilic syndrome: endomyocardial fibrosis. Heart 76:377–378

Ponsonnaille J, Citron B, Karsenty B, et al. (1986) Myocardite aiguë au cours d'un syndrome de Lyme. Intérêt de la scintagraphie myocardique au gallium 67. Arch Mal Coeur 13:1946–1950

Pykett IL (1982) NMR image in medicine. Sci Am 246:78–88

Rahimtoola SH (1993) The hibernating myocardium in ischaemia and congestive heart failure. Eur Heart J 14:22–26

Ramamurthy S, Talwar KK, Goswani KC, et al. (1993) Clinical profile of biopsy proven idiopathic myocarditis. Int J Cardiol 41:225–232

Redfield MM, Gersh BJ, Bailey KR, Rodeheffer RJ (1994) Natural history of incidentally discovered, asymptomatic idiopathic dilated cardiomyopathy. Am J Cardiol 74:737–742

Rehr RB, Peshock RM, Malloy CR, et al. (1986) Improved in vivo magnetic resonance imaging of acute myocardial infarction after intravenous paramagnetic contrast agent administration. Am J Cardiol 57:864–868

Reimer KA, Jennings RB (1979) The wavefront progression of myocardial ischemic cell death. II. Transmural progression of necrosis within the framework of ischemic bed size (myocardium at risk) and collateral flow. Lab Invest 40:633–644

Reimer KA, Lowe JE, Rasmussen MM, Jennings RB (1977) The wavefront phenomenon of ischemic cell death. I. Myocardial infarct size vs duration of coronary occlusion in dogs. Circulation 56:786–794

Remes J, Helin M, Vaino P, Rautio P (1990) Clinical outcome and left ventricular function 23 years after acute Coxsackie virus perimyocarditis. Eur Heart J 11:182–188

Revel D, Chapelon C, Mathieu D, et al. (1989) Magnetic resonance imaging of human orthotopic heart transplantation: correlation with endomyocardial biopsy. J Heart Transpl 8:139–146

Sardanelli F, Molinari G, Petillo A, et al. (1993) MRI in hypertrophic cardiomyopathy: a morphofunctional study. J Comput Assist Tomogr 17:862–872

Sasaguri S, LaRaia PJ, Fabri BM, et al. (1985) Early detection of cardiac allograft rejection with proton nuclear magnetic resonance. Circulation 72 (Suppl II) II-231–236

Sasaki H, Sada M, Nishimura T, et al. (1987) The expanded scope of effectiveness of nuclear magnetic resonance imaging to determine cardiac allograft rejection. Transplant Proc 19:1062–1064

Sasson Z, Rasooly Y, Chow CW, Marshall S, Urowitz MB (1992) Impairment of left ventricular diastolic function in systemic lupus erythematosus. Am J Cardiol 69:1629–1634

Schaper J, Froede R, Hein S, et al. (1991) Impairment of the myocardial ultrastructure and changes of the cytoskeleton in dilated cardiomyopathy. Circulation 83:504–514

Scott GE, Nath RL, Friedlich JA, Fallon JT, Erdmann AJ (1983) Usefulness of myocardial edema to assess heterotopic allograft rejection in dogs. Heart Transplant 2:232–237

Semelka RC, Tomei E, Wagner S, et al. (1990) Interstudy reproducibility of dimensional and functional measurements between cine magnetic resonance studies in the morphologically abnormal left ventricle. Am Heart J 119:1367–1373

Senocak F, Sarclar M, Ozkutlu S (1994) Echocardiographic findings in some metabolic storage diseases. Jpn Heart J 35:635–643

Shabetai R (1986) The pericardium and its diseases. McGraw-Hill, New York, pp 1249–1275

Shirey EK, Proudfit WL, Hawk WA (1980) Primary myocardial disease. Correlation with clinical findings, angiographic and biopsy diagnosis. Am Heart J 99:198–207

Siqueira-Filho AG, Cunha CLP, Tajik AJ, Seward JB, Schattenberg TT, Giuliani ER (1981) M-mode and two-dimensional echocardiographic features in cardiac amyloidosis. Circulation 63:188–196

Sivaram CA, Jugdutt BI, Amy RWM, Basualdo CA, Harapongsc M, Shnitkla TK (1985) Cardiac amyloidosis: combined use of two-dimensional echocardiography and electrocardiography in non-invasive screening before biopsy. Clin Cardiol 8:511–588

Smart FW, Young JB, Weilbaecher D, Kleiman NS, Wendt RIII, Johnston DL (1993) Magnetic resonance imaging for assessment of tissue rejection after heterotopic heart transplantation. J Heart Lung Transplant 12:403–410

Soler R, Rodriguez E, Rodriguez JA, Perez ML, Penas M (1997) Magnetic resonance imaging of apical hypertrophic cardiomyopathy. J Thorac Imaging 12:221–225

Stanek G, Klein J, Bittner R, Glogar D (1991) *Borrelia burgdorferi* as an etiologic agent in chronic heart failure? Scand J Infect Dis Suppl 77:85–87

Stark DD, Mosely ME, Bacon BR, et al. (1985) Magnetic resonance imaging and spectroscopy of hepatic iron overload. Radiology 154:137–142

Steward S, Mason D, Braunwald E (1968) Impaired rate of left ventricular filling in idiopathic hypertrophic subaortic stenosis and valvular aortic stenosis. Circulation 37:8–14

Suzuki J, Chang JM, Caputo GR, Higgins CB (1991a) Evaluation of right ventricular early diastolic filling by cine nuclear magnetic resonance imaging in patients with hypertrophic cardiomyopathy. J Am Coll Cardiol 18:120–126

Suzuki J, Caputo GR, Masui T, Chang JM, O'Sullivan M, Higgins CB (1991b) Assessment of right ventricular diastolic and systolic function in patients with dilated cardiomyopathy using cine magnetic resonance imaging. Am Heart J 122:1035–1040

Takahashi JC, Saiki M, Miyatake S, et al. (1997) Adenovirus-mediated gene transfer of basic fibroblast growth factor induces in vitro angiogenesis. Atherosclerosis 132:199–205

The TIMI Study Group (1985) The thrombolysis in myocardial infarction (TIMI) trial: phase I findings. N Engl J Med 312:932–936

Trevi GP, Sheiban I (1991) Chronic ischaemic ("hibernating") and postischaemic ("stunned") dysfunctional but viable myocardium. Eur Heart J 12:20–26

Tscholakoff D, Aherne T, Yee ES, Derugin N, Higgins CB (1985) Cardiac transplantations in dogs: evaluation with MR. Radiology 157:697–702

Tsukihashi H, Ishibashi Y, Shimada T, et al. (1994) Changes in gadolinium-DTPA enhanced magnetic resonance signal intensity ratio in hypertrophic cardiomyopathy. J Cardiol 24:185–191

van der Linde MR (1991) Lyme carditis: clinical characteristics of 105 cases. Scand J Infect Dis Suppl 77:81–84

Virmani R, Bures JC, Roberts WC (1980) Cardiac sarcoidosis: a major cause of sudden death in young individuals. Chest 77:423–428

von Kemp K, Beckers R, Vandenweghe J, Taeymans Y, Osteaux M, Block P (1989) Echocardiography and magnetic resonance imaging in cardiac amyloidosis. Acta Cardiol 44:29–36

Walpoth BH, Lazeyras F, Tschopp A, et al. (1995) Assessment of cardiac rejection and immunosuppression by magnetic resonance imaging and spectroscopy. Transplant Proc 27:2088–2091

Wang JZ, Mezrich RS, Scholz P, Als A, Douglas F (1990) MRI evaluation of left ventricular hypertrophy in a canine model of aortic stenosis. Invest Radiol 25:783–788

Weiss RG, Bottomley PA, Hardy CJ, Gerstenblith G (1990) Regional myocardial metabolism of high-energy phosphates during isometric exercise in patients with coronary artery disease. N Engl J Med 323:1593–1600

Weller PF, Bubley GJ (1994) The idiopathic hypereosinophilic syndrome. Blood 83:2759–2779

Wenger NK, Goodwin JF, Roberts WC (1986) Cardiomyopathy and myocardial involvement in systemic disease. McGraw-Hill, New York, pp 1181–1248

Wesbey G, Higgins CB, Lanzer P, Botvinick E, Lipton M (1984) Imaging and characterization of acute myocardial infarction in vivo by gated nuclear magnetic resonance. Circulation 69:125–130

White RD, Trohman RG, Flamm SD et al (1998). Right ventricular arrhythmia in the absence of arrhythmogenic dysplasia: MR imaging of myocardial abnormalities. Radiology 207:743-751

Wigle ED, Heimbecker RO, Gunton RW (1962) Idiopathic ventricular septal hypertrophy causing muscular subaortic stenosis. Circulation 26:325–340

Wisenberg G, Pflugfelder PW, Kostuk WJ, McKenzie FN, Prato FS (1987) Diagnostic applicability of magnetic resonance imaging in assessing human cardiac allograft rejection. Am J Cardiol 60:130–136

World Health Organization Expert Committee (1984) Chagas' disease. In: World Health Organization technical report series 697. Geneva: WHO 50–55

Young AA, Kramer CM, Ferrari VA, Axel L, Reichek N (1994) Three-dimensional left ventricular deformation in hypertrophic cardiomyopathy. Circulation 90:854–867

Zerhouni EA, Parish DM, Rogers WJ, Yang A, Shapiro EP (1988) Human heart: tagging with MR imaging – a new method for noninvasive assessment of myocardial motion. Radiology 169:59–63

6 Cardiac Function

F.E. Rademakers and J. Bogaert

6.1
Introduction

Global and regional ventricular performance remains an important prognostic factor in many disease states, and accurate, reproducible quantification of this performance has been the goal of many imaging modalities, i.e., ventriculography by contrast injection or radionuclide techniques, echocardiography, ultrafast CT scanning or electron beam tomography, and also magnetic resonance imaging (MRI). Although ejection fraction has the claim to be a simple universal parameter of left ventricular (LV) performance, it is largely dependent on preload and afterload and its accuracy and reproducibility are

only as good as the technique from which the cavity volumes are derived. In this respect MRI has much to offer since its provides a very accurate if not the most accurate measurement of cardiac volumes (Bloomgarden et al. 1997; van Rugge et al. 1993a); to be routinely used, however, the contouring and quantification have to be automated. Beside ejection fraction, end-diastolic and end-systolic volumes per se as well as stroke volume, cardiac output, wall thickening, and LV mass have prognostic importance (van der Wall et al. 1997).

In coronary heart disease global and regional evaluation of performance is necessary to identify ischemia, viability, and necrosis, both at rest and during stress, which in the magnet is mostly pharmacological stress although nonferrodynamic stress apparatus has been used (Schaefer et al. 1986). Good visualization of the epicardial and endocardial borders is essential to accurately quantify wall motion, thickness, and thickening; this can be most easily achieved with conventional or segmented gradient-echo (GE) sequences at different short-axis levels of the ventricle. The problems remain, however, of through-plane motion (Chai et al. 1997; Pattynama et al. 1992) and the need for an arbitrary reference point (often center of the ventricular cavity) for regional analysis, which can be very difficult in the case of dyskinesia. A possible solution is the use of myocardial tagging in combination with 3D reconstruction.

All the parameters described so far try to quantify performance and deformation, which are not equal to function. Both stress and strain have to be measured and it is only their relation under different hemodynamic circumstances which allows true quantification of intrinsic myocardial function or contractility.

Finally, a comprehensive analysis of function also includes the determination of perfusion, metabolism, and tissue characteristics, e.g., degree of fibrosis, myocardial disarray, vascularization, edema, necrosis. Many of these components of a complete functional analysis still elude quantification or can

F.E. Rademakers, MD, PhD, Department of Cardiology, University Hospitals Gasthuisberg, Catholic University of Leuven, Herestraat 49, B-3000 Leuven, Belgium
J. Bogaert, MD, PhD, Department of Radiology, University Hospitals Gasthuisberg, Catholic University of Leuven, Herestraat 49, B-3000 Leuven, Belgium

only be appraised by a combination of tests including positron emission tomography (PET) studies and biopsies; however, MRI combined with spectroscopy has the potential to make all this information available in one step.

6.2
Techniques for Quantification of Cardiac Function

6.2.1
Contrast Ventriculography

Several imaging techniques have been used to assess cardiac volumes and function; contrast ventriculography is often still considered as the gold standard but, beside being invasive, it uses geometric assumptions for the calculation of volumes and remains a projection technique in its evaluation of regional function (MANCINI et al. 1987); also it does not correct for rigid body motion and has to use a floating reference system which by itself introduces errors in nonhomogeneously contracting ventricles.

6.2.2
Echocardiography

All noninvasive modalities also have their specific advantages and disadvantages. Echocardiography is the most widely used technique for the determination of cardiac volumes and function, since it is real-time, relatively cheap, safe, mobile, and accessible (WAGGONER et al. 1996). The addition of Doppler has made it into a complete, noninvasive hemodynamic technique, and the use of stress imaging can help to differentiate dysfunctional but viable (stunned or hibernating) myocardium from infarcted tissue. In some 30% of patients, however, image quality is inferior, and the quantification of regional function, essential for the interpretation of dobutamine stress tests, remains extremely difficult, with a large interobserver variability. Since identification of the epicardial border is often difficult, accurate measurement of thickness and thickening is frequently elusive. Some of these difficulties, especially regarding image quality, have been overcome by transesophageal echocardiography, but due to the invasive nature of the technique its use for the study of ventricular function is mainly limited to intraoperative examinations and to intubated patients on intensive care (LIU et al. 1996).

6.2.3
Radionuclide Imaging

Radionuclide imaging using technetium-99m labeled tracers can provide information on both myocardial blood flow and function in one session (MIRON et al. 1996), but spatial resolution is poor and attenuation often makes interpretation difficult (BODEMHEIMER et al. 1980). Moreover sequential studies are limited due to radiation exposure for the patient. PET offers regional information on blood flow and metabolism (MAES et al. 1994, 1995, 1997) but has a limited spatial resolution and availability. The latter situation could be improved by using PET radiotracers on conventional gamma cameras (SANDLER and PATTON 1996).

6.2.4
Electron Beam Tomography

Electron beam tomography has a very high spatial and temporal resolution and can be used for volume, mass, and myocardial flow measurements (using passage of contrast medium) (FEIRING et al. 1985; GOULD 1992; WOLFKIEL and BRUNDAGE 1991; YAMAOKA et al. 1993). Need for calibration on a subject-to-subject basis and limited availability remain major drawbacks.

6.2.5
Magnetic Resonance Imaging

In comparison, MRI has sufficient spatial and temporal resolution using the older, more time-consuming sequences; with the newer, faster acquisition techniques a trade-off exists between temporal and spatial resolution (ATKINSON and EDELMAN 1991; GRISWOLD et al. 1997; MATTHAEI et al. 1990; STEHLING et al. 1991). Good delineation of epicardial and endocardial borders, completely free choice of imaging plane, capability of 3D reconstruction, availability of noninvasive tagging, and combination with flow and perfusion measurements are major advantages. Further evolution of hard- and software should make MRI real time, rendering it competitive in this respect with echocardiography.

6.3
Volumes and Ejection Fraction

As mentioned in Chap. 2 on normal anatomy, LV and right ventricular (RV) volumes can be measured on a stack of adjacent short-axis images by delineation of the endocardial contours, multiplication of the area by the thickness of the imaging plane and the interslice distance, and addition of these volumes (Simpson's rule) (Fig. 6.1) (BOGAERT et al. 1995; MOGELVANG et al. 1987; REHR et al. 1985; SOLDO et al. 1994; VAN ROSSUM et al. 1988a,b). A similar analysis can be performed on a set of transverse images but the potential problems of partial volume effects, mostly at the apex, and inability to define the mitral valve plane are even more pronounced than in the short-axis approach, although present with both incidences (BUSER et al. 1989). Through-plane motion at the base of the heart as a consequence of the long-axis shortening of about 15% has to be taken into account; a basal image plane at end diastole which contains only the ventricular cavity can slice entirely through the atrium at end systole, and when contoured and added to the end-systolic volumes would introduce major errors (Fig. 6.2) (see also Fig. 5.8). Usually this is easily recognized but sometimes the most basal ventricular slice cuts through the thin membranous interventricular septum and some misinterpretation can ensue. From the end-diastolic and end-systolic volumes, it is straightforward to calculate stroke volume, ejection fraction, and cardiac output.

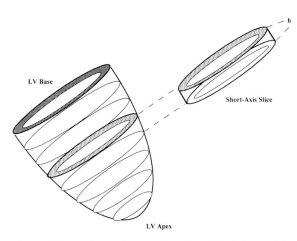

Fig. 6.1. True volumetric quantification of the left ventricle based on Simpson's rule. Contiguous short-axis images are positioned from the LV base to apex; volumes are calculated using slice thickness (h) and interslice distance

Spin-echo (SE) MRI can be used for this purpose and has high spatial resolution but it is time-consuming and the multislice technique is less convenient since the different slices are obtained at different phases of the cardiac cycle (CAPUTO et al. 1990). Turbo spin-echo (TSE), HASTE, GE (SECHTEM et al. 1987a), or echo-planar imaging (EPI) (HUNTER et al. 1994; LAMB et al. 1996) are therefore preferred (FORBAT et al. 1996; PATTYNAMA et al. 1993; SEMELKA et al. 1990a,b; SINHA et al. 1997). GE is most often used to provide deformation in one slice during the entire cardiac cycle; typically the repetition time is 30–40 ms, which provides an adequate temporal resolution (SECHTEM et al. 1987b,c). Acquisition of multiple k-space lines during one heart beat offers the possibility of breath-hold imaging but with some loss of temporal resolution (ATKINSON and EDELMAN 1991; BOGAERT et al. 1995; HERREGODS et al. 1994; SCHULEN et al. 1996) (Fig. 6.2).

Inclusion of the endocardial trabeculae at end systole but not at end diastole can contribute to small errors, more so in the right ventricle, as can the inclusion of slow-flowing blood near the endocardial border which mimics the tissue characteristics of myocardium. Overall reproducibility, however, is high, with low inter- and intraobserver variability (MARKIEWICZ et al. 1987a,b; PATTYNAMA et al. 1995; BOGAERT et al. 1995). Moreover, studies comparing LV and RV stroke volumes (which in the absence of intra- or extracardiac shunts should be equal) and others comparing flow in the great vessels by means of velocity mapping to ventricular volume measurements (which also should be equal) yielded near equal values, thus providing an elegant validation of the technique (CASALINO et al. 1996; CULHAM and VINCE 1988; KONDO et al. 1991).

Since the contouring of all the end-diastolic and end-systolic images still involves some manual intervention, several methods have been proposed to calculate volumes assuming some simpler ventricular geometry. In most normal ventricles this introduces only a small error but in regionally abnormal ventricles, the errors can be major and unpredictable (DEBATIN et al. 1992). By applying these simplifications one loses the major advantage of MRI volume calculation, which is precisely the absence of any assumption regarding geometry or symmetry; this is even more important for the right ventricle, which is asymmetrical in normal circumstances and whose contraction pattern is not concentric, as is the case for the left ventricle. Examples of the calculations used are: ellipsoid, starting from mono- or biplane

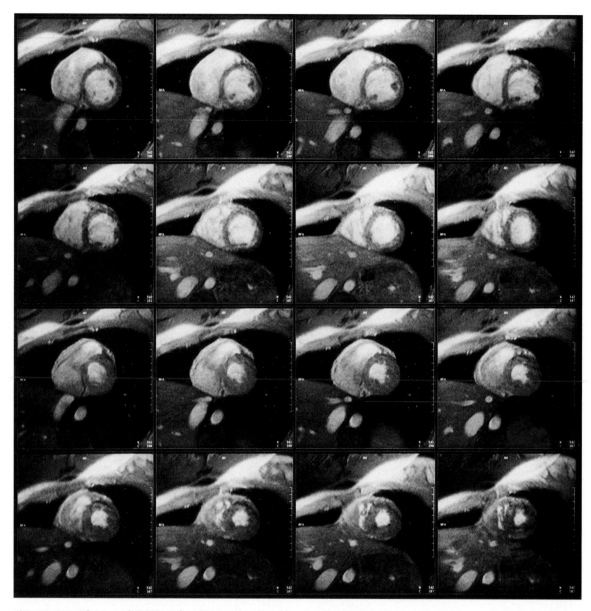

Fig. 6.2. Quantification of global LV function in a 25-year-old healthy female volunteer. Contiguous short-axis images are obtained from LV base to LV apex at end diastole (*upper two rows*) and end systole (*lower two rows*), using the segmented k-space cine MRI sequence. Each slice is studied in one breath-hold. This approach allows rapid and accurate quanti- fication of LV end-diastolic (EDV) and end-systolic volume (ESV), stroke volume (SV), ejection fraction (EF), cardiac output, and cardiac indices. Global LV parameters: EDV, 99.7 ml; ESV, 32.4 ml; SV, 67.3 ml; EF, 67.5%. Moreover, re- gional wall motion and wall thickening can be easily assessed on cine MRI

data, Teichholz, simplified Simpson (three volumes), etc.

In a similar way as for the ventricles, atrial vol- umes and changes from end diastole to end systole can be measured (JARVINEN et al. 1994a,b; LAUERMA et al. 1996; MOHIADDIN and HASEGAWA 1995).

6.4
Wall Thickness and Wall Thickening

From single-plane epicardial and endocardial con- tours or more accurately from 3D reconstructed volumes (LIMA et al. 1993), wall thickness can be measured and when images are acquired at end diastole and end systole, wall thickening or the absolute increase in wall thickness can be calculated (FISHER et al. 1985; RADEMAKERS et al. 1994). Preserved wall thickness is a good indicator of the presence of viable myocardium in the setting of a chronic infarction (BAER et al. 1994a), while thickening provides a powerful measure of regional LV performance, which is independent of any external reference point and can be used for assessment during pharmacological stress (Fig. 6.3). Some caution is needed, however. Left ventricular performance is characterized by the ejection of blood, which is dependent on adequate filling, preload, afterload, and contractility. The performance of the entire ventricle does not simply comprise the contribution of the different parts of the ventricle; rather it also depends on the correct interplay between these different segments. It is clear from studies with several techniques (echocardiography, radionuclide studies, MRI, use of invasive bead or transducer implants) that inhomogeneities in both the extent and the timing of deformation are also present to a large extent in the perfectly normal ventricle and can become exacerbated and pernicious in abnormal conditions such as ischemia or infarction. By using only a single end-systolic time point this temporal inhomogeneity cannot be appreciated and the maximal extent of deformation in a given segment can be underestimated. This is true not only for myocardial wall thickening but for every regional analysis of performance. Although there is one single time point where the ventricle reaches its smallest volume and ejection ends, maximal deformation for every segment of the ventricle does not necessarily occur at that specific time point. To appreciate this inhomogeneity and to be able to quantify it, multiple time points from mid ejection throughout isovolumic relaxation have to be acquired, since some segments start to relax and thin before aortic valve closure while others continue to thicken during isovolumic ventricular pressure fall.

Another issue in the regional contribution to ejection is the relative importance of wall thickening versus epicardial inward motion. Ejection of blood from the cavity is the result of a coordinated inward motion of the endocardium (Fig. 6.4). This can be accomplished by wall thickening while the epicardium remains stationary or, as in most normal conditions, moves slightly inwards; the latter, however, depends on the reference point that is used. Everyone is familiar with eccentric interventricular septal thickening after cardiac surgery where adequate septal thickening is obvious but the motion of the endocardium towards the LV cavity is diminished, absent, or even reversed. Sometimes, as in the postinfarct situation, wall thickening can be very reduced but partially compensated by increased subepicardial deformation and inward motion, resulting in a greater contribution of that segment to global ejection than could be expected from wall thickening alone. Even in the normal heart the relative contribution of wall thickening and epicardial inward motion to regional ejection differs from region to region, another example of ventricular inhomogeneity. A possible pitfall in this kind of analysis is the reference point in both time and space since motion has to be defined with regard to a certain point and both motion and thickening must be referenced to an end-diastolic situation; registration of the latter has to be very accurate as some segments perform one-third of their entire wall thickening during the 30 ms of early isovolumic contraction, meaning that even a slight misregistration of end diastole can result in significant alterations for the reference condition.

6.5
Circumferential and Longitudinal Shortening

With most techniques LV performance is assessed by evaluating the inward motion of the endocardium, usually in a short-axis plane, which corresponds to endocardial circumferential shortening. As mentioned above, this is the result of both wall thickening and epicardial inward motion (Fig. 6.4). According to the principle of conservation of mass, extensive wall thickening, as seen in a short-axis plane of the LV wall (50%–75%), can only occur when myocardial mass moves into the imaging plane, i.e., when substantial long-axis shortening is present. While long-axis shortening can easily be measured by echocardiography, it has principally been MRI that has contributed significantly to a better understanding of the importance of this phenomenon. A comprehensive evaluation of function, therefore, has to include both circumferential and long-axis shortening (CHAI et al. 1997), again stressing the need for 3D analysis of cardiac deformation. Segmental evaluation of circumferential and long-axis shortening necessitates the use of myocardial markers (such as MR tags); anatomical landmarks (RV insertions, papillary muscles) can also be used but only to a limited extent.

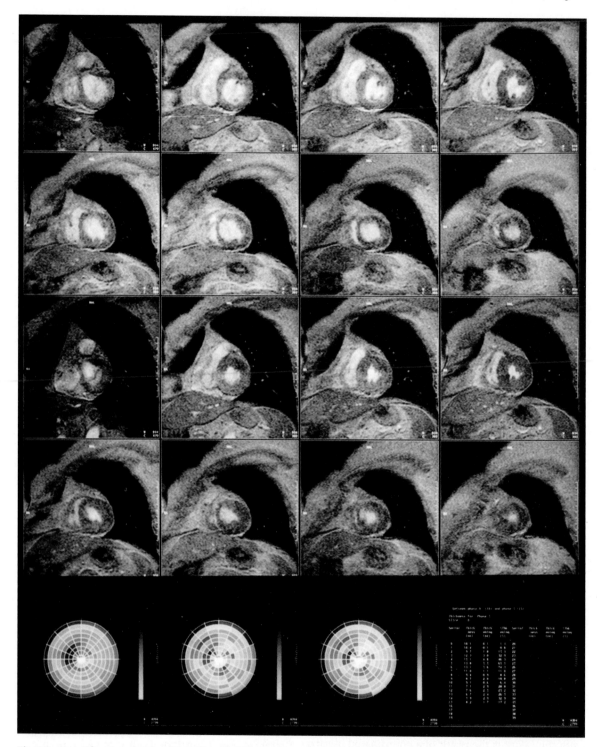

Fig. 6.3. Quantification of regional systolic wall thickening in a 59-year-old female patient with a previous myocardial infarction. In the *two upper rows* are shown the end-diastolic short-axis levels from LV base to LV apex. In the *third and fourth rows* are shown the corresponding end-systolic short-axis views. Note an important wall thinning in the apical part of the interventricular septum, showing not only an a- to dyskinetic wall motion pattern but also systolic wall thinning. In the *bottom row* are shown three bull's eye diagrams representing (*from left to right*): absolute wall thickness at end systole, absolute systolic wall thickening, and percentual systolic thickening. Abnormal low values (visible as dark gray regions) for both wall thickness and wall thickening are found in the apical portion of the interventricular septum (ARGUS, Siemens Erlangen, Germany)

6.6
Myocardial Tagging

During the cardiac cycle the heart deforms in a very complex pattern. It is also influenced by the attached and neighboring structures and it displays a whole body motion, including rotation and translation, beside its intrinsic deformation. To quantify only the latter, myocardial markers are essential. Implanted beads and coils were used for this purpose in animal models and post-transplant patients (HANSEN et al.

1988; WALDMAN et al. 1985, 1988), but their application was limited for obvious reasons. It was the introduction of MR tags which opened the way to noninvasive regional quantification of myocardial deformation.

6.6.1
Principles of Myocardial Tagging

Saturation of spins in a specific slab by means of excitation pulses prior to the imaging process is a technique that is routinely used in MRI in order to reduce artifacts (see Sect. 1.1.8). This same technique can also be used to destroy the MR signal of tissues at specific locations only. The creation of tags, as described by ZERHOUNI and colleagues in 1988, consists in the application of radiofrequency (RF) pulses in one or more planes perpendicular to the imaging plane, prior to the application of the RF pulses required for imaging (Fig. 6.5). In this way, the signal of the tissue in the tag planes is destroyed immediately prior to the imaging procedures (the tissue in the tag planes is said to be "saturated"). During the subsequent MRI procedure no signal is obtained from these protons, and they appear as hypointense or black areas. Since the crossing of two perpendicular planes is a line, tag lines can be imprinted on the myocardium. When imprinted at end diastole, the tags subsequently deform with the myocardium on which they were inscribed, and by measuring tag displacement and deformation, actual myocardial

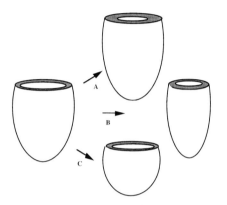

Fig. 6.4. Mechanisms of ventricular ejection. On the *left* is shown the ventricle at end diastole, and on the *right* the ventricle at end ejection: *A–C* represent three different hypothetical mechanisms of endocardial inward motion: *A*, pure wall thickening; *B*, circumferential shortening; *C*, longitudinal ventricular shortening. The normal ventricular ejection relies on a combination of these three mechanisms

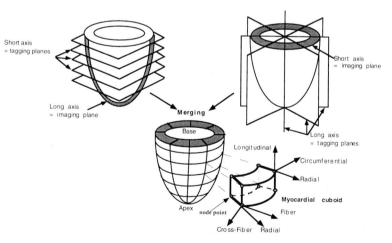

Fig. 6.5. Schematic representation of short- and long-axis images with corresponding tag planes. Merging the two 2D data sets yields a reconstruction of the left ventricle with cuboids, for which the node points are defined in 3D space. Their co-ordinates can be expressed in a local cardiac (radial-circumferential-longitudinal) or a fiber (radial-fiber-cross-fiber) coordinate system. When images are acquired at end diastole and other time points during the cardiac cycle, strains can be calculated

deformation can be analyzed (YOUNG and AXEL 1992; YOUNG et al. 1993). Tags are therefore truly noninvasive myocardial markers. Tag lines are a temporary phenomenon. Immediately after the tag preparation pulse, the fully saturated protons will gradually return to their normal energy level. This means that the difference between the tagged and the nontagged myocardium will progressively disappear in subsequent acquisitions later in the cardiac cycle. The rate of the loss of tag visibility is determined by the relaxation parameters of the myocardium (T1), and is a function of the imaging parameters used. With the most commonly used sequence parameters, myocardial tags persist up to 700 ms following the R wave of the QRS complex. The principle of presaturating pulses can and has been combined with different types of imaging modalities, i.e., beside SE, GE sequences, segmented GE sequences with acquisition of multiple k-space lines per heart beat, and EPI sequences. Differences in the persistence of tag lines also depend on the type and number of images that are acquired. Special techniques have been developed to improve the persistence so as to include fast filling, passive diastole, and atrial filling in the analysis.

In general two types of tags have been used, although some variations have been added over the years. A first type uses specific presaturation planes to define the tags and can use different geometric patterns [usually radial in the short-axis plane (Fig. 6.6) and parallel in the long-axis plane (Fig. 6.7)], provided this can be done in a sufficiently short period of time to avoid excessive deformation of the myocardium between putting down the first and last tag plane. In principle tags are put down just before end-diastole or mitral valve closure (MVC) but in practice the sequence is initiated by the onset of the QRS, which has a variable offset to MVC. The subsequent isovolumic contraction phase, during which the ventricle builds enough pressure to open the aortic valve, is far from isovolumetric, and a significant amount of deformation occurs. It is thus very important to be able to "inscribe" the tags during a very short period of time immediately followed by an end-diastolic image which is used as the reference image for all subsequent calculations. In practice the trigger of the sequence, i.e., usually the upslope of the QRS, just precedes actual MVC; the sequence has an internal delay of about 20 ms, then the tags are inscribed in 20–35 ms, followed immediately by an end-diastolic image which is thus very close to actual MVC.

The second type of tagging uses two perpendicular sets of parallel stripes which form a rectangular grid on the image that can be tracked through the cardiac cycle; this is termed the spatial modulation of magnetisation or SPAMM technique (Fig. 6.8). This method was developed by L. Axel et al. at the University of Pennsylvania, Philadelphia (AXEL and DOUGHERTY 1989a,b). The grid can be defined and inscribed in a very short time but its exact location on the heart is not as easily controlled.

Both of the aforementioned techniques have their advantages and disadvantages, and have greatly aided in our understanding of cardiac mechanics. Several adjustments and improvements to the sequences have been made which are beyond the scope of this chapter, but mainly involve faster implementation, improved persistence, and a finer grid (BOLSTER et al. 1990; BOSMANS et al. 1993, 1996; HENDRICH et al. 1994; McVEIGH and ATALAR 1992; MOORE et al. 1994; O'DELL et al. 1995; PERMAN et al. 1995; PIPE et al. 1991; ROGERS et al. 1991). Combinations of the two types of technique exist, e.g., use of striped radial tags where the radial tag planes are "SPAMM'd" to give a line composed of separate dots rather than a solid line; in this way information on radial inhomogeneity of deformation can be obtained which is otherwise impossible with radial tagging (BOLSTER et al. 1990; McVEIGH and ZERHOUNI 1991). Tagging can be applied to the right ventricle as well (NAITO et al. 1995).

Advantages of radial tagging are easier merging of short- and long-axis images in a truly 3D data set and more homogeneous distribution of markers or tagging points over the myocardium. Disadvantages are the absence of availability of radial tagging on commercial systems, longer duration of tag deposition, and more tedious contouring programs. The epicardial and endocardial contours are sometimes obscured by SPAMM tagging and a variable number of grid-crossings are available at different sites of the myocardium which are unevenly spread through the myocardial wall; however, the use of finite element analysis of images with SPAMM tagging has solved this problem.

6.6.2
Strain Analysis

Whatever the technique used, the final results are quantitative measures of cardiac deformation, i.e., normal, shear, and principal strains (WALDMAN

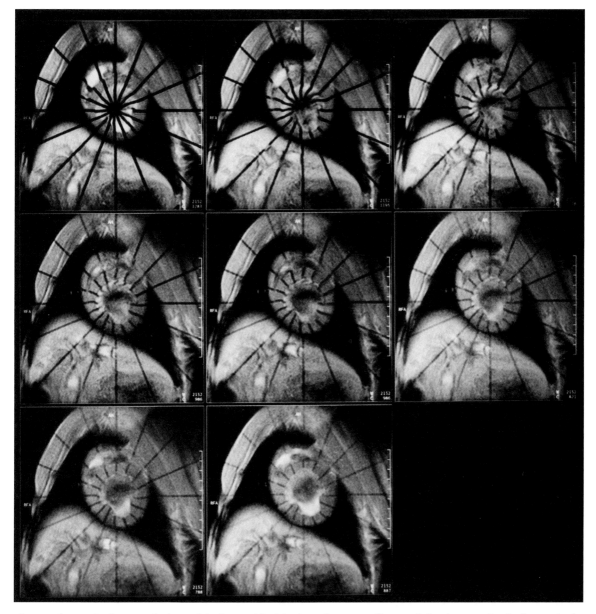

Fig. 6.6. Short-axis slice near the base of the heart with eight images during the cardiac cycle. Eight radially oriented tag lines create 16 intersections with epi- and endocardium. Note the changes in the position and shape of the tag lines inscribed on the myocardium, and the absence of such changes in the immobile thoracic and abdominal structures. On the end-diastolic image intracavitary blood is tagged as well; these tag lines disappear with the ejection of blood

et al. 1985, 1988). The examples in this chapter use radial tagging which divides the ventricle into 32–48 cuboidal volume elements; the corners or node points of these cuboids are known in 3D after merging the information from the short- and long-axis images (GOSHTASBY and TURNER 1996). The coordinate system for these node points and the subsequent strain analysis can be chosen, a first step involving selection of the external coordinate system of the magnet (XYZ). Since this does not contribute very much to our understanding of cardiac mechanics, strains are usually expressed in a cardiac coordinate system (RCL) (Fig. 6.5). Two of its axes are oriented tangential to the LV wall [circumferential (C) and longitudinal (L)] and the third axis is perpendicular to the LV wall [radial (R)]. R, C and L are

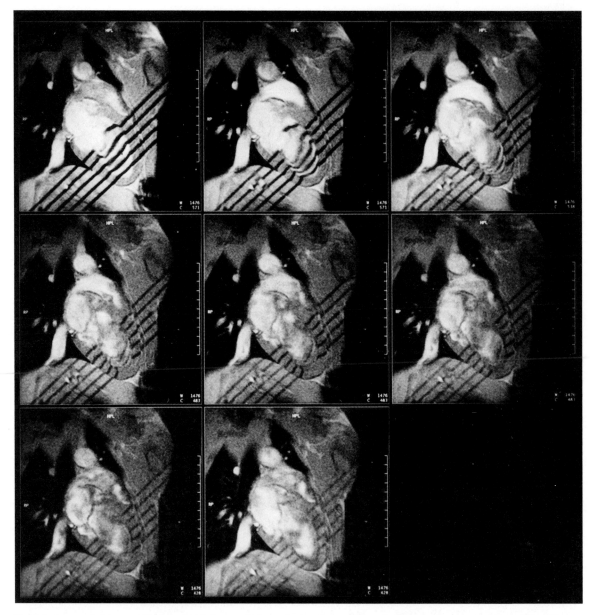

Fig. 6.7. Long-axis images of the heart with five parallel tags during the cardiac cycle. Note the important shift and tilt of the tag lines due to long-axis shortening

perpendicular to each other. This RCL coordinate system is thus specific for each epi- and endocardial location. Due to the taper of the apex, the radial axis points slightly down and the longitudinal axis slightly outward in this region.

In a further step to better understand myocardial function, one can use the fiber angles in the subepicardial and subendocardial regions to transform the local cardiac coordinate system (RCL) into a local fiber coordinate system (RFX) (Fig. 6.5). Fiber

angles obtained either from pathology examination in experimental animal studies or from autopsy series in human studies can be used; although the latter method is less accurate, the very stable fiber orientation from one subject to another in different regions of the left ventricle allows the use of a "standard set" of fiber orientations without significant loss of accuracy. The direction indicated by F is along the fiber direction parallel to the ventricular surface. The direction X is the cross-fiber direction, defined as the

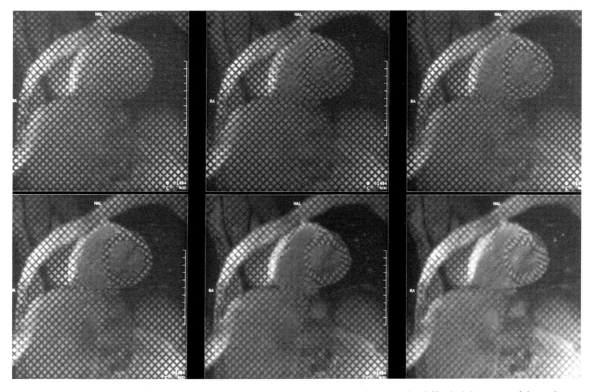

Fig. 6.8. Spatial modulation of magnetization (SPAMM) tagging technique. The grid which is placed on the short-axis image at end-diastole (*above left*) is deformed during the subsequent systole. Note the difficult delineation of the endocardial borders at end diastole

direction perpendicular to the fiber direction in a plane tangential to the ventricular surface. R (radial) remains the same as in the RCL coordinate system and is perpendicular to the fiber and cross-fiber axis. Noninvasive myocardial tagging thus permits quantification of the most basic component of myocardial deformation, i.e., fiber shortening.

As mentioned earlier, myocardial deformation can be best described by means of strains. The latter can be divided into normal and shear strains (Fig. 6.9) (MOORE et al. 1992; PIPE et al. 1991; RADEMAKERS 1991; YOUNG and AXEL 1992; YOUNG et al. 1993, 1994). Normal strains are defined as the displacements along a coordinate axis. Three normal strains are therefore defined for each coordinate system, three in the local cardiac coordinate system (RR, CC, LL) and three in the local fiber coordinate system (RR, FF, XX), in which the radial strain RR remains the same. Shear strains are defined in the plane between two axes of the coordinate system and describe the deformation of a square to a parallelogram. One of these, the circumferential-longitudinal shear strain or CL, describes the twisting motion

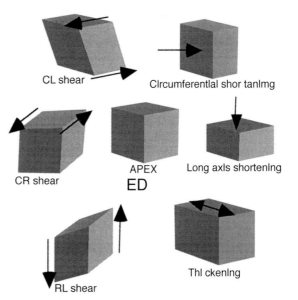

Fig. 6.9. Normal and shear strains referenced to the ED cuboid (*middle*). The normal strains are shown on the *right*, the shear strains on the *left*

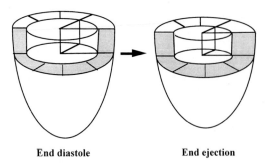

End diastole   **End ejection**

Fig. 6.10. Regional ejection fraction. Four adjacent radial tag lines on two adjacent levels describe an intracavitary triangle with the apex in the center of the left ventricle and the base on the endocardial surface. In this way, one cuboid describes a triangular volume which permits calculation and quantification of the regional ejection fraction for this cuboid

of the ventricle and is very closely related to torsion (AELEN et al. 1997; HANSEN et al. 1988; RADEMAKERS et al. 1992). Principal strains and their angle with a reference plane can also be obtained (AZHARI et al. 1993).

6.6.3
Regional Ejection Fraction

Magnetic resonance tagging also allows quantification of regional ejection fraction (Fig. 6.10). The amount of blood ejected by each cuboid during systole is expressed by the regional ejection fraction at the endocardium. Since the short-axis tags are radially oriented with the crossing of the tag lines in the center of the left ventricle, each cuboid defines an intracavitary triangular volume where the endocardial surface is the base of the triangle and the center of the left ventricle is the apex. The inward motion of the endocardium determines the changes in intracavitary triangular volume. Subtraction of the end-systolic triangular volume from the end-diastolic triangular volume divided by the end-diastolic volume gives the regional ejection fraction.

6.6.4
Radii of Curvature

Finally the circumferential and longitudinal radii of curvature, which are defined as the radius of the circle that best fits the contour of the segment under study, can be calculated and expressed in centimeters. A small radius of curvature denotes a curved

surface, while a large radius of curvature is representative of a flat surface. The radii of curvature can be computed for the subepicardium and subendocardium in both the longitudinal and the circumferential direction. Very similar longitudinal and circumferential radii of curvature represent a structure close to a sphere, whereas very different radii are typical for an ellipsoid. In a cylinder one of the radii of curvature is infinite. Changes in these radii of curvature during the cardiac cycle denote regional shape changes of the ventricle and can be used together with wall thickness to calculate wall stresses (BEYAR et al. 1993).

6.7
Wall Velocity Mapping

The basic principles of myocardial tagging also define its main limitations. By applying tag lines or a grid pattern on the myocardium, the myocardial signal is voluntarily destroyed in a part of the image. To increase the sensitivity of the technique, multiple tag lines have to be defined. The more tag lines are used, the more signal is omitted, and because tag lines possess a certain thickness, information is lost and not every point of the myocardial wall can be accounted for. Secondly, the life span of tag lines is unavoidably limited. As mentioned above, this poses certain limitations on this technique by inducing intensity variations in the images and sometimes leading to poorer image quality. Thirdly, notwithstanding considerable progress in automated analysis speed, delineation of data still remains a tedious task, reducing its clinical capability.

Phase imaging has been proposed as an alternative to tagging for quantification of myocardial deformation and motion (WEDEEN 1992; WEDEEN et al. 1995). Normally MR images are reconstructed from the magnitude of the received signal, but alternatively images can be calculated based on the phase of the spins in the imaging volume. It is possible to make these "phase images" sensitive to speed, so that the intensity of the voxels in the image is not directly proportional to the signal magnitude but rather to the velocity of the structure in that image point. This technique is routinely used for flow quantification in blood vessels and through the cardiac valves (FIRMIN et al. 1989; HIGGINS et al. 1992; KILNER et al. 1991). In a similar manner, the motion, speed, and direction of motion of solid organs such as the myocardium can be quantified (CONSTABLE et al. 1994).

With its specific properties, phase imaging overcomes the main limitations of myocardial tagging by persisting throughout the cardiac cycle, accounting for every point within the myocardium and maintaining signal. Nevertheless, this technique has not yet achieved a breakthrough in clinical cardiology, mainly because of its own major limitations. By giving up tag pulses, reference points within the myocardium are lost, the latter being the precise reason why tagging was created. Furthermore, velocity mapping measures wall speed. Assessing the position or displacement of a point in space with a reliable degree of accuracy requires multiplication of the velocity of that point by its time course. This implies that the accuracy of the calculation of the displacement is directly proportional to the accuracy of the velocity measurements. Velocity mapping only measures changes in speed along one axis, namely the axis perpendicular to the imaging plane. Given the complex rotational and multiaxial motion of myocardial tissue, several acquisitions have to be performed, increasing the duration of the measurement.

Phase imaging must certainly be considered a powerful and potentially useful diagnostic technique, but the laborious nature of the analysis and execution in measuring myocardial wall motion has extensively limited its clinical use. Its accuracy has nevertheless been effectively demonstrated in healthy subjects and in patients with cardiomyopathy.

6.8
Stress Testing

Regional or global myocardial ischemia has a cascade of consequences, starting with disturbed myocardial flow, followed by a reduction in diastolic and later systolic function and finally ECG changes and symptoms of angina. The use of an early manifestation of ischemia as a marker to increase the sensitivity of stress testing is appealing. Dobutamine and exercise echocardiography have been used for this purpose, but quantification of regional contractile function is often very difficult and not very reproducible. MRI could offer a major advantage in this field, which is expanding rapidly due to the need for evaluation of ischemia, stunning, and hibernation as indications for revascularization. For convenience most stress testing in the magnet is performed by pharmacological stress, e.g., using the β-agonist dobutamine or the vasodilator dipyridamole (BAER et al. 1993b). The former is preferred since it offers the possibility of both low- and high-dose examinations, needed for the differentiation of stunning and ischemia (CIGARROA et al. 1993; VAN RUGGE et al. 1993b, 1994).

In most instances one or two short-axis slices are imaged with a cine MR sequence to evaluate changes in LV performance. With the use of faster imaging it may become possible to image more slices and to proceed to a full 3D acquisition. This would increase the sensitivity of the technique and also allow the evaluation of changes in long-axis shortening which otherwise would be missed. In general, regional endocardial motion, wall thickening, and absolute increase in wall thickness are used as parameters of regional systolic performance, yielding sensitivity and specificity values of 70%–90% (BAER et al. 1992, 1993, 1994b,c, 1995; KLEINHANS et al. 1991; PENNELL et al. 1990, 1992; VAN RUGGE et al. 1993b, 1994). These stress test results could be enhanced by the simultaneous evaluation of regional perfusion (EICHENBERGER et al. 1994; HARTNELL et al. 1994). Aortic flow as a parameter of LV function has also been used with dobutamine stress (PENNELL et al. 1995).

6.9
Wall Stress

As outlined above, evaluation of intrinsic contractility necessitates the quantification of both stress and strain. While the latter can be obtained relatively easily, accurately, and noninvasively by myocardial tagging, wall stress is more difficult to quantify. One of the reasons is the absence of a gold standard, as exists for strain analysis by the use of albeit invasively implanted markers. No such devices have been accepted for stress measurements and until now most stress values are obtained by more or less complex calculations making major and mostly unacceptable assumptions about myocardial properties and ventricular geometry. MRI combined with tagging possibly offers a better solution since it provides detailed regional information about ventricular geometry, including wall thickness, radii of curvature in perpendicular directions, and cavity dimensions, but the problems with myocardial properties and the absence of a gold standard to test the results remain. Nevertheless a combined analysis of stress and strain could provide invaluable absolute and quantitative information about regional systolic function and help in the differentiation between infarcted and (overstressed) noncontractile myocardium.

6.10
Diastolic Function

As with other imaging modalities, diastolic function has retained less interest than systolic function in the analysis of cardiac function with MRI. A major reason is the absence of a simple parameter such as ejection fraction to try to quantify the overall diastolic performance (DENDALE et al. 1995; MATTER et al. 1996). Some of the known parameters of diastolic function from echo Doppler, i.e., mitral inflow characteristics (E and A wave velocities and their ratio), can also be obtained with MR flow measurements.

A novel parameter of diastolic performance which is related to elastic recoil of the ventricle is the rate, timing, and extent of untwisting, which can be measured with MR tagging (RADEMAKERS et al. 1992).

References

Aelen FW, Arts T, Sanders DG, et al. (1997) Relation between torsion and cross-sectional area change in the human left ventricle. J Biomech 30:207–212

Atkinson DJ, Edelman RR (1991) Cineangiography of the heart in a single breath hold with a segmented turboflash sequence. Radiology 178:357–360

Axel L, Dougherty L (1989a) Heart wall motion: improved method for spatial modulation of magnetization for MR imaging. Radiology 172:349–350

Axel L, Dougherty L (1989b) MR imaging of motion with spatial modulation of magnetization. Radiology 171:841–845

Azhari H, Weiss JL, Rogers WJ, Siu CO, Zerhouni EA, Shapiro EP (1993) Noninvasive quantification of principal strains in normal canine hearts using tagged MRI images in 3-D. Am J Physiol Heart Circ Physiol 264:33–41

Baer FM, Smolarz R, Jungehulsing M, et al. (1992) Feasibility of high-dose dipyridamole MRI for detection of coronary artery disease and comparison with coronary angiography. Am J Cardiol 69:51–56

Baer FM, Smolarz K, Theissen P, Voth E, Schicha H, Sechtem U (1993a) Identification of hemodynamically significant coronary artery stenoses by dipyridamole-magnetic resonance imaging and ⁹⁹ᵐTc-methoxyisobutyl-isonitrile-SPECT. Int J Cardiac Imaging 9:133–145

Baer FM, Theissen P, Smolarz K, et al. (1993b) Dobutamine versus dipyridamole-magnetic resonance imaging: safety and sensitivity for the diagnosis of coronary artery stenoses. Z Kardiol 82:494–503

Baer FM, Theissen P, Schneider CA, Voth E, Schicha H, Sechtem U (1994a) Magnetic resonance imaging techniques for the assessment of residual myocardial viability. Herz 19:51–64

Baer FM, Voth E, Theissen P, Schicha H, Sechtem U (1994b) Gradient-echo magnetic resonance imaging during incremental dobutamine infusion for the localization of coronary stenoses. Eur Heart J 15:218–225

Baer FM, Voth E, Theissen P, Schneider CA, Schicha H, Sechtem U (1994c) Coronary artery disease: findings with GRE MR imaging and technetium-99m methoxyisobuty-lisonitrile SPECT during simultaneous dobutamine stress. Radiology 193:203–209

Baer FM, Voth E, Schneider CA, Theissen P, Schicha H, Sechtem U (1995) Comparison of low-dose dobutamine-gradient-echo magnetic resonance imaging and positron emission tomography with [¹⁸F]fluorodeoxyglucose in patients with chronic coronary artery disease. A functional and morphological approach to the detection of residual myocardial viability. Circulation 91:1006–1015

Beyar R, Weiss JL, Shapiro EP, Graves WL, Rogers WJ, Weisfeldt ML (1993) Small apex-to-base heterogeneity in radius-to-thickness ratio by three-dimensional magnetic resonance imaging. Am J Physiol 264:H133–H140

Bloomgarden DC, Fayad ZA, Ferrari VA, Chin B, Sutton MGA (1997) Global cardiac function using fast breath-hold MRI: validation of new acquisition and analysis techniques. Magn Reson Med 37:683–692

Bodemheimer MM, Banka VS, Helfant RH (1980) Nuclear cardiology. I. Rradionuclide angiographic assessment of left ventricular contraction: uses, limitations and future directions. Am J Cardiol 45:661–673

Bogaert JG, Bosmans H, Rademakers F, et al. (1995) Left ventricular quantification with breath-hold MR imaging: comparison with echocardiography. MagMa 3:5–12

Bolster BJ, McVeigh ER, Zerhouni EA (1990) Myocardial tagging in polar coordinates with use of striped tags. Radiology 177:769–772

Bosmans H, Bogaert J, Rademakers F, Marchal G, Van Hecke P, Baert AL (1993) Optimization of a 3D tagging acquisition of the myocardium for improved time resolution. Eur Rad Suppl 3:165

Bosmans H, Bogaert J, Rademakers FE, et al. (1996) Left ventricular radial tagging acquisition using gradient-recalled-echo techniques: sequence optimization. MagMa 4:123–133

Buser PT, Auffermann W, Holt WW, et al. (1989) Noninvasive evaluation of global left ventricular function with use of cine nuclear magnetic resonance. J Am Coll Cardiol 13:1294–1300

Caputo GR, Suzuki JI, Kondo C, et al. (1990) Determination of left ventricular volume and mass with use of biphasic spin-echo MR imaging: comparison with cine MR. Radiology 177:773–777

Casalino E, Laissy JP, Soyer P, Bouvet E, Vachon F (1996) Assessment of right ventricle function and pulmonary artery circulation by cine MRI in patients with AIDS. Chest 110:1243–1247

Chai JW, Chen YT, Lee SK (1997) MRI assessment of regional heart wall motion in the longitudinal axis sections of left ventricle by spatial modulation of magnetization. Chung Hua I Hsueh Tsa Chih 60:13–30

Cigarroa CG, de Filippi C, Brickner ME, Alvarez LG, Wait MA, Grayburn PA (1993) Dobutamine stress echocardiography identifies hibernating myocardium and predicts recovery of left ventricular function after coronary revascularization. Circulation 88:430–436

Constable RT, Rath KM, Sinusas AJ, Gore JC (1994) Development and evaluation of tracking algorithms for cardiac wall motion analysis using phase velocity MR imaging. Magn Reson Med 32:33–42

Culham J, Vince DJ (1988) Cardiac output by MR imaging: an experimental study comparing right ventricle and left ventricle with thermodilution. J Can Assoc Radiol 39:247–249

Debatin JF, Nadel SN, Sostman HD, Spritzer CE, Evans AJ, Grist TM (1992) Magnetic resonance imaging-cardiac ejection fraction measurements: phantom study comparing four different methods. Invest Radiol 27:198–204

Dendale P, Franken PR, Waldman GJ, et al. (1995) Regional diastolic wall motion dynamics in anterior myocardial infarction: analysis and quantification with magnetic resonance imaging. Coron Artery Dis 6:723–729

Eichenberger AC, Schuiki E, Kochli VD, Amann FW, McKinnon GC, Von Schulthess GK (1994) Ischemic heart disease: assessment with gadolinium-enhanced ultrafast MR imaging and dipyridamole stress. J Magn Reson Imaging 4:425–431

Feiring AJ, Rumberger JA, Reiter SJ, et al. (1985) Determination of left ventricular mass in dogs with rapid-acquisition cardiac computed tomographic scanning. Circulation 72:1355–1364

Firmin DN, Klipstein RH, Hounsfield GL, Paley MP, Longmore DB (1989) Echo-planar high-resolution flow velocity mapping. Magn Reson Med 12:316–327

Fisher MR, Von Schulthess GK, Higgins CB (1985) Multiphasic cardiac magnetic resonance imaging: normal regional left ventricular wall thickening. Am J Roentgenol 145:27–30

Forbat SM, Sakrana MA, Darasz KH, El Demerdash F, Underwood SR (1996) Rapid assessment of left ventricular volume by short axis cine MRI. Br J Radiol 69:221–225

Goshtasby AA, Turner DA (1996) Fusion of short-axis and long-axis cardiac MR images. Comput Med Imaging Graph 20:77–87

Gould RG (1992) Perfusion quantitation by ultrafast computed tomography. Invest Radiol 27:S18–S21

Griswold MA, Sodickson DK, Jakob PM, Chen Q, Goldfarb JW, Edelman RR (1997) Resolution enhancement and artifact reduction in single shot MR imaging using simultaneous acquisition of spatial harmonics (SMASH) (abstract). Radiology 205:387

Hansen DE, Daughters G, Alderman EL, Ingels NJ, Miller DC (1988) Torsional deformation of the left ventricular midwall in human hearts with intramyocardial markers: regional heterogeneity and sensitivity to the inotropic effects of abrupt rate changes. Circ Res 62:941–952

Hartnell G, Cerel A, Kamalesh M, et al. (1994) Detection of myocardial ischemia, value of combined myocardial perfusion and cineangiographic MR imaging. Am J Roentgenol 163:1061–1067

Hendrich K, Xu Y, Kim S, Ugurbil K (1994) Surface coil cardiac tagging and (31)P spectroscopic localization with B-1-insensitive adiabatic pulses. Magn Reson Med 31:541–545

Herregods M, De Paep G, Bijnens B, et al. (1994) Determination of left ventricular volume by two-dimensional echocardiography: comparison with magnetic resonance imaging. Eur Heart J 15:1070–1073

Higgins CB, Caputo G, Wendland MF, Saeed M (1992) Measurement of blood flow and perfusion in the cardiovascular system. Invest Radiol 2:66–71

Hunter GJ, Hamberg LM, Weisskoff RM, Halpern EF, Brady TJ (1994) Measurement of stroke volume and cardiac output within a single breath hold with echo-planar MR imaging. J Magn Reson Imaging 4:51–54

Jarvinen VM, Kupari MM, Hekali PE, Poutanen VP (1994a) Assessment of left atrial volumes and phasic function using cine magnetic resonance imaging in normal subjects. Am J Cardiol 73:1135–1137

Jarvinen VM, Kupari MM, Hekali PE, Poutanen VP (1994b) Right atrial MR imaging studies of cadaveric atrial casts and comparisons with right and left atrial volumes and function in healthy subjects. Radiology 191:137–142

Kilner PJ, Firmin DN, Rees RSO, et al. (1991) Valve and great vessel stenosis: assessment with MR jet velocity mapping. Radiology 178:229–235

Kleinhans E, Altehoefer C, Arnold C, Buell U, vom Dahl J, Vebis R (1991) MRI measurements of left ventricular systolic wall thickening compared to regional myocardial perfusion as determined by ^{201}Tl SPECT in patients with coronary artery disease. Nuklearmedizin 30:61–66

Kondo C, Caputo GR, Semelka R, Foster E, Shimakawa A, Higgins CB (1991) Right and left ventricular stroke volume measurements with velocity-encoded cine MR imaging: In vitro and in vivo validation. Am J Roentgenol 157:9–16

Lamb HJ, Doornbos J, Van der Velde EA, Kruit MC, Reiber JH, de Roos A (1996) Echo planar MRI of the heart on a standard system: validation of measurements of left ventricular function and mass. J Comput Assist Tomogr 20:942–949

Lauerma K, Harjula A, Jarvinen V, Kupari M, Keto P (1996) Assessment of right and left atrial function in patients with transplanted hearts with the use of magnetic resonance imaging. J Heart Lung Transplant 15:360–367

Lima JAC, Jeremy R, Guier W, et al. (1993) Accurate systolic wall thickening by nuclear magnetic resonance imaging with tissue ragging: correlation with sonomicrometers in normal and ischemic myocardium. J Am Coll Cardiol 21:1741–1751

Liu N, Darmon PL, Saada M, et al. (1996) Comparison between radionuclide ejection fraction and fractional area changes derived from transesophageal echocardiography using automated border detection. Anesthesiology 85:468–474

Maes A, Flameng W, Nuyts J, et al. (1994) Histological alterations in chronically hypoperfused myocardium: correlation with PET findings. Circulation 90:735–745

Maes A, Van de Werf F, Nuyts J, Bormans G, Desmet W, Mortelmans L (1995) Impaired myocardial tissue perfusion early after successful thrombolysis. Impact on myocardial flow, metabolism, and function at late follow-up. Circulation 92:2072–2078

Maes A, Mortelmans L, Nuyts J, et al. (1997) Importance of flow/metabolism studies in predicting late recovery of function following reperfusion in patients with acute myocardial infarction. Eur Heart J 18:954–962

Mancini GB, De Boe SF, Anselmo E, Simon SB, Le Free MT, Vogel RA (1987) Quantitative regional curvature analysis: an application of shape determination for the assessment of segmental left ventricular function in man. Am Heart J 113:326–334

Markiewicz W, Sechtem U, Higgins CB (1987a) Evaluation of the right ventricle by magnetic resonance imaging. Am Heart J 113:8–15

Markiewicz W, Sechtem U, Kirby R, Derugin N, Caputo GC, Higgins CB (1987b) Measurement of ventricular volumes in the dog by nuclear magnetic resonance imaging. J Am Coll Cardiol 10:170–177

Matter C, Nagel E, Stuber M, Boesiger P, Hess OM (1996) Assessment of Systolic and diastolic LV function by MR myocardial tagging. Basic Res Cardiol 91 Suppl 2:23–28

Matthaei D, Haase A, Henrich D, Dühmke E (1990) Cardiac and vascular imaging with an MR snapshot technique. Radiology 177:527–532

McVeigh ER, Atalar E (1992) Cardiac tagging with breath-hold cine MRI. Magn Reson Med 28:318–327

McVeigh ER, Zerhouni EA (1991) Noninvasive measurement of transmural gradients in myocardial strain with MR imaging. Radiology 180:677–683

Miron SD, Finkelhor R, Penuel JH, Bahler R, Bellon EM (1996) A geometric method of measuring the left ventricular ejection fraction on gated Tc-99m sestamibi myocardial imaging. Clin Nucl Med 21:439–444

Mogelvang J, Thomsen C, Mehlsen J, Bräckle G, Stubgaard M, Henriksen O (1987) Evaluation of left ventricular volumes measured by magnetic resonance imaging. Eur Heart J 1986:1016–1021

Mohiaddin RH, Hasegawa M (1995) Measurement of atrial volumes by magnetic resonance imaging in healthy volunteers and in patients with myocardial infarction. Eur Heart J 16:106–111

Moore CC, O'Dell WG, McVeigh ER, Zerhouni EA (1992) Calculation of three-dimensional left ventricular strains from biplanar tagged MR images. J Magn Reson Imaging 2:165–175

Moore CC, Reeder SB, McVeigh ER (1994) Tagged MR imaging in a deforming phantom: photographic validation. Radiology 190:765–769

Naito H, Arisawa J, Harada K, Yamagami H, Kozuka T, Tamura S (1995) Assessment of right ventricular regional contraction and comparison with the left ventricle in normal humans: a cine magnetic resonance study with presaturation myocardial tagging. Br Heart J 74:186–191

O'Dell WG, Moore CC, Hunter WC, Zerhouni EA, McVeigh ER (1995) Three-dimensional myocardial deformations: calculation with displacement field fitting to tagged MR images. Radiology 195:829–835

Pattynama PM, Doornbos J, Hermans J, van der Wall EE, de Roos A (1992) Magnetic resonance evaluation of regional left ventricular function. Effect of through-plane motion. Invest Radiol 27:681–685

Pattynama PM, Lamb HJ, van der Velde EA, van der Wall EE, de Roos A (1993) Left ventricular measurements with cine and spin-echo MR imaging: a study of reproducibility with variance component analysis. Radiology 187:261–268

Pattynama PM, Lamb HJ, Van der Velde EA, Van der Geest RJ, Van der Wall EE, De Roos A (1995) Reproducibility of MRI-derived measurements of right ventricular volumes and myocardial mass. Magn Reson Imaging 13:53–63

Pennell DJ, Underwood SR, Ell PJ, Swanton RH, Walker JM, Longmore DB (1990) Dipyridamole magnetic resonance imaging: a comparison with thallium-201 emission tomography. Br Heart J 64:362–369

Pennell DJ, Underwood SR, Manzara CC, et al. (1992) Magnetic resonance imaging during dobutamine stress in coronary artery disease. Am J Cardiol 70:34–40

Pennell DJ, Firmin DN, Burger P, et al. (1995) Assessment of magnetic resonance velocity mapping of global ventricular function during dobutamine infusion in coronary artery disease. Br Heart J 74:163–170

Perman WH, Creswell LL, Wyers SG, Moulton MJ, Pasque MK (1995) Magnetic resonance imaging during dobutamine stress in coronary artery disease. Am J Cardiol 70:34–40

Pipe JG, Boes JL, Chenevert TL (1991) Method for measuring three-dimensional motion with tagged MR imaging. Radiology 181:591–595

Rademakers FE (1991) Three-dimensional strain analysis of the left ventricle. Proefschrift tot het behalen van de graad van geaggregeerde voor het hoger onderwijs. Universitaire instelling, Antwerpen

Rademakers FE, Buchalter MB, Rogers WJ, et al. (1992) Dissociation between left ventricular untwisting and filling: accentuation by catecholamines. Circulation 85:1572–1581

Rademakers FE, Rogers WJ, Guier WH, et al. (1994) Relation of regional cross-fiber shortening to wall thickening in the intact heart. Three-dimensional strain analysis by NMR tagging. Circulation 89:1174–1182

Rehr RB, Malloy CR, Filipchuk NG, Peshock RM (1985) Left ventricular volumes measured by MR imaging. Radiology 156:717–719

Rogers WJ, Shapiro EP, Weiss JL, et al. (1991) Quantification of and correction for left ventricular systolic long-axis shortening by magnetic resonance tissue tagging and slice isolation. Circulation 84:721–731

Sandler MP, Patton JA (1996) Fluorine 18-labeled fluorodeoxyglucose myocardial single-photon emission computed tomography: an alternative for determining myocardial viability. J Nucl Cardiol 3:342–349

Schaefer S, Peshock RM, Parkey RW, Willerson JT (1986) A new device for exercise MR imaging. Am J Roentgenol 147:1289–1290

Schulen V, Schick F, Loichat J, et al. (1996) Evaluation of K-space segmented cine sequences for fast functional cardiac imaging. Invest Radiol 31:512–522

Sechtem U, Pflugfelder PW, Gould RG, et al. (1987a) Measurement of right and left ventricular volumes in healthy individuals with cine MR imaging. Radiology 163:697–702

Sechtem U, Pflugfelder PW, White RD, et al. (1987b) Cine MR imaging: potential for the evaluation of cardiovascular function. Am J Roentgenol 148:239–246

Sechtem U, Plugfelder P, Higgins CB (1987c) Quantification of cardiac function by conventional and cine magnetic resonance imaging. Cardiovasc Intervent Radiol 10:365–373

Semelka RC, Tomei E, Wagner S, et al. (1990a) Interstudy reproducibility of dimensional and functional measurements between cine magnetic resonance studies in the morphologically abnormal left ventricle. Am Heart J 119:1367–1373

Semelka RC, Tomei E, Wagner S, et al. (1990b) Normal left ventricular dimensions and function: interstudy reproducibility of measurements with cine MR imaging. Radiology 174:763–768

Sinha S, Mather R, Sinha U, Goldin J, Fonarow G, Yoon HC (1997) Estimation of the left ventricular ejection fraction using a novel multiphase, dark-blood, breath-hold MR imaging technique. Am J Roentgenol 169:101–112

Soldo SJ, Norris SL, Gober JR, Haywood LJ, Colletti PM, Terk M (1994) MRI-derived ventricular volume curves for the assessment of left ventricular function. Magn Reson Imaging 12:711–717

Stehling MK, Turner R, Mansfield P (1991) Echo-planar imaging: magnetic resonance imaging in a fraction of a second. Science 254:43–50

van der Wall EE, van Rugge FP, Vliegen HW, Reiber JH, de Roos A, Bruschke AV (1997) Ischemic heart disease: value of MR techniques. Int J Card Imaging 13:179–189

van Rossum AC, Visser FC, Sprenger M, Van Eenige MJ, Valk J, Roos JP (1988a) Evaluation of magnetic resonance imaging for determination of left ventricular ejection fraction and comparison with angiography. Am J Cardiol 1988:628–633

van Rossum AC, Visser FC, van Eenige MJ, Valk J, Roos JP (1988b) Magnetic resonance imaging of the heart for determination of ejection fraction. Int J Cardiol 18:53–63

van Rugge FP, Holman ER, van der Wall EE, De Roos A, van der Laarse A, Bruschke AVG (1993a) Quantitation of global and regional left ventricular function by cine magnetic resonance imaging during dobutamine stress in normal human subjects. Eur Heart J 14:456–463

van Rugge FP, Van der Wall EE, de Roos A, Bruschke AVG (1993b) Dobutamine stress magnetic resonance imaging for detection of coronary artery disease. J Am Coll Cardiol 22:431–439

van Rugge FP, Van der Wall EE, Spanjersberg SJ, et al. (1994) Magnetic resonance imaging during dobutamine stress for detection and localization of coronary artery disease:

quantitative wall motion analysis using a modification of the centerline method. Circulation 90:127–138

Waggoner AD, Harris KM, Braverman AC, Barzilai B, Geltman EM (1996) The role of transthoracic echocardiography in the management of patients seen in an outpatient cardiology clinic. J Am Soc Echocardiogr 9:761–768

Waldman LK, Fung YC, Covell JW (1985) Transmural myocardial deformation in the canine left ventricle. Normal in vivo three-dimensional finite strains. Circ Res 57:152–163

Waldman LK, Nosan D, Villarreal F, Covell JW (1988) Relation between transmural deformation and local myofiber direction in canine left ventricle. Circ Res 63:550–562

Wedeen VJ (1992) Magnetic resonance imaging of myocardial kinematics. Technique to detect, localize, and quantify the strain rates of the active human myocardium. Magn Reson Med 27:52–67

Wedeen VJ, Weisskoff RM, Reese TG, et al. (1995) Motionless movies of myocardial strain-rates using stimulated echoes [published erratum appears in Magn Reson Med 1995; 33:743]. Magn Reson Med 33:401–408

Wolfkiel CJ, Brundage BH (1991) Measurement of myocardial blood flow by UFCT: towards clinical applicability. Int J Card Imaging 7:89–100

Yamaoka O, Yabe T, Okada M, et al. (1993) Evaluation of left ventricular mass: comparison of ultrafast computed tomography, magnetic resonance imaging, and contrast left ventriculography. Am Heart J 126:1372–1379

Young AA, Axel L (1992) Three-dimensional motion and deformation of the heart wall: estimation with spatial modulation of magnetization – a model-based approach. Radiology 185:241–247

Young AA, Axel L, Dougherty L, Bogen DK, Parenteau CS (1993) Validation of tagging with MR imaging to estimate material deformation. Radiology 188:101–108

Young AA, Kramer CM, Ferrari VA, Axel L, Reichek N (1994) Three-dimensional left ventricular deformation in hypertrophic cardiomyopathy. Circulation 90:854–867

Zerhouni EA, Parish DM, Rogers WJ, Yang A, Shapiro EP (1988) Human heart: tagging with MR imaging – a new method for noninvasive assessment of myocardial motion. Radiology 169:59–63

7 Myocardial Viability

Y. Ni

CONTENTS

7.1 Introduction

There are three stages in the history of every medical discovery. When it is first announced, people say that it is not true. Then, a little later, when its truth has been borne in on them, so that it can no longer be denied, they say it is not important. After that, if its importance becomes sufficiently obvious, they say that anyhow it is not new.

Sir James Mackenzie, 1853–1925

Myocardial viability represents one of the most challenging topics in clinical and experimental cardiology. Identification of irreversible necrotic from dysfunctional but viable and potentially salvageable myocardium after a heart attack is of paramount importance for the management of cardiac patients. In particular, revascularization of an infarcted area by percutaneous transluminal coronary angioplasty (PTCA) or coronary artery bypass grafting is justified only if functional recovery is predictable following the surgery. A tremendous number of research studies, published papers, reviews, editorials, and books have addressed different aspects of this topic. The current chapter is intended not only to convey the main messages from previously published work but also to introduce some of the most recent advances in cardiac MRI which may impact on our understanding of myocardial viability and eventually on clinical decision-making in respect of ischemic heart disease.

7.2 Physiopathological Aspects of Myocardial Viability

The heart is virtually a segment of the blood vessel, but highly specialized as a double pump made of striated muscle capable of spontaneous rhythmical contractions for propulsion of circulating blood flow in the body. Its right and left ventricles are responsible for the pulmonary and systemic circulations respectively. The inner, middle, and outer layers of cardiac wall are termed the endocardium, myocardium, and epicardium. The particularly differentiated myocardium represents the main mass of the organ. However, it has been demonstrated that the inner one-fifth of the left ventricular (LV) wall thickness, or subendocardial myocardium, predominantly contributes to the wall thickening during systolic contraction at rest (Myers et al. 1986). The rest of the muscle increases wall thickening only when there is catecholamine stimulation (Sklenar et al. 1994). The heart is provided with its own nutrient vessels called coronary arteries which are characterized by strengthened vascular wall as a result of adaptation to the high blood pressure near the origin of the aorta. The overall density of the microvascular bed in myocardium is 2–3 times greater than in skeletal muscle. The amount of blood passing through coronary arteries is about 250 ml/min (or about 1 ml/min/g), i.e. approximately 5% of normal cardiac output. Coronary flow is greater during dias-

Y. Ni, MD, PhD, Department of Radiology, University Hospitals Gasthuisberg, Catholic University of Leuven, Herestraat 49, B-3000 Leuven, Belgium

tole than during systole, in contrast to the situation in other parts of the circulation. Capillaries in myocardium are more permeable than those in skeletal muscle despite their morphological similarities.

Myocardial viability (the ability to survive) is affected when different pathological factors cause ischemia or hypoxia in myocardium as a result of restricted coronary perfusion. In some cases, this represents a broader etiology including inadequate blood volume, valvular or congenital heart diseases, cardiac arrhythmias, and myocardial or pericardial diseases. In a large majority of cases, however, reduced coronary perfusion is more limited, being present only at a local or regional level.

Coronary arteries are particularly vulnerable to atherosclerosis, which is the main cause of coronary artery disease (CAD). CAD is by far the most common health-threatening problem among adults in modern society. It causes myocardial ischemia and may ultimately result in myocardial infarction (MI), which is the most frequent cause of death in industrialized countries (COOPER 1993). The time course of acute myocardial ischemia has been clinically recognized and well documented in animal experiments. Myocardium may cease its aerobic metabolism within 10s after the interruption of coronary blood flow, which is soon followed by an inhibition of anaerobic metabolism due to the accumulation of lactate and other acidic metabolites (WHITEMAN et al. 1983). The systolic contraction is markedly inhibited within 10–15s to preserve limited high-energy phosphate or ATP storage, which is anyhow depleted by the ongoing cell membrane activities (JENNINGS et al. 1978). By 40 min of ischemia, the chemogradients of the membrane can no longer be maintained. The consequent influx of calcium and sodium causes intracellular edema, which, together with accumulation of toxic metabolites, finally leads to myocardial death. The infarction almost always occurs earlier and more prominently in subendocardial than in subepicardial muscles, since the systolic wall stress and the resulting oxygen consumption are greater at the endocardium than at the epicardium. As a matter of fact, the size of the infarct evolves over time transmurally, with a wave front of necrotic myocardium from endocardium towards epicardium. Usually the maximal infarct size has been achieved by 6h. However, the presence of even a small fraction of perfusion to the infarct bed, for instance more than 20% of the normal coronary supply, from either antegrade or collateral flow would significantly delay necrosis and limit infarct size (RIVAS et al. 1976). This is true especially in chronic

CAD patients. Coronary collateral circulation usually takes time to become functional (PATTERSON et al. 1993) and plays an important role in maintaining the viability of myocardium distal to coronary occlusion. When collateral flow is insufficient to prevent a marked fall in coronary perfusion pressure for a prolonged period, e.g., above 1h, infarction inevitably happens (FUSTER et al. 1979).

Clinically, the functional status of the left ventricle, as represented by the LV ejection fraction at rest, is known to be a predictor for cardiac death after acute myocardial infarction (AMI). The prognosis of such patients depends upon many interrelated factors including the duration or extent of coronary occlusion, the presence or absence of collateral circulation, the timeliness and effectiveness of reperfusion, cardioelectrical stability, and eventually the recovery of LV function.

The pathophysiological understanding of myocardial ischemia and infarction has been evolving over time. In the past, LV dysfunction was exclusively attributed to myocardial death (HERMAN and GORLIN 1968). It has gradually been recognized that areas of poor or no contractility after AMI are not always associated with necrosis; instead they may represent areas of potentially reversible damage which can improve spontaneously or after intervention to reestablish coronary blood flow (LEWIS et al. 1991).

As illustrated in the flow chart of Fig. 7.1, coronary occlusion yields different outcomes of ischemia. The most severe consequence is myocardial cell death, which is absolutely nonviable and irreversible in terms of metabolic and contractile function. This may result from complete and persistent coronary occlusion or from reperfusion after prolonged and severe ischemia. The latter condition has been termed "reperfusion damage," which is associated with vascular injury, interstitial hemorrhage, release of lysosomal enzymes, disruption of membranes, influx of calcium, and cessation of functional activity (FISHBEIN et al. 1980).

In acute ischemia after spontaneous or therapeutic reperfusion and in chronic ischemia prior to revascularization intervention, several forms of myocardial viability have been characterized in clinical patients and experimental animals. The best outcome is an instantaneous normalization of contractility in the affected myocardium. However, due to the prior ischemic insult, the recovery of contraction more frequently occurs after a considerable delay, a condition called *"stunned myocardium"* (BRAUNWALD and KLONER 1982). Stunning is de-

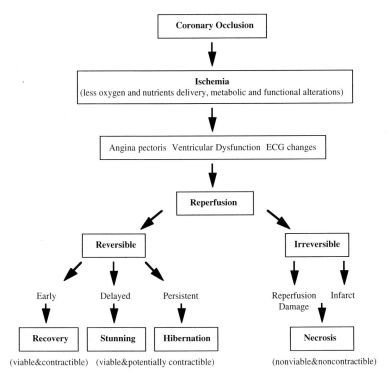

Fig. 7.1. Simplified flow chart of ischemic events after coronary occlusion and reperfusion

scribed as a transient LV dysfunction that persists after reperfusion despite restored coronary flow and the absence of necrosis. Excessive oxygen free radicals and cytosolic calcium imbalance are claimed to be the mechanisms of the impaired contraction (Bolli 1990).

When a certain degree of ischemia persists for weeks, months, or years, myocytes may still remain viable but dysfunctional by downregulating their energy consumption through a lower level of aerobic and/or anaerobic metabolism. However, the areas of LV that are dyskinetic (either hypokinetic or akinetic) may restore normal contractile function after effective reperfusion interventions with angioplasty or bypass surgery. This type of ischemia associated with a chronic and reversible LV dysfunction has been termed *"hibernating myocardium"* (Rahimtoola 1989). Acute hibernation has also been observed in more recent studies (Downing and Chen 1992). Increased glucose utilization and decreased free fatty acid metabolism are features of energy consumption in ischemic myocardium (Liedtke 1981), and have been exploited for metabolic cardiac imaging (Camici et al. 1989). The mechanisms of contractile and metabolic "downregulation" underlying myocardial hibernation have been mainly hypothesized rather than experimentally defined (Ferrari et al. 1996; Ross 1991).

Although the simplistic classification of stunning and hibernating myocardium is derived from clinical observations and imperfect animal experiments with many exceptions and overlaps (Bashour and Mason 1990; Neill et al. 1986; Nienaber et al. 1991), it is at least conceptually of clinical significance. If reliable and precise diagnostic methods become available, recognition of stunning will be helpful in assessing the prognosis and adjusting the treatment of the AMI, while evidence of hibernating myocardium will indicate a need for angioplasty or coronary bypass grafting surgery.

7.3
Definition of Myocardial Viability

To give a definition of myocardial viability can be complicated and controversial (Conti 1993; Goldstein 1991; Gould 1991; Gropler and Bergmann 1991b; Kaul 1995; Lindner and Kaul 1996). From a biological point of view, viability implies the presence of structural integrity together with the metabolic activities that are essential for survival of the organism. In this state, specialized functions such as muscular contraction and glandular excretion may fully or partially occur or may simply not occur. In compliance with this concept, the triphenyltetrazolium chloride (TTC) histochemical staining technique was validated for macroscopic discrimination between viable and acute nonviable myocardium (FISHBEIN et al. 1981; KLEIN et al. 1981; KLONER et al. 1981; NACHLAS and SHNITKA 1963). The reddish or TTC positively stained area is considered to be viable, whereas the pale or negatively stained area is regarded as nonviable and irreversible myocardium. The loss of active respiratory enzymes and coenzymes due to disruption of cellular integrity during ischemic insult underlies the negative staining of necrotic myocardium (KLEIN et al. 1981). This in vitro method has been routinely used in laboratory research as a gold standard for determination of myocardial necrosis, but it is virtually inapplicable in the clinic because of its destructive nature.

From a clinical point of view, the most prominent feature of a viable heart is its pump function and cardiac management ultimately aims at restoring synergic contractility. Therefore, the following plausible interpretation based on functional recovery has been widely accepted. Jeopardized myocardium that manifests improved contractile function after appropriate therapy is considered viable, while myocardium that is persistently dysfunctional, as typically seen in completed infarction, is regarded as nonviable. (GROPLER and BERGMANN 1991a,b). However, this definition only reflects the diagnostic capability of that time. The reason why only functional recovery is taken here as an indicator for myocardial viability is at least partially due to the fact that an in vivo technique which enables clear-cut distinction between viable and nonviable myocardium, as seen with ex vivo TTC staining, has not yet become available. Obviously, this kind of expedient definition is mainly of significance for retrospective diagnosis, since it relies on the eventual outcome of cardiac contractility. In reality, whether, when, and how the jeopardized myocardium recovers contractile function remains an unsolved multifactorial problem. Even if inotropic stimulation is applied, the viability cannot be absolutely ascertained or excluded with currently available techniques (FERRARI et al. 1996).

The foregoing clinical definition of myocardial viability has recently been disputed within cardiological circles (KAUL 1995; LINDNER and KAUL 1996). After disproving the validity of defining myocardial viability as recovery in regional function following revascularization, it was stated in the editorial of a recent issue of *Circulation* that "Ideally, the definition of viability should be as simple as that in the Oxford English Dictionary (viable means

capable of living). It should be also independent of the result of an intervention.... The ideal imaging method for assessing viability should be able to delineate infarcted from noninfarcted tissue with the same resolution as shown in Fig. 2 (which is a hand-drawn diagram of the infarcted heart)" (KAUL 1995). This aspiration has now probably been fulfilled due to recent advances in the search for infarct-avid contrast media (NI and MARCHAL et al. 1994–1998) in conjunction with the rapid development of new cardiac MRI techniques, to be addressed later in this chapter. It is now entirely possible to identify in vivo irreversible, necrotic from reversible, viable myocardium at an early stage of infarction by means of specifically enhanced high-resolution MRI. The eventual clinical application of this technique would greatly benefit coronary patients by providing unambiguous diagnosis and optimized therapy so that the myocardium at risk might be salvaged and reperfusion damage minimized. Only by this means will it be possible to define myocardial viability according to a single principle which integrates both biological and clinical considerations.

7.4
Techniques Other than MR
for Detecting Myocardial Viability

Endeavors to find a reliable method for the detection of myocardial viability can be traced back a long time and continue today. Besides recently emerging MR techniques, which will be discussed later in the chapter, the following methods have been developed, investigated, and clinically used, with each playing an indispensable role in the overall effort to resolve the clinical problems related to myocardial viability.

7.4.1
Symptomatology

Assessment of symptoms is usually the primary step in outpatient cardiology. The occurrence of myocardial ischemia and infarction is suggested by evidence of angina or chest pain and heart failure together with a typical history of CAD. The relief or improvement of these symptoms often suggests a benign alteration that has occurred either spontaneously or after therapeutic intervention. However, cardiac ischemia is not always symptomatic, and silent events are not uncommon; furthermore, and on the other hand, collection of data is not possible from critically ill patients with abrupt onset of a cardiac event. In addition, symptoms alone are insufficient for characterizing or localizing specific segments with jeopardized viability

7.4.2
Electrocardiography

Throughout this century, despite the advent of more sophisticated methods, the electrocardiogram (ECG) has been applied by clinicians as a "first-line" tool to determine whether, when, and where myocardial death has occurred. Universal availability, low cost, objective criteria of interpretation, and freedom from adverse effects are apparent advantages of this technique. With characteristic changes in the QRS complex, ST segment, and T wave, ECG is routinely used in clinical practice for the diagnosis of MI, though it is unable to quantify the extent of myocardial loss. Variables that affect the diagnostic accuracy of ECG include the location of the infarct, the longitudinal dimension of the infarct, the thickness of myocardium involved, the presence of multiple infarcts (either prior or concurrent), the presence of other ventricular anomalies (e.g., conductive defects, hypertrophy, and other myocardial diseases), and metabolic imbalances. The overall sensitivity, specificity, and positive predictive value of ECG for the detection of infarction are about 70%, 80%, and 60% respectively (PARKER et al. 1996).

Electrocardiography is more accurate at diagnosing acute than healed MI. The ease with which the location of the MI can be approximated by ECG varies: MI at the anterior wall is easiest to locate, and MI at the lateral wall most difficult. Although indicative in some cases, "Q-wave" or "non-Q-wave" does not absolutely mean transmural or subendocardial MI (ANTALOCZY et al. 1988). The potential of the ECG to identify viable and still salvageable myocardium has been explored by coupling with stress testing (MARGONATO and CHIERCHIA 1996). Transient ST segment elevation, T wave pseudonormalization, and ventricular arrhythmias elicited by exercise testing or dobutamine (a synthetic catecholamine) infusion are major predictors of reversible perfusion, postinfarction functional recovery, and residual viability in a previous MI (LOMBARDO et al. 1996). Obviously, ECG cannot provide information on the metabolic activity of the heart and is unable to accurately localize or delineate the extent of irreversible

damage which may coexist with dysfunctional yet viable tissue.

7.4.3
Myocardial Biochemistry

A variety of biochemical markers released from necrosing myocardial cells into the peripheral blood are recognized to be of value for the detection and stratification of myocardial injury. They are categorized as enzymatic markers such as lactate dehydrogenase, creatine kinase (CK), and glycogen phosphorylase; nonenzymatic cytoplasmic markers such as myoglobin and the fatty acid-binding protein heart isoform (hFABP); and nonenzymatic noncytoplasmic markers such as myosin chains and troponins. These laboratory tests are more economical and easier to perform than other more complicated techniques. Under most circumstances, they provide interpretable parameters to confirm the diagnosis of AMI, monitor its evolution, and estimate infarct size. However, these markers do have limitations. Usually they are insensitive within the first 3–4 h after the onset of AMI or are not sensitive enough to detect minor myocardial damage due to the analytical imprecision of activity measurements and wide range of normal values. In addition, most of these markers are rather nonspecific, since they are also released after skeletal muscle damage and surgical intervention (BIRDI et al. 1997). Therefore, many new markers, most of which are isoenzymes or isoforms of the above-mentioned substances, have been identified in order to improve the sensitivity and cardiac specificity (HAMM and KATUS 1995). For instance, the cardiac isoenzyme CK-MB and its subforms CK-MB$_1$ and CK-MB$_2$ as well as cardiac isoform troponin I were reported to be useful for earlier and more precise diagnosis of myocardial injury, although the results appeared controversial (BAKKER et al. 1993). Similarly, glycogen phosphorylase isoenzyme BB has recently been shown to hold promise for the clinical assessment of the severity of myocardial ischemia, because it is released earlier in the course of reversible ischemic injury (KRAUSE et al. 1996). Nevertheless, the ECG (if informative) is still considered superior to detection of these markers because it is quicker, simpler, and more reliable for the early diagnosis of the AMI (MAIR et al. 1995; TIMMIS 1990). In general, biochemical markers only provide nonvisual, nonlocalizing, and somewhat delayed information in the assessment of myocardial viability.

7.4.4
Coronary Angiography

It has been 40 years since Sones et al. first visualized atherosclerotic CAD in vivo by performing selective coronary angiography in 1957 (SONES and SHIREY 1962). Today, this method is still considered by most physicians to be the "gold standard" for definition of coronary anatomy. Myocardial viability can be suggested by the presence of antegrade or collateral flow, especially when ventriculography reveals recovered ventricular hypokinetics after administration of pharmacological vasodilators. Capillary filling in the infarct-related area is also indicative for viability (CONTI 1993), although its visibility on angiography is still questionable (ROBLES et al. 1994).

The accuracy and reproducibility of coronary angiography have always been questioned by investigators (GRODIN et al. 1974; TOPOL and NISSEN 1995). The major limitations of this method are high intraobserver and interobserver variability, inferior spatial resolution for visualization of structures smaller than 0.2 mm (e.g., capillaries), and misleading depiction of coronary lumen due to the overlapping two-dimensional projection (TOPOL and NISSEN 1995). The information gained is insufficient to differentiate between viable and nonviable myocardium. For example, a patent coronary artery may perfuse a region of necrotic myocardium or scar; this is especially true early after a reperfused AMI (DEWOOD et al. 1980).

Coronary intravascular ultrasound is a similar approach which provides more precise information on pathological changes of the main branches of the coronary artery (NISSEN and GURLEY 1991). However, the interventional risk and the high cost prevent application of this technique for clinical diagnosis.

7.4.5
Echocardiography

Being a widely available, noninvasive, inexpensive technique that can be performed at the bedside, two-dimensional echocardiography (2-DE) shares the highest temporal resolution with coronary angiography and has been by far the most popular diagnostic imaging tool in cardiology. Since the dysfunctional myocardium may contain both viable and necrotic components, the mere detection of regional contractility with conventional 2-DE is insufficient

for predicting reversibility. Accordingly the 2-DE assessment of myocardial viability can be based on two methods: (1) evaluation of myocardial motion or wall thickening after inotropic stimulation (CIGARROA et al. 1993), and (2) evaluation of coronary or collateral perfusion, using myocardial contrast echocardiography (SABIA et al. 1992).

Dobutamine stress 2-DE compares wall motion or thickening at baseline and during intravenous infusion of incremental doses of dobutamine. Whether contractile function improves or not may suggest the presence or absence of viable myocardium. This technique can be used to demonstrate reversibility of resting dysfunction in hypoperfused areas which are viable (SMART 1994). The sensitivity, specificity, and positive or negative predictive value of dobutamine stress 2-DE have all been reported to be above 80% (LA CANNA et al. 1994; BONOW 1995). On the other hand, contrast 2-DE involves intracoronary injection of air microbubbles and has to be performed together with coronary angiography. Since the air bubbles remain transiently in the vascular bed, the coronary flow (antegrade or collateral) and microvascular perfusion, which may reflect myocardial viability, can be appreciated (CAMARANO et al. 1995). The invasiveness of this approach does not favor its wide clinical use unless suitable intravenous contrast agents can be developed.

Use of stress 2-DE may be limited by an unacceptable acoustic window due to the high prevalence of smoking and obesity among CAD patients and by strong dependence on subjective interpretation of results by the operators who vary in experience (FRAGASSO et al. 1993). Several measures may help to improve the diagnostic accuracy and ease of interpretation. First, transesophageal echocardiography yields better image quality due to an improved acoustic window, though at a price of increased invasiveness. Second, use of quantification techniques may provide more objective grading in respect of ventricular function reserve (PEREZ et al. 1992). Another possible approach is to exploit integrated ultrasonic backscatter for complementary documentation of wall motion in relation to the physical status of myocardium (MILUNSKI et al. 1989).

7.4.6
Nuclear Scintigraphy

Up to now, nuclear cardiology has been one of the major domains of radionuclide imaging. The equipment used has evolved from the conventional gamma camera for planar imaging to more sophisticated tomographic imagers such as single-photon emission computer tomography (SPECT) and positron emission tomography (PET) with improved image quality.

Many techniques are available for global assessment of myocardial viability on the basis of myocardial perfusion, cell membrane integrity, and metabolic activity. These methods are believed to provide greater precision than information obtained with above-mentioned modalities, such as that regarding coronary patency, regional function, or the presence or absence of Q waves. The principle of myocardial perfusion imaging is that the tracers distribute proportionally in the myocardium according to regional blood flow. However, CAD patients usually demonstrate normal myocardial perfusion at rest, unless the coronary stenosis is already severe, which causes resting ischemia or even myocardial infarction. This situation calls for stress tests. The physiological basis of stress myocardial perfusion test is production of an increase in coronary flow in the territory of normal, but not stenosed, vessels by means of exercise or pharmacological vasodilatation so that on the perfusion image, the territory with coronary stenosis appears as a "cold" area due to lower regional uptake of the tracer. In clinical practice, a number of stressors such as dobutamine, dipyridamole, and adenosine are currently used, especially in patients whose exercise capability is inadequate (PENNELL 1994).

Among the nuclide tracers, thallium-201 (^{201}Tl) has been most widely used in myocardial perfusion imaging for more than 20 years. Since ^{201}Tl also acts as a potassium analogue, after its initial blood pool effect, this tracer redistributes to viable myocytes. This feature has formed the basis for a unique stress-redistribution ^{201}Tl imaging method. In this technique, defects on early stress images that resolve or improve on delayed redistribution images, i.e., "reversible defects," indicate myocardial ischemia and therefore potentially salvageable myocardium, while "fixed defects" that do not resolve on the delayed redistribution images may indicate absence of viable myocardium. However, it was found that standard stress-redistribution ^{201}Tl imaging underestimated the extent of viable myocardium and this has led to a further ^{201}Tl reinjection protocol (HENDEL 1994). Fixed defects that persist on redistribution images may resolve on reinjection images, suggesting myocardial viability. For chronic CAD patients who are potential candidates for coronary revascularization,

^{201}Tl myocardial scintigraphy with rest-redistribution or reinjection is regarded as an established, proven, and cost-effective way of detecting viable myocardium, while ^{201}Tl myocardial SPECT is a method of choice (SCHOEDER et al. 1993). The inconvenience of ^{201}Tl due to its limited half-life after being produced in a cyclotron has led to the introduction of alternative agents such as technetium-99m sestamibi (^{99m}Tc-MIBI) and ^{99m}Tc-tetrafosmin, which have an advantage over ^{201}Tl in terms of reduced radiation to patients and improved image quality despite a lack of redistribution capability (BERMAN et al. 1994).

Performance of PET needs a dedicated scanner with cyclotron-produced short-life tracers including blood flow agents such as rubidium-82 (^{82}Rb), nitrogen-13 (^{13}N)-ammonia, and oxygen-15 (^{15}O)-water and metabolic agents such as fluorine-18-labelled fluorodeoxyglucose (^{18}F-FDG). Despite being expensive, PET scanning has been considered the best proven method for determination of the presence of viable myocardium, e.g., a perfusion-metabolism mismatch demonstrated by combined use of ^{13}N-ammonia and ^{18}F-FDG is suggested to be diagnostic of hibernating myocardium.

The high sensitivity and specificity with quantifiable results are apparent strong points of nuclide imaging, especially in tomographic techniques such as SPECT and PET. However, these advantages are largely offset by the poor spatial resolution, which together with the dependence on external radioactive tracers for imaging consitute the major intrinsic drawbacks of the techniques. The black-and-white or color-coded cardiac images created with both conventional and tomographic methods are usually appreciated as somewhat horseshoe-like or doughnut-like figures without clear marginal demarcation and local anatomical information (DILSIZIAN and BONOW 1993). Their spatial resolution in the order of 1 cm is obviously insufficient to display detailed anatomy of the ventricular wall, the normal thickness of which is only about 2 cm (MORGUET et al. 1996). Imagination, manual contouring, and experience are frequently necessary for imaging interpretation, giving rise to inaccuracy, subjectivity, and uncertainty. The loss of detail concerning the presence or absence of subendocardial and subepicardial uptake could cause incorrect assessment of the transmural extent of the infarct, which is a crucial indicator of future functional recovery (MYERS et al. 1986).

7.5
Incremental Role of MR in the Determination of Myocardial Viability

As briefly reviewed above, indicators of myocardial viability with various non-MR techniques are often nonlocalizing, nonspecific, invasive, and inaccurate. An optimal modality has not yet been defined despite intensive investigation (DILSIZIAN and BONOW 1993). Lack of detailed topography in ventricular wall layers and of distinction between viable and nonviable myocardium are common problems even among the "gold standard" cardiac imaging techniques in the assessment of myocardial viability. Indeed, spatial resolution is a sine qua non for interpretation of transmural events such as those that occur in acute myocardial infarction (BIANCO and ALPERT 1997). The capability to label specifically either viable or nonviable myocardium represents another key factor in tackling the problems.

Magnetic resonance (MR) has emerged as a new and rapidly growing methodology. Its versatile strengths are superb spatial resolution in the range of 1–2 mm, nonionizing safety, noninvasiveness, intrinsic contrast exploitable for tissue characterization, inherent 3-D data acquisition with unlimited orientation, sensitivity to blood flow and cardiac wall motion, and potential for in vivo measurement of myocardial metabolism (VAN DER WALL et al. 1996). All these features may make MR techniques advantageous over other imaging modalities. Although it is more difficult to image an ever-moving heart than any other stationary body structure, cardiac MR has become technically possible by gating collection of imaging information with ECG signals. Cardiac MR can be applied to acquire either images (MRI) or spectroscopic data (MRS). The latter is mainly used for studies on myocardial metabolism (WEISS et al. 1990). Unlike coronary angiography and echocardiography, MRI does not provide real-time images, but its temporal resolution has been markedly improved by the recent development of rapid acquisition techniques such as ultrafast echo planar imaging (EPI). These make it possible to acquire images within milliseconds and, therefore, to eliminate cardiac as well as respiratory motion artifacts. Choice of appropriate MRI techniques permits acquisition of almost all pertinent information related to myocardial viability, such as myocardial morphology, cardiac function, myocardial perfusion, and coronary flow. All of these aspects have been covered in different chapters of this book.

Experimentally, sodium (^{23}Na) cardiac MRI has been investigated to distinguish viable from nonviable myocardium (CANNON et al. 1986; KIM et al. 1997). This interesting approach explores intrinsic contrast between normal and ischemic segments due to disruption of the sodium concentration gradient across the cell membrane of myocytes after ischemic injury. However, its clinical application relies on the resolution of multiple theoretical and technical obstacles (KIM et al. 1997).

Currently, the clinical use of MRI in ischemic heart disease is still limited in comparison with other cardiac imaging techniques. However, given the potential of MRI to overcome the limitations of other imaging modalities, this situation will soon be changed by the active research in this field. In general, cardiac MR is suitable for the following clinical purposes.

1. *Localization of MI.* Myocardial edema (or increase in tissue water content), cellular infiltration, capillary proliferation, and collagen formation are histopathological features in the process of MI that may result in altered tissue T1 (or longitudinal) and T2 (or transverse) relaxation times. With T2-weighted MRI, the prolonged T2 relaxation time, especially during the acute phase, can be translated into regional hyperintense signals, although such signals are not necessarily related to loss of viability (WISENBERG et al. 1988). T1-weighted MRI yields better image quality of the heart, but is insensitive to such inherent histological changes or reveals only negligible signal intensity changes in the same area. Therefore, for improved contrast between normal and abnormal myocardium on T1-weighted images, paramagnetic contrast agents are needed to shorten the T1 relaxation time.

2. *Functional evaluation.* The regional contractile function is impaired even prior to ECG changes and angina in an ischemic event. This fact has led to increased use of stress echocardiography in the clinic. For visualization of global and regional cardiac wall motion in a more standardized manner, cine or tagging MRI is superior to echocardiography, which is limited by the acoustic window. Both pharmacological stress and physical exercise (with an accessory device fitted outside the bore of the unit) are now feasible with MRI (see Chap. 2).

3. *Perfusion study.* The development of faster MRI sequences has made it possible to image and quantify regional myocardial blood volume and flow by detecting the first pass of the contrast bolus through myocardium and perfusion defects (WILKE et al. 1995) (see Chap. 8).

4. *Coronary angiography (MRA).* Although still at an experimental stage, noninvasive coronary MRA

may soon enter clinical use as a result of fast image acquisition and 3-D image reconstruction (MULLER et al. 1997) (see Chap. 12).

5. *Myocardial metabolism.* Changes in high-energy phosphate metabolism caused by ischemia or infarction can be studied with ^{31}P-MRS. A few reports on the use of MRS in man to study myocardial phosphorus metabolism have revealed a decrease in the phosphocreatine/ATP ratio in ischemia (WEISS et al. 1990). In addition, the concentrations and kinetics of some important metabolites can be determined, intracellular pH can be measured, and the fate of exogenous tracers can be followed. However, a major technical breakthrough is needed before the technique can be widely used in clinical practice (see Chap. 9).

It is of note that the excellent image quality of cardiac MRI has been utilized to correct or to re-evaluate the performance of other "gold standard" cardiac imaging techniques (MORGUET et al. 1996).

7.6
Magnetopharmaceuticals as Magic Bullets for Targeting Necrotic Myocardium?

One of the most difficult clinical issues is how to determine viability of injured myocardium, especially when regional contraction has ceased. Theoretically, there are two possible strategies, i.e., either to point out the viable or to rule out the dead. Unfortunately, so far all current imaging modalities have failed to detect any intrinsic features distinctive for these two types of myocardium. In this regard, the use of more specific diagnostic pharmaceuticals may yield a solution. Although plain MRI can provide superb soft tissue contrast, unenhanced T1-weighted images are unable to visualize ischemic lesions (VAN DIJKMAN et al. 1991; MARCHAL et al. 1996). On the other hand, optimized T2-weighted images reveal all ischemic lesions as regions of increased signal intensity without distinction between reversibly injured and irreversibly infarcted myocardium (JOHNSTON et al. 1986). Similarly, the use of nonspecific extracellular agents such as Gd-DTPA and albumin-(Gd-DTPA) aids in the diagnosis of myocardial injury but fails to definitely differentiate reversible from irreversible changes (MCNAMARA et al. 1984; SCHMIEDL et al. 1987; SAEED et al. 1992).

Shortly after intravenous injection, commercially available Gd-chelates nonspecifically enhance the injured myocardium for at least 30 min, followed by a progressive diminution in contrast (VAN ROSSUM et al. 1990; DE ROOS et al. 1991). This enhancement is unstable in terms of both the size of the enhanced region and the degree of signal increase. In theory, the enhanced area accurately matches the necrotic myocardium only at a certain "optimal" post-contrast phase. Outside this phase, the infarct size is either overestimated or underestimated. However, as it is influenced by multiple factors, such as the extent of ischemia or infarction, the degree and duration of myocardial injury, arterial patency, and collateral circulation, as well as the dose, timing, and nature of contrast delivery, this "optimal" phase is individually variable and therefore practically uncatchable. To solve this problem, protocols combining a bolus and constant infusion of Gd-DTPA were applied both in clinical practice (FEDELE et al. 1994) and in animal experiments (TONG et al. 1993; PEREIRA et al. 1996) with the aim of maintaining a favorable equilibrium necessary for prolonged enhancement of myocardial infarcts. However, the excessive dose of contrast medium used and the nonspecific distribution between reversibly and irreversibly injured areas remain major concerns in the application of this protocol.

Another strategy has been to develop infarct-specific MRI contrast agents (WEISSLEDER et al. 1992; ADZAMLI et al. 1993). Due to their affinity for calcium-rich tissues, phosphonate-modified Gd-DTPA complexes cause strong enhancement in the infarcted myocardium. This effect has been shown in rats with diffuse and occlusive MI present for at least 24 h. However, these agents may result in a disorder of calcium homeostasis and subsequent impairment of ventricular contractility (ADZAMLI et al. 1993). Besides, studies with technetium-99m pyrophosphate, a scintigraphic analogue of this type, showed a lack of specificity between ischemic and necrotic myocardium (BIANCO et al. 1983) and a significant overestimation of the infarct size (KHAW et al. 1987).

Magnetopharmaceuticals labelled with antimyosin-antibody represent appealing infarct-selective agents. However, the possible immunogenic side-effects and the complexity in preparation and handling make it questionable whether their clinical use is feasible (WEISSLEDER et al. 1992).

The discovery of another type of infarct-avid contrast agent is a story with three episodes. Porphyrin derivatives have been investigated for a long time for the diagnosis and treatment of malignant tumors (PASS 1993; GOMER 1989; KESSEL 1984; NELSON et al. 1990). The rationale for porphyrin-mediated photodynamic therapy of cancer is based on the "tumor-localizing" and photosensitizing properties of the agents. By analogy, the tumoral "preferential uptake" of porphyrins has been exploited to develop paramagnetic metalloporphyrins as "tumor-seeking" MRI contrast agents (CHEN et al. 1984; OGAN et al. 1987; FURMANSKI and LONGLEY 1988; VAN ZIJL et al. 1990; FIEL et al. 1990; BOCKHORST et al. 1990; NELSON and SCHMIEDL 1991; PLACE et al. 1992; HINDRÈ et al. 1993; YOUNG et al. 1994; SAINI et al. 1995). However, recent research in our laboratories in collaboration with the Institut für Diagnostikforschung, Berlin, Germany has dramatically converted metalloporphyrins from tumor-seeking agents into markers of myocardial infarction (NI et al. 1996a). We started with an investigation in primary and secondary liver tumors and found that the observed "specific" enhancement could be attributed only to nonviable tumoral components (NI et al. 1995). To support this finding, more metalloporphyrins were assessed in animals with a variety of induced "benign" necroses and a phenomenon similar to the so-called "tumor-localizing" effect was reproduced (NI et al. 1997). Eventually, a novel application of metalloporphyrins was developed for accurate visualization of acute MI with T1-weighted MRI (NI and MARCHAL et al. 1994–1998; HERIJGERS et al. 1997).

Models of occlusive and reperfused MI or ischemia were induced in rats and dogs. Two paramagnetic metalloporphyrins, gadolinium mesoporphyrin (Gd-MP or Gadophrin-2, a proposed generic name) and manganese tetraphenylporphyrin (Mn-TPP), were studied initially with intravenous doses varying from 0.01 to 0.1 mmol/kg (MARCHAL et al. 1996). Gadophrin-2 was preferred in later dog experiments due to its stronger contrast-enhancing efficacy and less skin-coloring effects. Considering clinical situations in cardiac patients, who may or may not receive percutaneous transluminal coronary angioplasty (PTCA), both intracoronary (i.c.) and intravenous (i.v.) administrations of Gadophrin-2 at 5 µmol/kg and 50 µmol/kg were studied (HERIJGERS et al. 1997, NI et al. 1998). Nonspecific Gd-DTPA at 0.1 mmol/kg and 0.2 mmol/kg for intracoronary and intravenous injection was compared with necrosis-avid Gadophrin-2 in the same or different dogs with acute MI. In i.c. administration, both fast bolus and slow infusion were tested for the enhancing effects. Intracoronary injections of normal saline and Gadophrin-2 were also compared to identify any cardiovascular side-effects through parameters such as ECG, heart rate, and systolic and diastolic ventricular pressures.

Ventilator-controlled breath-held and ECG-triggered MRI was conducted with a T1-weighted segmented turbo FLASH sequence to observe contrast-enhancing effects, and with a T2-weighted segmented HASTE sequence to document any intrinsic signal changes after ischemia and reperfusion events. The heart was scanned apex-to-base perpendicular to the long axis and slice-by-slice, with a slice thickness of 6 mm. Cine and tagging MRI were also performed to evaluate functional changes. To facilitate more precise MRI-histochemistry morphometric correlation, a bridging technique was developed.

Briefly, after in vivo MRI, the dog was sacrificed and the heart excised and cooled in ice-cold saline to preserve the intracellular enzymes essential for later histochemical staining. The heart was then filled with and embedded in 3% agar solution in a plastic container and cooled again at −20°C for 15 min. High-resolution T1-weighted (TR/TE: 450 ms/12 ms; FOV: 75 × 100; matrix: 192 × 256) and T2-weighted (TR/TE: 3000 ms/90 ms; FOV: 68 × 136; matrix: 120 × 256) spin-echo MR scans were performed in multiple thin slices of 2 mm to encompass the entire left ventricle. The embedded heart was then sectioned into 6-mm short-axis slices using a calibrated slicer, and stained with 1% buffered triphenyltetrazolium chloride (TTC) solution. With this staining technique, normal myocardium appeared brick red, whereas the infarcted area appeared pale gray with dark brown in hemorrhagic foci (if there were any). These stained specimens were photographed with colored-slide films from which the images were digitized and stored on the Kodak Photo CD for later computer-assisted quantification.

Every three consecutive 2-mm slices in ex vivo MRI corresponded to one 6-mm slice in vivo MRI and TTC staining. With this intermediate step, the partial volume artifacts due to the discrepancy between information derived from voxel-based (3-D) 6-mm-thick in vivo MRI tomography and that acquired from pixel-based (2-D) TTC surface staining were minimized.

The contrast between infarcted and normal myocardium was calculated from the signal intensities (SIs) obtained with the monitor-defined region of interest (ROI), and expressed as the contrast ratio ($CR = SI_{infarct}/SI_{normal}$). The colored photo-CD images of TTC staining and the black-and-white MR images were transferred to a PC for planimetric analysis using a commercial program Adobe Photoshop 3.0. The reddish left ventricular wall and the discolored infarct regions were contoured manually on the computer screen and the number of pixels (representing the area) were determined automatically. The black-and-white MR images were processed similarly, but the contouring was based on signal intensities of the normal myocardium, the enhanced area on T1-weighted images, and the hyperintense area on T2-weighted images.

The infarct size was expressed as a percentage of the infarcted area over the entire area of the left ventricle, i.e., $S_{infarct}(\%) = Pixels_{infarct}/Pixels_{left\ ventricle} \times 100\%$. The infarct sizes derived from in vivo and ex vivo, T1-weighted and T2-weighted MRI were correlated with those derived from TTC staining using linear regression analysis (Microsoft Excel 7.0).

For the measurement of tissue concentrations of contrast agent, both infarcted and normal myocardium were sampled and gadolinium concentration was measured with the inductively coupled plasma atomic emission spectroscopy (ICP-AES) technique to gain an insight into the local distribution of the agent.

These studies demonstrated that neither intravenous nor intracoronary infusion of porphyrin agents caused detectable side-effects. Obvious greenish and slightly reddish colors appeared in animals after doses above 50 mmol/kg of Mn-TPP and Gadophrin-2, respectively, but faded considerably over 24 h.

Although indiscernible with unenhanced T1-weighted MRI (Figs. 7.2a, 7.3a), both ischemic injury and myocardial infarction (caused by 20 and 180 min of coronary occlusion respectively) appeared hyperintense on T2-weighted images (CR ≈ 1.5), but the borderline between the lesion and normal myocardium was unclear, which made it more difficult to delineate (Fig. 7.4.b,b′). Shortly after intravenous injection of Gadophrin-2, the occlusive MI appeared on T1-weighted MRI as a perfusion defect (Fig. 7.2b) but progressively evolved into a doughnut sign as a result of binding of the agent to the peripheral part of the necrotic myocardium (Fig. 7.2c). Irreversible infarcts as confirmed by TTC staining, but not ischemic injury as defined by T2-weighted MRI, could be strongly and specifically enhanced by infarct-avid agents (Figs. 7.2c, 7.3b,c, 7.4a,a′). The optimal doses of Gadophrin-2 tended to be 50 μmol/kg and 5 μmol/kg for intravenous and

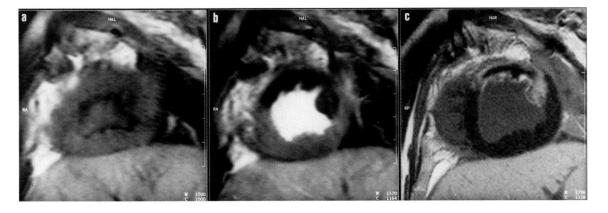

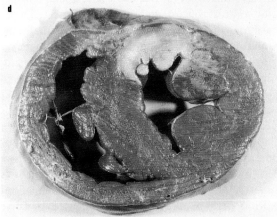

Fig. 7.2. Short-axis T1-weighted MR images before (a) and 10 min (b) and 24 h (c) after intravenous injection of Gadophrin-2 at 50 μmol/kg in a dog with occlusion of the left anterior descending artery (LAD) for 10 h, and corresponding TTC stained specimen (d). Before contrast, the infarct was virtually indiscernible (a). Shortly after Gadophrin-2 injection, the cavity and LV wall were enhanced by the circulating contrast agent (nonspecific enhancement), whereas the LAD-supplied area appeared as a filling defect due to a lack of perfusion (b). During the delayed phase when signal intensities elsewhere had largely diminished, a nicely delineated rim enhancement indicated an occlusive transmural MI (c). The MR images matched very well with the histochemically stained specimen (d). Note that partial involvement of the anterior papillary muscle can be seen on both enhanced MR images (b, c) and the specimen (d)

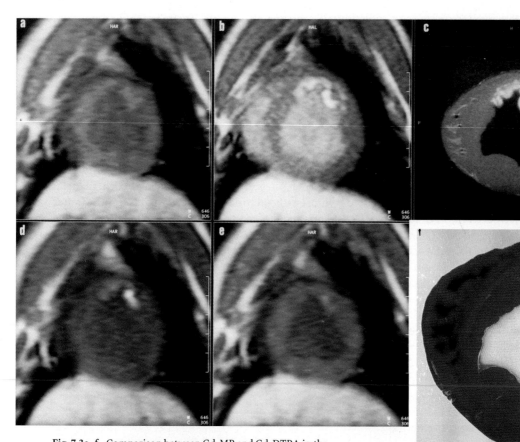

Fig. 7.3a–f. Comparison between Gd-MP and Gd-DTPA in the same dog with reperfused MI in the LAD-supplied anterior LV wall. Before contrast administration, the infarct was undetectable with T1-weighted MRI (**a**). Twelve hours after intravenous injection of Gadophrin-2 at 50 μmol/kg, a scattered subendocardial MI was clearly depicted on both in vivo and ex vivo T1-weighted MR images (**b, c**). Two hours prior to Gadophrin-2 study but 30 min after intracoronary injection of Gd-DTPA at 0.1 mmol/kg in the same dog, the infarcted area was also enhanced although less sharply demarcated (**d**). However, 1 h later the enhancement had almost completely disappeared as a result of local washout of this nonspecific agent (**e**). The TTC-stained heart section (**f**) only matched Gadophrin-2-enhanced MR images (**b, c**), not Gd-DTPA-enhanced MR images (**d, e**). Note the similarities of every detail of the infarct on the Gadophrin-2-enhanced MR images (**b, c**) and the TTC-stained specimen (**f**)

intracoronary injection respectively. The contrast ratios were 200%–300% and 150%–170% on in vivo and ex vivo T1-weighted MR images respectively, leading to sharp contrast between the infarct and surrounding myocardium and easy manual contouring of the infarct territory. Visually, metalloporphyrin-enhanced T1-weighted MRI mirrored in detail TTC histochemical staining regarding all topographic features such as transmural, subendocardial, patchy or scattered, and small infarcts, as well as involvement of papillary muscles (Figs. 7.2–7.4). This was consistent with the outcome of MRI-histochemical correlation. The enhanced areas on both ex vivo and in vivo T1-weighted MRI correlated perfectly to the TTC-negatively stained areas (Fig. 7.5a,b).

Gd-DTPA could also enhance the infarcted region in animals with reperfused MI as a result of increased distribution space and capillary permeability, but the infarct size was always exaggerated initially and underestimated or indiscernible later due to nonspecific contrast wash-in and wash-out in affected myocardium (Fig. 7.3d,e). In reperfused MI, usually the larger the infarct size and the dosage, the longer regional enhancement can be seen. In the experiment, the enhancement after intracoronary injection of Gd-DTPA persisted for many hours if the catheter was kept in the coronary artery, but quickly disappeared after withdrawal of the catheter, indicating an important role of coronary flow in the observed nonspecific enhancement (Ni et al. unpublished data, 1997). From a clinical point of view, though it is unstable and not very precise, Gd-DTPA enhanced MRI is perhaps already good enough to visualize acute MI since it has apparently outperformed other

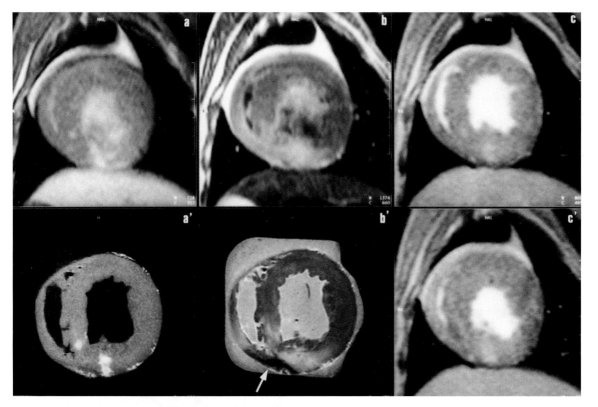

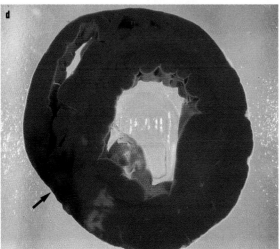

Fig. 7.4a–d. Comparison between T1- and T2-weighted and cine MR images and TTC-stained specimen of a dog with reperfused mini MI in the posterior LV wall supplied by the left circumflex artery. Five hours after intracoronary bolus injection of Gadophrin-2 at 5 µmol/kg, the mini infarcted foci could be seen with both in vivo (**a**) and ex vivo (**a′**) T1-weighted MRI. However, the hyperintense area with both in vivo (**b**) and ex vivo (**b′**) T2-weighted MRI was much larger than the real infarct and matched quite well with the dyskinetic LV region, as could be deduced from the diastolic (**c**) and systolic (**c′**) phases of cine MRI. The TTC-stained specimen (**d**) only matched with Gadophrin-2-enhanced T1-weighted MR images (**a, a′**), not with T2-weighted MR images (**b, b′**). This example indicates the comprehensive capability of MRI in the evaluation of myocardial viability. The dark area (*arrow*) on both the TTC-stained specimen (**d**) and ex vivo T2-weighted MRI (**b′**) represents the interstitial hemorrhage caused by vascular injury during coronary catheterization

preexisting techniques including echocardiography and cardiac scintigraphy owing to its higher spatial resolution and better morphological definition. For this application, the wide availability and proven safety may further make this agent preferable to other agents, including current infarct-avid agents. However, from a scientific point of view, only when either irreversible infarct or reversible injury is unambiguously indicated, as when Gadophrin-2 is used, can the issue of myocardial viability be resolved. Nonspecific enhancement may always lead to false or inaccurate diagnosis.

Although the lesion sizes on ex vivo and in vivo T2-weighted MRI were also positively correlated to the infarct size defined with TTC, T2-weighted MRI overestimated infarct size by more than twofold (Fig. 7.4), as reflected by intercepts larger than 16 and slopes higher than 1.023 in the linear regression tests

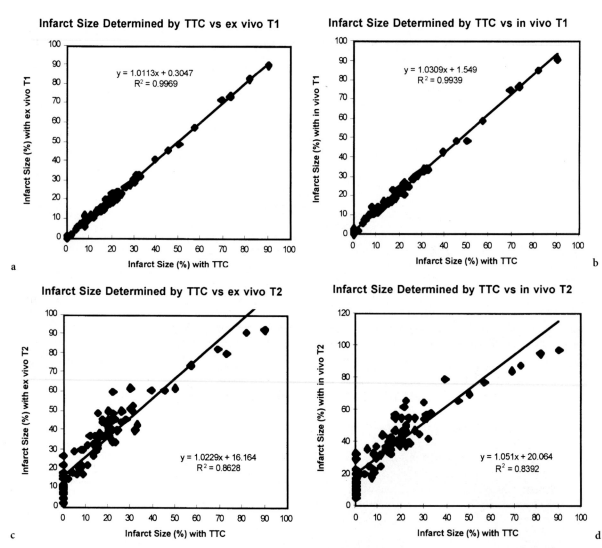

Fig. 7.5. The scatter graphs of the planimetric correlation between TTC staining and ex vivo T1 (**a**), in vivo T1 (**b**), ex vivo T2 (**c**), and in vivo T2 (**d**) weighted MRI, with the results of linear regression analysis

(Fig. 7.5c,d). The LV wall with regional dysfunction showed quite a good match with the hyperintense area on T2-weighted MRI; such a match was not evident with infarct-avid agent-enhanced T1-weighted MRI (Fig. 7.4). Disregarding irreversible infarcts, the observed hyperintense area on T2-weighted MRI and the dyskinetic area on cine or tagging MRI were likely due to myocardial edema, as suggested by our preliminary results regarding tissue water content measurement (Ni et al. unpublished data, 1996). These phenomena imply that the edematous areas surrounding necrotic myocardium are stunned but viable, and that impaired contractile function is potentially reversible.

So far, TTC staining is the only widely accepted gold standard for macroscopic identification and quantification of acute MI. But it is a post-mortem technique and not clinically applicable. Therefore, cardiologists are eagerly calling for in vivo markers of intact cellular function such as preserved metabolic activity or cell membrane integrity, something similar to ex vivo TTC staining (HENDEL and BONOW 1993). As demonstrated in our series of studies, both i.v. and i.c. injected infarct-avid agents can specifically label acute myocardial infarcts, which in turn can be precisely visualized with T1-weighted MRI. Despite the different principles of the two techniques, actually what had been labelled by the infarct-avid agent on MRI was just what TTC dye failed to stain on excised heart specimen, yielding the same accuracy in the delineation of necrotic myocardium (Figs. 7.2–7.5a,b). Although negligible from a practical point of view, the difference in calculated infarct size between TTC preparations and T1-weighted MR images can be attributed to the discrepancy between tomographic MRI with partial volume effects and the TTC color reaction recorded only on the tissue surface. Since the presence and extent of irreversible infarcts can be ascertained by means of infarct-avid agent-enhanced MRI, further experiments should be aimed at linking later functional recovery with the nonnecrotic but abnormal areas on MRI. Thereafter the viable and salvageable myocardium could be estimated by subtracting infarct-avid agent-enhanced T1-weighted MRI from T2-weighted MRI. In combination with cine and tagging MRI for functional assessment, this approach may lead to a final solution to the issue of myocardial viability.

The impact of such a clear-cut in vivo technique cannot be overestimated. In experimental research, it can be used as an in vivo substitute for postmortem TTC staining or a virtual "gold standard" to monitor the natural evolution of myocardial infarction and to evaluate the effects of mechanical or pharmaceutical reperfusion therapies under development. In clinical practice, it can be helpful for early determination of myocardial viability of the region which fails to show ventricular motion or wall thickening. The local delivery of a minimal amount of infarct-avid agent is particularly interesting in those patients for whom PTCA has been chosen as primary treatment for acute MI. A postprocedure MRI scan performed after stabilization of the patient's condition may justify the therapeutic intervention and assist in the evaluation of the prognosis.

The measured tissue content of gadolinium was over 10 and 7 times higher in the infarcted myocardium than in normal myocardium with intravenous and intracoronary injection respectively, suggesting the avidity of the agent for necrotic myocardium. The striking and prolonged contrast enhancement of infarcts caused by one intravenous dosage or only one pass of the agent delivered locally provides further insight into the strong affinity of the agent for necrotic areas. The following hypothesis may explain the mechanisms of such a unique targeting mode (NI et al. 1997). After intracoronary or systemic administration, the necrosis-avid agent approaches the reperfused infarcts by perfusion, extravasation, and diffusion. The occlusive infarcts can be stained only from the periphery of the lesion by the agent circulating in adjacent viable myocardium, e.g., rim enhancement (Fig. 7.2c). The loss of cell membrane integrity during postinfarct autolysis and the long

plasma half-life (~2.5 h) of the agent facilitate massive and persistent contact and physicochemical interaction or binding with the denatured tissue debris. As a result of this binding, the relaxivity (the magnetic efficiency of the agent on local proton relaxation) can be augmented. Like commercial gadolinium chelates, the nonspecific enhancing property of this type of necrosis-avid agent also can be utilized for the assessment of organ blood perfusion, for instance, in first-pass myocardial perfusion MRI.

7.7
Cardiac MR: a "One-Stop Shop" for Determination of Myocardial Viability?

As indicated in previous sections, the availability of more reliable and accurate methods for detecting viable or excluding nonviable myocardium may simplify the clinical and experimental issues related to myocardial viability. Eventually, comprehensive cardiac MR techniques in combination with the use of an infarct-avid contrast agent may prove to be a "one-stop shop" not only for the detection of myocardial infarction, but also for anatomical, functional, and metabolic assessment of myocardial viability. Clinically, determination of myocardial viability is crucial in two groups of patients: (1) those with known or suspected MI, and (2) those with chronic CAD and global LV dysfunction. In the *former*, the questions to be answered are: Has any nonviable or necrotic myocardium already developed? If yes, what is its location, size, and extent? Is it subendocardial or transmural? Is the remaining myocardium still subject to ischemia? If not, what is the status of coronary perfusion and flow? How about the type and degree of coronary stenosis? In the *latter group*, it is important to distinguish between viable myocardium and areas of myocardial fibrosis and to assess functional and metabolic reserves of the myocardium. Viable myocardium may benefit from revascularization, whereas fibrotic myocardium cannot recover contractile function (ISKANDRIAN et al. 1987). These questions are critical in deciding upon therapeutic regimens, preventing postinfarct complications, and selecting candidates for reperfusion therapies.

As illustrated in Fig 7.6, T1-weighted MRI and combined use of an infarct-avid agent may pinpoint necrotic myocardium on the basis of detailed cardiac anatomical structure and differentiate reperfused and occlusive MI. T2-weighted MRI may reveal all injured areas (whether edematous or necrotic) in

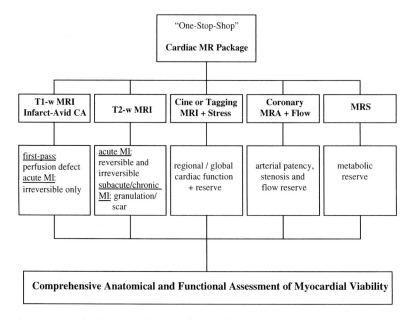

Fig. 7.6. "One-stop shop" strategy for diagnosis of myocardial viability. *CA*, Contrast agent; *MRI*, magnetic resonance imaging; *MRA*, magnetic resonance angiography; *MRS*, magnetic resonance spectroscopy; *MI*, myocardial infarction

acute cases and fibrotic or scarring tissue in chronic cases. Quantitative cine and tagging MRI with or without stress test may provide indexes of global and regional myocardial function, including the LV mass index, end-diastolic and end-systolic volume indexes, cardiac output, ejection fraction, and functional reserve. Jeopardized but viable (including stunned and hibernating) myocardium can be estimated by cross-reference between contrast-enhanced T1-weighted MRI, T2-weighted MRI, and cine or tagging MRI. Infarct artery patency or the presence/absence of coronary stenosis and its extent can be evaluated with noninvasive coronary MRA. Lastly, metabolic reserve can be assessed with MR spectroscopy.

Since the MR modality alone provides all these necessary elements, it is most likely that we are now entering a historical period which may generate a "one-stop shop" as a final solution in the diagnosis of myocardial viability. However, we should bear in mind that current MRI also has its drawbacks and its performance is still far from optimal. The closed design of MRI scanners and the noise generated may increase the stress for cardiac patients. Some patients may become claustrophobic in the scanner. Although geographic quantification can be perfectly achieved, there is no straightforward link between contrast uptake and measured signal intensities. As with TTC staining, the current infarct-avid agents are effective only for acute MI, not for subacute or

early healing MI where necrosis has been replaced by viable granulation tissue. Therefore, for the time being, the presently available cardiac imaging modalities should be deployed in a complementary manner, rather than being regarded as exclusive alternatives.

Before MR techniques can be routinely practiced as a "one-stop shop" in cardiac patients, strenuous efforts must be made to achieve technical refinements. These tasks include optimization of both hardware and software to achieve a more patient-friendly cardiac MR unit, the development of safer or more effective infarct-avid MRI contrast media, and the conduct of extensive preclinical and clinical trials in order to validate such a diagnostic setting and to elucidate morphological, functional, and metabolic interrelationships of MR phenomena. Recent preliminary study has demonstrated that in patients with AMI, comprehensive assessment of LV structure and function, infarct artery patency, and regional myocardial contrast uptake is safe and feasible with MRI of <1h (KRAMER et al. 1997). Further improvement is undoubtedly possible and necessary.

Acknowledgements. This work has been supported in part by an NFWO grant (project number 3.0132.94). The author thanks Prof. Dr. A.L Baert and Prof. Dr. G. Marchal for their leadership and supervision as well as financial and infrastructural support; the Institut für Diagnostik Forschung, Berlin, Germany for providing contrast media; Dr. Y. Miao,

Prof. Dr. H. Bosmans, Prof. Dr. J. Bogaert, and Dr. S. Dymarkowski for their technical collaboration; Dr. P. Herijgers, Prof. Dr. W. Flameng, Dr. S. Pislaru, Dr. C. Pislaru, and Prof. Dr. F Van de Werf for making open and close-chest models of myocardial infarction in rats and dogs; and Mr. W. Desmedt for the production of illustrations

References

Adzamli IK, Blau M, Pfeffer MA, Davis MA (1993) Phosphonate-modified Gd-DTPA complexes. III. The detection of myocardial infarction by MRI. Magn Reson Med 29:505–511

Antaloczy Z, Barcsak J, Magyaar E (1988) Correlation of electrocardiologic and pathologic findings in 100 cases of Q wave and non-Q wave myocardial infarction. J Electrocardiol 2:331–338

Bakker A, Koelemay M, Georgels J, et al. (1993) Failure of new biochemical markers to exclude acute myocardial infarction at admission. Lancet 342:1220–1222

Bashour TT, Mason D (1990) Myocardial hibernation and "embalment". Am Heart J 119:706–708

Berman DS, Kiat HS, van Train KF, Germano G, Maddahi J, Friedman JD (1994) Myocardial imaging with technetium-99m-sestamibi: comparative analysis of available imaging protocols. J Nucl Med 35:681–688

Bianco JA, Kemper AJ, Taylor A, Lazewatsky J, Tow DE, Khuri SF (1983) Technetium-99m(Sn^{2+}) pyrophosphate in ischemic and infarcted dog myocardium in early stages of acute coronary occlusion: histochemical and tissue-counting comparisons. J Nucl Med 24:485–491

Bianco JA, Alpert JS (1997) Physiologic and clinical significance of myocardial blood flow quantification: what is expected from these measurements in the clinical ward and in the physiology laboratory? Cardiology 88:116–126

Birdi I, Angelini GD, Bryan AJ (1997) Biochemical markers of myocardial injury during cardiac operations. Ann Thorac Surg 63:879–884

Bockhorst K, Hohn-Berlage M, Kocher M, Hossmann KA (1990) Proton relaxation enhancement in experimental brain tumors: in vivo NMR study of manganese (III) TPPS in rat brain gliomas. Magn Reson Imaging 8:499–504

Bolli R (1990) Mechanism of myocardial stunning. Circulation 82:723–738

Bonow RO (1995) The hibernating myocardium: implication for management of congestive heart failure. Am J Cardiol 75:17A–25A

Braunwald E, Kloner RA (1982) The stunned myocardium: prolonged, postischemic ventricular dysfunction. Circulation 66:1146–1149

Camarano G, Ragosta M, Gimple GW, Powers ER, Kaul S (1995) Identification of viable myocardium with contrast echocardiography in patients with poor left ventricular systolic function caused by recent or remote myocardial infarction. Am J Cardiol 75:215–219

Camici P, Ferrannini E, Opie LH (1989) Myocardial metabolism in ischemic heart disease: basic principles and application to imaging by positron emission tomography. Prog Cardiovasc Dis 32:217–238

Cannon PJ, Maudsley AA, Hilal SK, Simon HE, Cassidy F (1986) Sodium nuclear magnetic resonance imaging of myocardial tissue of dogs after coronary artery occlusion and reperfusion. J Am Coll Cardiol 7:573–579

Chen C, Cohen J, Myers C, Sohn M (1984) Paramagnetic metalloporphyrins as potential contrast agents in NMR imaging. FEBS Lett 168:70–74

Cigarroa CG, DeFillippi CR, Brickner ME, Alvarez LG, Wait MA, Grayburn PA (1993) Inotropic contractile reserve during dobutamine stress echocardiography predicts recovery of regional left ventricular function after coronary revascularization. Circulation 88:430–436

Conti CR (1993) Myocardial hypokinesis, coronary angiography, and myocardial viability. Clin Cardiol 16:847–848

Cooper ES (1993) Prevention: the key to progress. Circulation AHA Medical/Scientific Statement. 24:629–632

De Roos A, Matheijsen NA, Doornbos J, Van Dijkman PR, Van Rugge P, Van de Wall EE (1991) Myocardial infarct sizing and assessment of reperfusion by magnetic resonance imaging: a review. Int J Card Imaging 7:133–138

DeWood MA, Spores J, Notske R, et al. (1980) Prevalence of total coronary occlusion during the early hours of transmural myocardial infarction. N Engl J Med 303:891–902

Dilsizian V, Bonow RO (1993) Current diagnostic techniques of assessing myocardial viability in hibernating and stunned myocardium. Circulation 87:1–20

Downing SE, Chen V (1992) Acute hibernation and reperfusion of the ischemic heart. Circulation 82:699–707

Fedele F, Montesano T, Ferro-Luzzi M, et al. (1994) Identification of viable myocardium in patients with chronic coronary artery disease and left ventricular dysfunction: role of magnetic resonance imaging. Am Heart J 128:484–489

Ferrari R, Ceconi C, Curello S, Benigno M, La Canna G, Visioli O (1996) Left ventricular dysfunction due to the new ischemic outcomes: stunning and hibernation. J Cardiovasc Pharmacol 28 (Suppl 1):18–26

Fiel RJ, Musser DA, Mark EH, Mazurchuk R, Alletto JJ (1990) A comparative study of manganese meso-sulphonatophenyl porphyrins: contrast enhancing agents for tumors. Magn Reson Imaging 8:255–259

Fishbein M, Rit J, Lando U, Kanmatsuse K, Mercier JC, Granz W (1980) The relationship of vascular injury and myocardial hemorrhage to necrosis after reperfusion. Circulation 62:1274–1279

Fishbein M, Meerbaum S, Rit J, et al. (1981) Early phase acute myocardial infarct size quantification: validation of the triphenyl tetrazolium chloride tissue enzyme staining technique. Am Heart J 101:593–600

Fragasso G, Margonato A, Chierchia SL (1993) Assessment of viability after myocardial infarction: clinical relevance and methodological problems. Int J Cardiac Imaging 9:3–10

Furmanski P, Longley C (1988) Metalloporphyrin enhancement of magnetic resonance imaging of human tumor xenografts in nude mice. Cancer Res 48:4604–4610

Fuster V, Frye RL, Kennedy MA, Connolly DC, Makin HT (1979) The role of collateral circulation in the various coronary syndromes. Circulation 59:1137–1144

Goldstein RA (1991) Myocardial viability. J Nucl Med 32:1315

Gomer C (1989) Photodynamic therapy in the treatment of malignancies. Semin Hematol 26:27–34

Gould KL (1991) Myocardial viability, what does it mean and how do we measure it? (editorial comment). Circulation 83:333–335

Grodin CM, Dyrda I, Pasternac A, Campeu L, Bourassa MG (1974) Discrepancies between cineangiographic and postmortem findings in patients with coronary artery disease and recent myocardial revascularization. Circulation 49:703–709

Gropler RJ, Bergmann SR (1991a) Myocardial viability – what is the definition? J Nucl Med 32:10–12

Gropler RJ, Bergmann SR (1991b) Reply. J Nucl Med 32:1315–1316

Hamm CW, Katus HA (1995) New biochemical markers for myocardial cell injury. Curr Opin Cardiol 10:355–360

Hendel RC, Bonow RO (1993) Disparity in coronary perfusion and regional wall motion: effect on clinical assessment of viability. Coronary Artery Dis 4:512–520

Hendel RC (1994) Single-photon perfusion imaging for the assessment of myocardial viability. J Nucl Med 35:23S–31S

Herijgers P, Laycock SK, Ni Y, et al. (1997) Localization and determination of infarct size by Gd-mesoporphyrin enhanced MRI in dogs. Int J Cardiac Imaging 13:499–507

Herman MV, Gorlin R (1968) Implications of ventricular asynergy. Am J Cardiol 23:538–574

Hindré F, LePlouzennec M, de Certained JD, Foultier MT, Patrice T, Simonneaux G (1993) Tetra-*p*-aminophenylporphyrin conjugated with Gd-DTPA: tumor-specific contrast agent for MR imaging. J Magn Reson Imaging 3:59–65

Iskandrian AS, Heo J, Helfant RH, Segal BL (1987) Chronic myocardial ischemia and left ventricular function. Ann Intern Med 107:925–927

Jennings RB, Hawkins HK, Lowe JE, Hill ML, Klotman S, Reimer KA (1978) Relation between high-energy phosphate and lethal injury in myocardial ischemia in the dog. Am J Pathol 92:187–214

Johnston D, Thompson R, Liu P (1986) Magnetic resonance imaging during acute myocardial infarction. Am J Cardiol 58:214–219

Kaul S (1995) Dobutamine echocardiography for determining myocardial viability after reperfusion: experimental and clinical observations. Eur Heart J 16 (Suppl M):17–23

Kessel D (1984) Porphyrin localization: a new modality for detection and therapy of tumors. Biochem Pharmacol 33:1389–1393

Khaw BA, Strauss HW, Moore R, et al. (1987) Myocardial damage delineated by indium-111 antimyosin Fab and technetium-99m pyrophosphate. J Nucl Med 28:76–82

Kim RJ, Lima JAC, Chen E-L, Reeder SB, Klocke FJ, Zerhouni EA, Judd RM (1997) Fast ^{23}Na magnetic resonance imaging of acute reperfused myocardial infarction: potential to assess myocardial viability. Circulation 95:1877–1885

Klein HH, Puschmann S, Schaper J, et al. (1981) The mechanism of the tetrazolium reaction in identifying experimental myocardial infarction. Virchows Arch A Pathol Anat 393:287–297

Kloner RA, Darsee JR, DeBoer LWV, Carlson N (1981) Early pathologic detection of acute myocardial infarction. Arch Pathol Lab Med 105:403–406

Kramer CM, Rogers WJ, Geskin G, et al. (1997) Usefulness of magnetic resonance imaging early after acute myocardial infarction. Am J Cardiol 80:690–695

Krause EG, Rabitzsch G, Noll F, Mair J, Puschendorf B (1996) Glycogen phosphorylase isoenzyme BB in diagnosis of myocardial ischemic injury and infarction. Mol Cell Biochem 160–161:289–295

La Canna G, Alfieri O, Giubbini R, Gargano M, Ferrari R, Visioli O (1994) Echocardiography during infusion of dobutamine for identification of reversible dysfunction in patients with chronic coronary artery disease. J Am Coll Cardiol 23:617–626

Lewis S, Sawada S, Ryan T, et al. (1991) Segmental wall motion abnormalities in the absence of clinically documented myocardial infarction: clinical significance and evidence of hibernating myocardium. Am Heart J 121:1088–1094

Liedtke AJ (1981) Alteration of carbohydrate and lipid metabolism in the acutely ischemic heart. Prog Cardiovasc Dis 23:321–336

Lindner JR, Kaul S (1996) Assessment of myocardial viability with two-dimensional echocardiography and magnetic resonance imaging. J Nucl Cardiol 3:167–182

Lombardo A, Loperfido F, Pennestri F, et al. (1996) Significance of transient ST-T segment changes during dobutamine testing in Q wave myocardial infarction. J Am Coll Cardiol 27:599–605

Mair J, Smidt J, Lechleitner P, Dienstl F, Puschendorf B (1995) A decision tree for the early diagnosis of acute myocardial infarction in non-traumatic chest pain patients at hospital admission. Chest 108:1502–1509

Marchal G, Ni Y, Herijgers P, et al. (1996) Paramagnetic metalloporphyrins: infarct avid contrast agents for diagnosis of acute myocardial infarction by magnetic resonance imaging. Eur Radiol 6:1–8

Margonato A, Chierchia SL (1996) Old tools for sophisticated diagnosis: electrocardiography for the assessment of myocardial viability. Q J Nucl Biol Med 40:17–19

McNamara MT, Higgins CB, Ehman RL, Revel D, Sievers R, Brasch RC (1984) Acute myocardial ischemia: magnetic resonance contrast enhancement with gadolinium-DTPA. Radiology 153:157

Milunski MR, Mohr GA, Perez JE, et al. (1989) Ultrasonic tissue characterization with integrated backscatter: acute myocardial ischemia, reperfusion, and stunned myocardium in patients. Circulation 80:491–503

Morguet AJ, Kögler A, Schmitt H-A, Emrich D, Kreuzer H, Munz DL (1996) Assessment of myocardial viability in persistent defects on thallium-201 SPECT after reinjection using gradient-echo MRI. Nuklearmedizin 35:146–152

Muller MF, Fleisch M, Kroeker R, Chatterjee T, Meier B, Vock P (1997) Proximal coronary artery stenosis: three-dimensional MRI with fat saturation and navigator echo. J Magn Reson Imaging 7:644–651

Myers JH, Stirling MC, Choy M, Buda AJ, Gallagher KP (1986) Direct measurement of inner and outer wall thickening dynamics with epicardial echocardiography. Circulation 74:164–172

Nachlas MM, Shnitka TK (1963) Macroscopic identification of early myocardial infarcts by alterations in dehydrogenase activity. Am J Pathol 42:379–385

Neill W, Ingwall J, Andrews E, et al. (1986) Stabilization of the derangement in adenosine triphosphate metabolism during sustained, partial ischemia in the dog heart. J Am Coll Cardiol 8:894–900

Nelson J, Schmiedl U (1991) Porphyrins as contrast media. Magn Reson Med 22:366–371

Nelson J, Schmiedl U, Shankland E (1990) Metalloporphyrins as tumor-seeking MRI contrast media and as potential selective treatment sensitizers. Invest Radiol 25:S71–S73

Ni Y, Marchal G, Petré C, et al. (1994) Metalloporphyrin enhanced magnetic resonance imaging of acute myocardial infarction (abstract). Circulation 90 (Suppl): I-468

Ni Y, Marchal G, Yu J, et al. (1995) Localization of metalloporphyrin induced "specific" enhancement in experimental liver tumors: comparison of magnetic resonance imaging, microangiographic and histologic findings. Acad Radiol 2:687–699

Ni Y, Marchal G, Herijgers P, et al. (1996a) Paramagnetic metalloporphyrins: from enhancers for malignant tumors to markers of myocardial infarcts. Acad Radiol 3:S395–S397

Ni Y, Pislaru C, Bosmans H, et al. (1996b) Intracoronary administration of gadolinium mesoporphyrin for determination of myocardial viability with magnetic resonance imaging (abstract). Circulation 94 (Suppl):I-542

Ni Y, Petré C, Miao Y, et al. (1997). Magnetic resonance imaging – histomorphologic correlation studies on paramagnetic metalloporphyrins in rat models of necrosis. Invest Radiol 32:770–779

Ni Y, Pislaru C, Bosmans H, et al. (1998) Validation of intracoronary delivery of metalloporphyrin as an in vivo "histochemical staining" for myocardial infarction with MR imaging. Acad Radiol 5 (Suppl 1):537–541

Nienaber CA, Brunken RC, Sherman CT (1991) Metabolic and functional recovery of ischemic human myocardium after coronary angioplasty. J Am Coll Cardiol 18:966–978

Nissen SE, Gurley JC (1991) Application of intravascular ultrasound to detection and quantification of coronary atherosclerosis. Int J Cardiac Imaging 6:165–177

Ogan M, Revel D, Brasch R (1987) Metalloporphyrin contrast enhancement of tumors in magnetic resonance imaging. A study of human carcinoma, lymphoma, and fibrosarcoma in mice. Invest Radiol 22:822–828

Parker III AB, Waller BF, Gering LE (1996) Usefulness of the 12-lead electrocardiogram in detection of myocardial infarction: electrocardiaographic-anatomic correlations. Clin Cardiol 19:55–61, 141–148

Pass H (1993) Photodynamic therapy in oncology: mechanisms and clinical use (review) J Natl Cancer Inst 85:443–456

Patterson RE, Jones-Collins BA, Aamodt R, Ro YM (1993) Differences in collateral myocardial blood flow following gradual vs abrupt coronary occlusion. Cardiovasc Res 17:207–213

Pennell DJ (1994) Pharmacological cardiac stress: when and how? Nucl Med Commun 15:578–585

Pereira RS, Prato FS, Wisenberg G, Sykes J (1996) The determination of myocardial viability using Gd-DTPA in a canine model of acute myocardial ischemia and reperfusion. Magn Res Med 36:684–693

Perez JE, Waggoner AD, Davila-Roman VG, Cardona H, Miller JG (1992) On-line quantification of ventricular function during dobutamine stress echocardiography. Eur Heart J 13:1669–1676

Place DA, Faustino JP, Berghmans KK, van Ziji PCM, Chesnick AS, Cohen JS (1992) MRI contrast-dose relationship of manganese (III) tetra (4-sulfonatophenyl) porphyrin with human xenograft tumors in nude mice at 2.0 T. Magn Reson Imaging 10:919–928

Rahimtoola SH (1989) The hibernating myocardium. Am Heart J 117:211–220

Rivas F, Cobb FR, Bache RJ, Greenfield JC (1976) Relationship between blood flow to ischemic regions and extent of myocardial infarction. Circ Res 38:439–447

Robles HB, Lawson MA, Johnson LL (1994) Role of imaging in assessment of ischemic heart disease. Curr Opin Cardiol 9:435–447

Ross J Jr (1991) Myocardial perfusion-contraction matching: implications for coronary heart disease and hibernation. Circulation 83:1076–1082

Sabia P, Powers ER, Ragosta M, Sarenbock IJ, Burwell LR, Kaul S (1992) An association between collateral blood flow and myocardial viability in patients with recent myocardial infarction. N Eng J Med 327:1825–1831

Saeed M, Wendland M, Takehara Y, Masui T, Higgins C (1992) Reperfusion and irreversible myocardial injury: identification with a nonionic MR imaging contrast medium. Radiology 182:675–683

Saini SK, Jena A, Dey J, Sharma AK, Singh R (1995) MnPcS4: a new MRI contrast enhancing agent for tumor localization in mice. Magn Reson Imaging 13:985–990

Schmiedl U, Moseley M, Sievers R, et al. (1987) Magnetic resonance imaging of myocardial infarction using albumin-(Gd-DTPA), a macromolecular blood-volume contrast agent in a rat model. Invest Radiol 22:713–721

Schoeder H, Friedrich M, Topp H (1993) Myocardial viability: what do we need? Eur J Nucl Med 20:792–803

Sklenar J, Villanueva FS, Glasheen WP, Ismail S, Goodman NC, Kaul S (1994) Dobutamine echocardiography for determining the extent of myocardial salvage after reperfusion: an experimental evaluation. Circulation 90:1503–1512

Smart SC (1994) The clinical utility of echocardiography in the assessment of myocardial viability. J Nucl Med 35:49S–58S

Sones FM, Shirey EK (1962) Cine coronary arteriography. Mod Concepts Cardiovasc Dis 31:735–738

Timmis AD (1990) Early diagnosis of acute myocardial infarction: electrocardiography is still best [editorial]. Br Med J 301:941–942

Tong CY, Prato FS, Wisberg G, et al. (1993) Techniques for the measurement of the local myocardial extraction efficiency for inert diffusible contrast agents such as gadopentate dimeglumine. Magn Reson Med 30:332–336

Topol EJ, Nissen SE (1995) Our preoccupation with coronary luminology: the dissociation between clinical and angiographic findings in ischemic heart disease. Circulation 92:2333–2342

van der Wall EE, Vliegen HW, de Roos A, Bruschke AVG (1996) Magnetic resonance techniques for assessment of myocardial viability. J Cardiovasc Pharmacol 28 (Suppl 1):S37–S43

Van Dijkman PRM, van der Wall EE, de Roos A (1991) Acute, subacute, and chronic myocardial infarction: quantitative analysis of gadolinium-enhanced MR images. Radiology 180:147–151

Van Rossum AC, Visser FC, Van Eenige MJ, et al. (1990) Value of gadolinium-diethylene-triamine pentaacetic acid dynamics in magnetic resonance imaging of acute myocardial infarction with occluded and reperfused coronary arteries after thrombolysis. Am J Cardiol 65:845–851

Van Zijl PCM, Place DA, Cohen JS, Faustino PJ, Lyon RC, Patronas NJ (1990) Metalloporphyrin magnetic resonance contrast agents: feasibility of tumor-specific magnetic resonance imaging. Acta Radiol Suppl 374:75–79

Weiss RG, Bottomly PA, Hardy CJ, Gerstenblith G (1990) Regional myocardial metabolism of high energy phosphates during isometric exercise in patients with coronary artery disease. N Engl J Med 323:1593–1600

Weissleder R, Lee A, Khaw B, Shen T, Brady T (1992) Antimyosin-labeled monocrystalline iron oxide allows detection of myocardial infarct: MR antibody imaging. Radiology 182:381–385

Whiteman G, Kieval R, Wetstein L, Seeholzer S, McDonald G, Harken A (1983) The relationship between global myocardial redox state and high energy phosphate profile: a phosphorous-31 nuclear magnetic resonance study. J Surg Res 35:332–339

Wilke N, Kroll K, Merkle H, et al. (1995) Regional myocardial blood volume and flow: first-pass MR imaging with polylysine-Gd-DTPA. J Magn Reson Imaging 5:227–237

Wisenberg G, Prato FS, Carroll SE, Turner KL, Marshall T (1988) Serial nuclear magnetic resonance imaging of acute myocardial infarction with and without reperfusion. Am Heart J 115:510–518

Young SW, Sidhu MK, Qing F, et al. (1994) Preclinical evaluation of gadolinium (III) texaphyrin complex: a new paramagnetic contrast agent for magnetic resonance imaging. Invest Radiol 29:330–338

8 Myocardial Perfusion

J. Bogaert, S. Dymarkowski, and H. Bosmans

CONTENTS

8.1
Introduction

Coronary artery disease (CAD) remains the leading cause of death in the Western world (National Heart Lung and Blood Institute 1990). Moreover, about one-half of all deaths from CAD occur suddenly without warning (Kannel et al. 1976). One of the great challenges in the last decades has been the search for the ultimate noninvasive test to detect CAD. Not only would this reduce the number of (unnecessary) invasive angiographic procedures, but because CAD is the most important potentially preventable cause of congestive heart failure, it would lead to a better patient outcome and a decrease in the cost of care for cardiovascular disease.

Accurate assessment of CAD includes visualization of the coronary artery anatomy (see Chap. 13), quantification of regional and global ventricular function during rest and stress (see Chap. 6), and assessment of myocardial viability (see Chap. 7), and metabolism (see Chap. 9), and finally myocardial perfusion. With the advent of faster magnetic resonance (MR) techniques in the early 1990s, assessment of myocardial perfusion by means of MR has become feasible (Atkinson et al. 1990). This chapter aims to provide a general review of current techniques used for assessing myocardial perfusion, to situate the position of MR in relation to the other modalities, to describe the requisites for performance of an MR myocardial perfusion study; to discuss the results in both animals and humans; and to stress the strengths and current limitations of MR myocardial perfusion.

8.2
Pathophysiology of Myocardial Perfusion

A unique feature of the myocardium is its oxidative metabolism with a limited and short-lived capacity for anaerobic metabolism. Therefore, any consideration of myocardial perfusion needs to stress the pivotal relationship between myocardial oxygen requirements and coronary blood flow. In normal conditions, there is a balance between oxygen demand and oxygen supply. Oxygen demand is primarily influenced by wall stress, heart rate, and contractility, while oxygen supply is determined by the coronary blood flow and the oxygen extraction. The oxygen extraction in the myocardial microcirculation is high under basal conditions (i.e., with an oxygen saturation of coronary sinus blood of only 20%–30%). Therefore, it is mandatory that changes in myocardial oxygen demand result from similar changes in coronary flow.

The increase in coronary blood flow primarily relies on vasodilation. A normal coronary circulation may increase its flow in resting conditions by a factor of 4–6. Wilke and colleagues (1993)

J. Bogaert MD, PhD, Department of Radiology, University Hospitals Gasthuisberg, Catholic University of Leuven, Herestraat 49, B-3000 Belgium
S. Dymarkowski, MD, Department of Radiology, University Hospitals Gasthuisberg, Catholic University of Leuven, Herestraat 49, B-3000 Belgium
H. Bosmans, PhD, Department of Radiology, University Hospitals Gasthuisberg, Catholic University of Leuven, Herestraat 49, B-3000 Belgium

showed a baseline myocardial blood flow of 0.5–1.1 ml min^{-1}g^{-1} while the flow in the hyperemic myocardium was 3.7–6.7 ml min^{-1} g^{-1}. The capacity to increase the coronary flow or the "coronary flow reserve" is defined by the ratio of flow during maximum vasodilation to flow under resting conditions. There are also transmural differences in oxygen demand. The oxygen demand is greater in the subendocardium than in the subepicardium, with a greater flow and oxygen extraction in the inner myocardial layers. Therefore, the subendocardial layers are much more vulnerable to ischemia, and myocardial necrosis starts in the inner layers with a variable transmural spread (REIMER and JENNINGS 1979).

Conditions with an imbalance between oxygen demand and oxygen supply are primarily the result of coronary atheromatosis with one or several stenoses on the coronary arteries. This imbalance causes myocardial ischemia, and, if prolonged, myocardial necrosis. Perturbations in the myocardial microcirculation with angiographically normal coronary arteries (i.e., syndrome X), may also lead to myocardial ischemia but are much less frequent. The flow profile across a stenosis has a close relation with the degree of stenosis. A narrowing below 70% has only a minimal influence on the flow resistance. Above 70% the resistance increases sharply, leading to a significant pressure drop across the stenosis. The effects of a coronary artery stenosis on the myocardial perfusion are closely related to the flow hemodynamics in the coronary arteries. In resting conditions, the myocardial perfusion is not altered until the coronary artery has an 85%–90% stenosis. This is the result of the coronary vasodilator reserve which compensates for the effects of coronary stenoses under basal conditions. Progressive arteriolar vasodilation allows coronary flow to be maintained (KLOCKE 1990). However, during stress conditions the coronary reserve cannot be induced by vasodilatory stimulus. Under these circumstances, the myocardium distal to less severe coronary stenosis (i.e., between 50% and 85%) may become ischemic and the coronary artery stenosis can be considered as hemodynamically significant (GOULD 1978). Thus, stress testing is generally considered as a prerequisite for assessment of hemodynamically significant stenoses (see Sect. 8.4.4)

8.3
Modalities to Assess Myocardial Perfusion

Numerous techniques have been developed for measuring coronary flow and myocardial perfusion in experimental and clinical settings; these include electromagnetic flowmeters, coronary sinus indicator dilution techniques, velocity probes, inert gas washout analysis, labeled particles administered into the coronary arteries or the left ventricle (radioactive microspheres), and radionuclides trapped in the myocardium (WILKE et al. 1993). In the clinical setting, only radionuclide imaging is routinely used to assess myocardial perfusion. More recently, new clinically useful techniques such as contrast echocardiography and MR myocardial perfusion have become available (Table 8.1).

Table 8.1. Modalities used to assess myocardial perfusion

Nuclear medicine
Single-photon emission computed tomography (SPECT) (rest - stress) (with attenuation correction)
    Thallium-201 (^{201}Tl)
    Technetium-99m (^{99m}Tc) sestamibi (MIBI)
    Others (such as ^{99m}Tc-teboroxime)
Positron Emission Tomography (PET) (rest - stress)
    Rubidium -82
    Nitrogen -13 ammonia
    Carbon -11 acetate
    Oxygen -15H$_2$O

Contrast echocardiography (rest-stress)

Magnetic resonance (MR) (rest-stress)
    Extracellular contrast agents
    Intravascular contrast agents

8.3.1
Nuclear Medicine

Nuclear medicine is currently a cornerstone in the assessment of myocardial perfusion in patients with CAD. Most cardiologists are well aware of the possibilities of this technique. Most often the single-photon emission computed tomography (SPECT) technique is used to diagnose and evaluate the severity of CAD, while positron emission tomography (PET) is more accurate but also more expensive and less available.

8.3.1.1
Single-Photon Emission Computed Tomography

Following intravenous administration of radio-nuclides[such as thallium201(^{201}Tl), technetium 99m (^{99m}Tc) sestamibi (MIBI), and ^{99m}Tc Teboroxime] the relative myocardial distribution of these radionuclides is measured. Different protocols are used for ^{201}Tl and ^{99m}Tc-MIBI because in contrast to ^{201}Tl, ^{99m}Tc- MIBI exhibits little or no redistribution within the first 1–2 h after administration. ^{201}Tl is injected during stress, while redistribution of the tracer is measured at rest after a delay (e.g., 4 h). MIBI SPECT is performed by means of an injection of tracer during stress and a second injection at rest (or vice versa). In regions with an abnormal myocardial perfusion this will result in a lower number of counts (i.e., a defect) compared with normally perfused regions. The myocardial perfusion, however, remains unchanged unless the coronary artery has a stenosis of more than 85%. To detect less severe stenoses (between 50% and 85%), stress protocols (e.g., exercise, dipyridamole, dobutamine) are used. In these conditions, the stenosis will limit an increase

in perfusion and decrease counts in the abnormal region. Thus, the defect on stress that is absent at rest identifies an ischemic region that is usually supplied by a coronary artery with a 50%–85 % reduction in lumen diameter (i.e., redistribution on ^{201}Tl SPECT; Fig. 8.1). Fixed defects (i.e., no redistribution at rest) are interpreted as myocardial necrosis. The severity of the defect (i.e., reduction in counts) is related to the severity of the stenosis while the area of the defect is related to the mass of myocardium dependent on the stenotic artery (PATTERSON et al. 1994).

Although SPECT is widely used in clinical practice, certain pitfalls should be mentioned. It has been demonstrated that in patients with severe coronary artery stenosis a lesion may appear as a fixed defect even though there is still viable, hibernating myocardium. This suggests that ^{201}Tl scintigraphy can fail to distinguish viable from nonviable myocardium. Furthermore, the correlations between ^{201}Tl defect severity score and the descriptors of coronary stenosis were shown to improve when patients with collateral vessels were excluded. (HADJIMILTIADES et al. 1989). This suggests that ^{201}Tl scintigraphy may

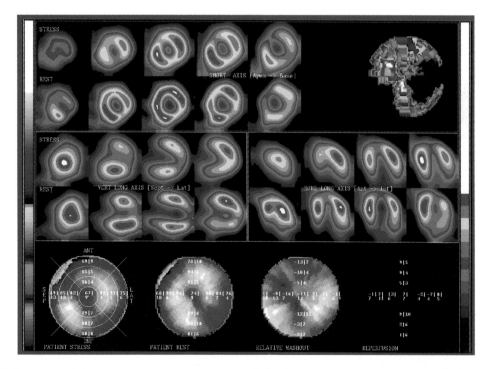

Fig. 8.1. ^{201}Tl SPECT study during stress and rest obtained in a 68-year-old male patient with complaints suggestive for CAD. Short-axis (above), vertical long-axis (middle left) and horizontal long-axis (middle right) images show an anteroseptal defect during stress with redistribution at rest, indicating a coronary artery stenosis on the left anterior descending coronary artery. (Courtesy of A. Maes, MD, PhD and J. Nuyts, PhD, Department of Nuclear Medicine, University Hospitals Leuven, Belgium)

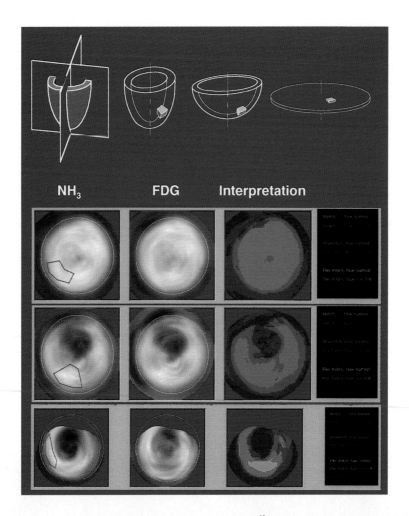

Fig. 8.2. PET myocardial viability study. The above drawings illustrate how the data obtained from the left ventricle are "compressed" into a bull's eye or polar map. The center of the polar map represents the left ventricular (LV) apex, while the periphery contains the data measured at the LV base. Myocardial blood flow is assessed by means of nitrogen-13 ammonia, and myocardial glucose metabolism by means of fluorine-18 deoxyglucose ([18]FDG). A flow index is calculated as the ratio of [13]NH$_3$ uptake in each region over the [13]NH$_3$ uptake in the region with the highest uptake (reference region indicated in red). The same anatomical region is used as the reference region for [18]FDG. A metabolic index is defined as the ratio of the glucose utilization in each region over that in the reference zone. Regions with a flow index > 0.8 are considered to be normal *(above)*. In the remaining regions, a flow-metabolism match pattern is assumed if the ratio of metabolism to flow was ≤ 1.2 *(middle)* and a mismatch pattern if this ratio is > 1.2 *(below)*. A mismatch pattern is considered as viable but ischemic myocardium, while a match pattern on PET is considered as infarcted myocardium. (Courtesy of A. Maes, MD, PhD and J. Nuyts, PhD, Department of Nuclear Medicine, University Hospitals Leuven, Belgium).

not be sensitive enough for the detection of low-range collateral flow in ischemic myocardium, although the potential of ^{201}Tl for detection of extensive collateral flow cannot be dismissed (NIENHABER et al. 1987).

Compared with MR first-pass studies, the interpretation of [210]Tl scintigraphy scans requires substantial expertise and experience (HENKIN et al. 1994). False-positive studies are common as thallium depends very much on body habitus. It is not uncommon for the female breast shadow to be interpreted as a septal defect. Incorrect selection of the long axis of the left ventricle during reconstruction may result in areas of decreased activity which do not correspond to anatomic lesions (HENKIN et al. 1994).

False-negative results from ^{201}Tl scintigraphy may occur when a lesion appears to cause significant luminal narrowing but is not hemodynamically significant. In patients with multivessel disease, hypoperfusion of the entire myocardium may mask regional abnormalities resulting from a fall in blood flow below a critical threshold to maintain viability. Since there has to be at least a 30%–40% blood flow reduction to be detectable with ^{210}Tl scintigraphy, mild perfusion changes cannot be discerned. By contrast, we could demonstrate (KIVELITZ et al. 1997a,b) in patients that changes of 20% in rest blood flow can be detected with MR perfusion imaging, and this may explain the smaller rate of false-positive results compared with ^{201}Tl scintigraphy. Wackers et al. reported substantial interobserver variability due to a lack of uniformly accepted standards for quantification of myocardial perfusion with ^{201}Tl scintigraphy. The reproducibility of quantitative planar ^{201}Tl scintigraphy was inversely related to the size of perfusion abnormalities (SIGAL et al. 1991), a finding shared with other imaging modalities and pointing to the importance of good spatial resolution.

8.3.1.2
Positron Emission Tomography

Positron emission tomography is very useful for assessing myocardial perfusion and metabolism (GOULD 1990). Assessment of myocardial perfusion with PET can be performed with nitrogen-13 ammonia, oxygen-15 H$_2$0, rubidium-82, or carbon-11 acetate. PET has several advantages over SPECT, such as a higher spatial resolution. Moreover, the absolute myocardial blood flow (MBF) can be measured (ml min^{-1} g^{-1}) while SPECT can only measure the relative blood flow. This is advantageous in patients with balanced ischemia caused by left main or three-vessel CAD in which the maximal MBF is reduced in all regions of the left ventricle, or in patients in whom the myocardial ischemia is not caused by large-vessel CAD such as syndrome X. It is furthermore considered the method of choice for determining the extent of viable myocardium (Fig. 8.2). The drawbacks of PET are that the patient is exposed to radiation, PET is costly, the spatial resolution of cardiac PET images is less than that presently achievable with myocardial perfusion MR imaging, and it is not likely that PET scanners will be widely available in the near future.

8.3.2
Myocardial Contrast Echocardiography

Another means to obtain quantitative information on myocardial perfusion is contrast echocardiography. Intravenous or intracoronary injection of microbubbles provides good estimates of coronary blood flow and can be used to detect CAD (MEZA et al. 1996). Advantages of contrast echocardiography are the real-time mode, the absence of injection of radioactive tracers, and the good spatial resolution. Its role in the clinical setting, however, needs to be established. Recently, KAUL and colleagues (1997) compared myocardial contrast echocardiography with SPECT in patients with known or suspected CAD. The information obtained by myocardial contrast echocardiography on the location of perfusion abnormalities and their physiologic relevance (reversible or irreversible) is similar to that provided by SPECT. However, the determination of endocardial-to-epicardial blood flow ratios during myocardial ischemia not associated with infarction has been characterized as very problematic with myocardial contrast echocardiography by one of the pioneers in this field (VATNER 1980). Different semiquantitative parameters such as curve width and height and the time constant for contrast washout have been proposed for the assessment of perfusion with myocardial contrast echocardiography (UNGER et al. 1994), not all of which are good measures of blood flow changes. The determination of the myocardial flow reserve has therefore relied on ratios of the intensity curve areas or amplitudes for two myocardial regions (VERNON et al. 1996). Nevertheless it is the determination of blood flow changes which forms the basis for measurement of the myocardial perfusion reserve. With myocardial contrast echocardiography the quality of regional intensity time courses is compromised by shadowing artifacts, which impose the need to use very low dosages of echo contrast agent. Both gated imaging and second harmonic imaging have led to improvements in this respect, but it has not been demonstrated that capturing an adequate arterial input function for modeling is feasible.

8.3.3
Magnetic Resonance (MR)

Compared with the radionuclide techniques, myocardial MR perfusion has several advantages, including higher spatial resolution, no radiation exposure, and no attenuation problem related to overlying breast shadow, elevated diaphragm, or obesity (Saeed et al. 1995). Fast gradient-echo and echo planar imaging (EPI) are the techniques currently used for myocardial perfusion. Fast gradient-echo imaging has the potential to acquire tomographic images at 1- to 3-s intervals, whereas EPI needs minimally 30–50 ms for each slice. These MR pulse sequences can be either T1- (inversion recovery pulse) or T2-sensitive (driven equilibrium). Contrast media for these studies are T1-enhancing contrast agents and magnetic susceptibility agents (T2* contrast agents), respectively. Perfusion studies for detection of regional ischemia are accomplished using low doses of MR contrast media and multislice measurements along different axes of the heart (WENDLAND et al. 1993a,b). Using inversion recovery and gradient recalled EPI, respectively, the ischemic area is identified as a zone of either low "cold-spot" or high "hot-spot" signal (WENDLAND et al. 1993a,b; YU et al. 1992).

While quantification of absolute myocardial blood flow is extensively validated by means of PET (KIVELITZ et al. 1997a,b; KLOCKE 1983; KLONER et al. 1992; KRAITCHMAN et al. 1996), this is true to a much lesser degree for MR imaging. However, the superior spatial and temporal resolution of MR first-pass imaging and the use of stable and well-tolerated MR contrast agents provide compelling reasons for the study of transmural variations in blood flow and the detection perfusion deficits confined to the subendocardium (KROLL et al. 1996; LAUB and SIMONETTI 1996).

8.4
Techniques for MR Myocardial Perfusion

8.4.1
Principles and Assumptions

Most techniques applied to measure myocardial perfusion are based on the indicator-dilution theory as described by W. F. Hamilton and colleagues in 1932 (WILKE et al. 1993). The general theory relies on the law of conservation of mass: by measuring the indicator content at the entry and exit of an organ, perfusion can be quantified. This theory, however, cannot readily be applied because MR techniques do not measure the absolute quantity of contrast medium either in the myocardium or in the blood; rather, MRI measures the signal intensity, which is not necessarily proportional to the concentration of the agent (MAUSS et al. 1985; BURSTEIN et al. 1991; WENDLAND et al. 1994; DONAHUE et al. 1994; JUDD et al. 1995a). Moreover, to attempt myocardial perfusion quantification from dynamic tomographic MR images: (a) the kinetics of the tracer in the tissue must be known and described with an appropriate model of distribution, and (b) the blood pool input function must be correctly defined. At the present time, MR perfusion imaging research makes several

assumptions (SAEED et al. 1995): (a) myocardial water is freely diffusible between the different compartments (intravascular, interstitial, and intracellular); (b) extravascular gadolinium agents enhance myocardial signal mono-exponentially (i.e., the regional signal intensity time courses change linearly with the amount of contrast agent injected); (c) MR contrast media behave as a blood component of physiologic interest in its flow patterns; (d) MR contrast agents do not perturb the physiologic parameters being measured; (e) the measured parameters are constant in the MR images used for calculation. WEDEKING and co-workers (1992) noted that at low contrast agent concentration, the concentration of the contrast agent can be calculated from the signal intensity. Increasing the dose leads to a saturation of signal enhancement and extravasation of the contrast agents which obscures the clearance phase of the first pass (WENDLAND et al. 1994). In practice, at concentrations between 0.2 mmol/l and 1.2 mmol/l, the signal intensity displays a linear progression compared with the Gd-DTPA concentrations. Above this limit, the signal increase becomes nonlinear as full relaxation is approached due to ever-decreasing T1 and due to signal loss induced by the T2* effect. Above 5.0 mmol/l, increasing Gd-DTPA concentrations result in a drop in signal intensity as the signal losses induced by the T2* effect become dominant (WILKE et al. 1993).

8.4.2
MR Myocardial Perfusion Sequence Design

Any MR myocardial perfusion sequence designed to monitor the first pass of a contrast medium must meet several requirements. It must: (a) simultaneously collect data of the entire heart, (b) provide adequate temporal resolution to characterize wash-in and wash-out kinetics, (c) render sufficient spatial resolution for accurate localization of perfusion deficits, and (d) be sensitive to the signal changes brought about by the bolus (SCHWITTER et al. 1997). A bolus injection of MR contrast media is necessary for perfusion studies to obtain pure first-pass transit of contrast through the myocardium. Currently, assessment of myocardial perfusion can be obtained by means of fast gradient-echo techniques and EPI techniques.

Fast gradient-echo technique sequences have image acquisition times between 160 ms and 1s. Due to short TR/TE or inversion preparatory pulses, they usually provide T1-weighted images. This fast acquisition mode allows the imaging of dynamic phenomena such as the firstpass of contrast through the heart. The longer the total acquisition time in comparison with the length of the heart beat, the more the images will be blurred by cardiac motion. Further shortening of the acquisition time can be obtained by means of acquisition where only a part of the k-space is filled during every heart beat, known as segmented k-space acquisitions, or by "keyhole" imaging (WALSH et al. 1995; WILKE et al. 1997). The latter technique samples only a limited segment of the k-space corresponding to the low spatial frequencies during the first-pass of contrast medium, thus significantly reducing the acquisition time. To null the signal of the myocardium and to obtain an improved T1 weighting, different strategies are available. Best known is the use of an inversion recovery (180°) preparation pulse with a subsequent delay (e.g. 300 ms) to null the signal of myocardium (this technique is called turbo-FLASH). In patients with a constant heart rate, the extent of T1 relaxation between images is constant. However, in patients with arrhythmias, the change in R-R interval allows a different amount of T1 relaxation to occur between images. As a consequence, the signal intensity and contrast detected as a function of time are modulated by sources other than the passage of the contrast agent. TSEKOS and co-workers (1995) introduced the AICE (i.e., arrhythmia-insensitive contrast enhancement) technique to produce T1 weighting that is independent of the magnitude of longitudinal magnetization at the moment of the ECG trigger pulse. The magnetization preparation is started with a non-section-selective 90° RF pulse that nulls the longitudinal magnetization followed by a gradient crusher pulse that dephases the transverse magnetization (WILKE et al. 1997). JUDD and co-workers (1995b) replaced the inversion pulse in the inversion recovery turbo-FLASH sequence by a train of preparatory RF pulses. These nonselective preparatory RF pulses drive the magnetization to a steady state prior to the image acquisition. Several experimental and clinical studies have demonstrated the capability of fast gradient-echo in detecting regions of ischemia (ATKINSON et al. 1990; HARTNELL et al. 1994; EICHENBERGER et al. 1994; KRAITCHMAN et al. 1996). The same type of acquisitions can also be used with other preparation pulses, such as 90°–180°–90° triplets (ANDERSON and BROWN 1993). In this case, the images have T2 weighting.

Echo planar imaging is most frequently used for T2-weighted perfusion studies. EPI acquires all the data for an image after a single excitation pulse, which reduces the acquisition times to between 50 and 100 ms for each image (MANSFIELD 1977). EPI has the potential to image the heart with sufficient temporal resolution and is therefore perfectly suited to study fast and dynamic phenomena such as the myocardial perfusion following bolus injection of contrast media. The spatial resolution can be improved, and the spatial distortion reduced, by using a multishot data acquisition (WETTER et al. 1995). Recently, SCHWITTER and colleagues (1997) reported the use of this multishot EPI to assess myocardial perfusion in normal volunteers. The complete heart could be covered, with five to seven contiguous axial slices, every two heartbeats. Similarly to fast gradient-echo sequences, the spatial and temporal resolution with EPI are sufficient to evaluate perfusion of the subendocardial, midepicardial, and subepicardial layer of the heart distinctly (WILKE et al. 1993; EDELMAN and LI 1994). While T2*-weighted gradient-echo EPI suffers from bolus-induced susceptibility problems, contrast dynamics can be best studied with T1-weighted spin-echo EPI using an inversion recovery preparation pulse to induce T1 weighting in the subsequent signals and dephasing gradients to null the contribution from the cavity (EDELMAN and LI 1994). An obvious drawback of EPI is the need for extensive hardware modifications that only recently have become commercially available.

8.4.3
Contrast Media for MR Myocardial Perfusion

Most techniques for assessing myocardial perfusion with MR rely on the administration of exogenous contrast media (e.g., paramagnetic gadolinium chelates, manganese gluconate, iron oxide particles, deuterium, or magnetic susceptibility agents such as dysprosium) (SCHAEFER et al. 1989; ATKINSON et al. 1990; MITCHEL and OSBAKEN 1991; CANET et al. 1993; KANTOR et al. 1994). Alternative techniques include the use of endogenous tracers, such as deoxyhemoglobin (i.e., BOLD technique) or spin tagging of arterial water (ATALAY et al. 1993; WILLIAMS et al. 1993; BERR and MAI 1998). Exogenous contrast media are usually classified according to their distribution pattern (i.e., extracellular and intravascular contrast media) (Table 8.2) or to their effects on the longitudinal or transverse relaxation (T1-enhancing contrast agents and magnetic susceptibility agents (T2* contrast agents), respectively).

Table 8.2. Extracellular versus intravascular contrast agents

	Extracellular	Intravascular
Examples		
T1-enhancing	Gd-DTPA Gd-DOTA Gd-BOPTA	Dextran-(Gd-DTPA) Albumin-(Gd-DTPA) Polylysine-(Gd-DTPA) USPIO
Magnetic susceptibility (T2*)	Dy-DTPA	Albumin-(Dy-DTPA) MION SPIO USPIO
Molecular weight (daltons)	< 1000	> 50000
Distribution	Intravascular Interstitial	Intravascular
Distribution volume	30%–40%	5%–10 %
Intravascular Half-life	20 min	180 min (MION)
Excretion	Renal	Renal / MPS*
Application(s)		
T1-enhancing CM	Most widely and clinically used MR contrast agent	– Blood volume – Tissue perfusion – Capillary integrity – MR angiography
T2* CM	Detection of ischemia and early infarction and differentiation between occlusive and reperfused myocardial infarction	– See T1-enhancing CM
MR perfusion imaging	First-pass imaging	First-pass imaging Steady-state imaging

CM, Contrast media; DTPA, diethylene-triamine penta-acetic acid; Dy, dysprosium; Gd, gadolinium; MION, monocrystalline iron oxides; MPS, mononuclear phagocytic system; SPIO, superparamagnetic iron oxides; USPIO, ultrasmall superparamagnetic iron oxides; *, iron oxide molecules are accumulated into the MPS system

8.4.3.1
Extracellular Contrast Media

Extracellular contrast agents or low molecular weight contrast agents (e.g., Gd-DTPA and Gd-DOTA) are small molecules (< 1000 daltons) that rapidly diffuse through the capillary walls into the

interstitium (WEINMANN et al. 1983). Their kinetic modeling is complex and has to take into account various flow- and tissue-dependent variables such as extraction fraction and partition coefficient (BURSTEIN et al. 1991; DIESBOURG et al. 1992; WENDLAND et al. 1994). Because of the rapid redistribution of extracellular contrast agents, rapid imaging techniques are required to image the inflow of the contrast agent following a bolus injection (i.e., first-pass study) (see Sect. 8.4.2) (SCHAEFER et al. 1992). Bolus injection of extracellular contrast media results in typical first-pass effects, i.e., a sudden signal increase in the right ventricular blood pool, followed by a similar signal intensity increase in the left ventricular blood pool and subsequently a slower signal intensity increase in the left ventricular myocardium. This increase is followed by a delayed decrease in signal intensity which may be attributed to the extravasation of Gd-DTPA through the capillary bed (WENDLAND et al. 1994). On the first pass through the capillary bed, 50% of circulating Gd-DTPA diffuses from the intravascular compartment into the extravascular compartments (BRASCH 1992). The optimum contrast dose for Gd-DTPA is 0.03–0.05 mmol/kg body weight with an injection time of 3–5s (SCHAEFER et al. 1992; MATHEIJSSEN et al. 1996; SCHWITTER et al. 1997). Above this dose, the maximal relative increase in signal intensity begins to saturate (SCHWITTER et al. 1997). Furthermore, saturation also affects the down-slope of the signal intensity versus time curve and obscures the wash-out phase of the contrast medium, and may result in a plateau-shaped curve. At the present time, clinical assessment of myocardial perfusion is largely restricted to the use of these extravascular contrast media because the use of most intravascular contrast agents is still not allowed in humans.

8.4.3.2
Intravascular Contrast Media

Intravascular contrast agents (also called blood-pool agents, macromolecular MR contrast media, or nondiffusible agents) are typically gadolinium molecules bound to large molecules such as albumin, polylysine, and dextrans (> 5 0000 daltons). The relatively large size of these molecules confines them to the intravascular space for a significant period. A second type of intravascular contrast media are molecules that are removed from the vascular space by the mononuclear phagocytic system, such as superparamagnetic iron oxide particles (CANET et al.

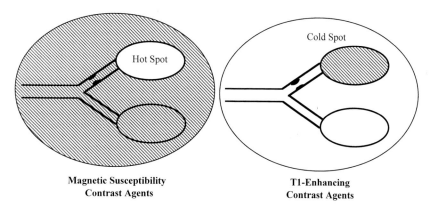

Magnetic Susceptibility
Contrast Agents

T1-Enhancing
Contrast Agents

Fig. 8.3. T1-enhancing versus magnetic susceptibility contrast agents. This figure shows the differences in myocardial signal intensity after administration of magnetic susceptibility contrast agents *(left)* and T1-enhancing contrast agents *(right)*. Following bolus injection of magnetic susceptibility MR contrast agents, such as dysprosium or iron oxide particles, the normally perfused myocardium *(below)* will show a drop in signal intensity; this is not the case for the hypoperfused myocardium *(above)*, which therefore appears as a bright area or "hot" spot. In contrast, T1-enhancing contrast agents (e.g., gadolinium) show an enhancement of the normal myocardium that is absent in hypoperfused myocardial regions; the latter thus appear as a "cold" spot

1993; REVEL et al. 1996). These contrast media allow an easier kinetic modeling and have significant advantages over extracellular fluid space MR contrast media. They can be used for accurate assessment of tissue perfusion, measurement of relative blood volume, and the detection of abnormal capillary leakage (ROSEN et al. 1990; WEISKOFF et al. 1993; TONG et al. 1993; WENDLAND et al. 1994; ARTEAGA et al. 1994). Unfortunately, most of these intravascular contrast agents are currently not available for clinical use. Recently, JOHANSSON et al. (1998) and PANTING et al. (1998) reported initial results using an ultrasmall paramagnetic iron oxide (USPIO) in humans to study myocardial perfusion. A distinct advantage of intravascular contrast agents over extracellular contrast agents in the assessment of myocardial perfusion is that first-pass imaging is not strictly required because these contrast agents remain much longer in the vascular compartment (i.e., steady state myocardial perfusion instead of first-pass myocardial perfusion). For instance, PANTING et al. (1998) performed their MR perfusion studies 30 min after the administration of the contrast agent.

8.4.3.3
T1-Enhancing and Magnetic Susceptibility MR Contrast Media

Magnetic resonance contrast media act by influencing the relaxation times of the neighboring resonating protons. Several magnetic materials, such as manganese, gadolinium, dysprosium, and iron, are used. Their effect can be either a shortening of the longitudinal relaxation (i.e., T1 enhancing), a shortening of the transversal relaxation (i.e., magnetic susceptibility), or a combination of both. For example, gadolinium chelates at low doses are strong relaxivity (T1) enhancing agents, causing a myocardial signal enhancement on T1-sensitive sequences, whereas at higher doses susceptibility effects become dominant and can be detected as signal loss on either $T2^*$- or T2-sensitive sequences (SAEED et al. 1995). Thus on MR myocardial perfusion imaging, hypoperfused myocardial regions will be visible as dark areas or "cold spots" using T1-enhancing contrast agents and as bright areas or "hot spots" using magnetic susceptibility MR contrast agents (YU et al. 1993) (Fig. 8.3). While gadolinium (Gd) is most frequently used as a T1-enhancing contrast agent, dysprosium (Dy) is a typical magnetic susceptibility contrast agent (WENDLAND et al. 1993b). Ultrasmall superparamagnetic iron oxide particles (USPIO) can be used for both T1-weighted and $T2^*$-weighted MR myocardial perfusion studies (PANTING et al. 1998).

8.4.4
Stress Imaging

Stress imaging is essential to accurately assess hypoperfused myocardium. The basis is that a hemodynamically significant stenosis is present when coronary reserve cannot be induced by vasodilatory stimulus (GOULD 1978). In the presence of a critical stenosis, the area in jeopardy may not be evident during the first pass in the basal state. When the flow is challenged by infusion of a vasodilator, the area in jeopardy becomes visible during the first pass of gadolinium chelates (SAEED et al. 1994) (Fig. 8.4). In clinical practice, dipyridamole is the most commonly used pharmacological vasodilator. It indirectly causes coronary vasodilatation by increasing the interstitial levels of adenosine, which activate the α^2 receptors (PENNELL 1994). The infusion regimen commonly used is 0.56 mg/kg intravenously, spread over 4 min. The increase in coronary flow after dipyridamole reaches its zenith approximately 2 min after the end of the 4-min infusion, and it is at this time that a myocardial contrast agent should be given (Fig. 8.5). It is well known that with maximal vasodilation, coronary blood flow in healthy subjects increases four- to fivefold over the baseline value of approximately 0.8–1.2 ml min^{-1} g^{-1} (WILSON et al. 1990), and there is an average blood volume increase of ~50% in the myocardium (WILKE et al. 1993). The hemodynamic response is prolonged and the half-life of reduction in coronary flow is of the order of 30 min. Side-effects (e.g., chest pain, headache, dizziness, and nausea) and ischemia are reversible with aminophylline. An alternative to dipyridamole is adenosine. Adenosine is infused at 0.140μgkg^{-1}min^{-1} for 6 min (0.84 mg/kg total dose). After 2–3 min, the adenosine reaction peaks and the heart rate increases. Coronary flow velocity returns to basal levels within 1–2 min. Both pharmacologic stressors are approved by the US FDA for inducing coronary hyperemia (SIEBERT et al. 1998).

8.4.5
Coverage of the Entire Ventricle

One of the main limitations of MR myocardial perfusion imaging in comparison with radionuclide imaging has been the restricted coverage of the myocardium. Although three-dimensional MR sequences have been developed, such as for imaging of the coronary arteries, MR myocardial perfusion sequences are still two-dimensional. Taking into account the rapid extravasation of extracellular contrast agents and the necessity for MR imaging during the first pass of the bolus, usually only a single slice is measured. To cover a much larger part of the myocardium, different strategies have been developed. Either multislice imaging or multiple injections can be used, but clearly the former is both more elegant and time efficient, particularly during stress imaging (TAYLOR and PENNELL 1996). MATHEIJSSEN and colleagues (1996) showed that a double-slice approach enhanced the detection of coronary artery lesions in five of ten patients. WALSH and colleagues (1995) used a modification of "keyhole" imaging by sampling a limited segment of the center of the k-space for a series of slices, such that after each two heart beats, the center of k-space could be completed for all the slices, while WILKE and co-workers (1997) used an ultrafast saturation recovery gradient-echo acquisition. In this fashion up to five slices through the heart can be simultaneously obtained in a patient with a heart rate of 65 beats/minute (or less). With the advent of ultrafast EPI techniques the entire ventricle can be studied

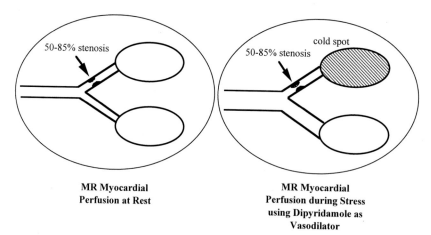

MR Myocardial
Perfusion at Rest

MR Myocardial
Perfusion during Stress
using Dipyridamole as
Vasodilator

Fig. 8.4. Stress MR myocardial perfusion imaging using dipyridamole. Hemodynamically significant stenosis (50%–85% lumen narrowing) may be undetected during resting conditions (**left**). During stress conditions, such as after the administration of dipyridamole, the myocardium supplied by the stenotic coronary artery becomes hypoperfused and will be visible as a cold spot using T1-enhancing contrast agents

MR Myocardial Perfusion Study during Stress Imaging

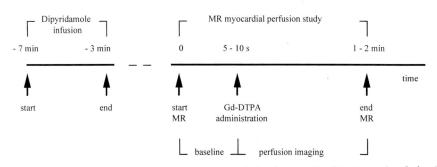

Fig. 8.5. Typical stress protocol for MR myocardial perfusion. An infusion regimen of dipyridamole 0.56 mg/kg body weight intravenously spread over 4 min is used, starting 7 min before the start of MR myocardial perfusion study. After a series of prebolus images (baseline images), a bolus injection of Gd-DTPA (commonly 0.04–0.05 mmol/kg body weight) is given. Fast MR imaging is continued during the next 1–2 min

following a single injection of contrast medium. SCHWITTER and colleagues (1997) were able to obtain seven slices through the left ventricle. A drawback in comparison with SPECT is that the cardiac short-axis, which is most frequently used to assess myocardium perfusion, does not provide information on the perfusion of the left ventricular apex. Ideally one has to use a combination of both cardiac short-axis and long-axis views, which is difficult in practice. At the intersection of both planes, the signal in the tissue will recover less completely in between successive acquisitions.

importance. The time of inflow of contrast medium is typically in the range of 7–12 s. If the sampling rate is too low, this will result in a large variation in measured up-slope or maximum signal enhancement.

During hyperemia there is a shortening of the rise time to peak signal intensity, higher peak signal intensity, and a clear descending limb after the peak signal, reflecting the higher perfusion rate due to dipyridamole-induced vasodilation and hyperemia. In addition to the coronary flow reserve (see Sect. 8.2), the myocardial perfusion reserve can also be determined, being defined as the ratio of regional

8.4.6
Analysis of Signal Intensity-Versus-Time Curves

The analysis of signal intensity-versus-time curves can be performed in different ways. The signal intensities before injection of the agent at the time T_{null} are averaged and used as offset (Fig. 8.6). The following parameters can easily be calculated: (a) the rate of increase in signal intensity after the bolus injection of contrast agent, using a linear fit; (b) the maximum signal intensity increase; (c) the time from T_{null} to the maximum signal intensity increase; (d) the signal intensity decrease after the peak signal intensity using an exponential fit (MATHEIJSSEN et al. 1996).

As the up-slope and maximum signal enhancement after contrast agent administration are accepted parameters describing myocardial perfusion (MANNING et al. 1991; WILKE et al. 1993), the sampling rate (i.e., the number of time points on the up-slope or from the onset of signal enhancement to maximum signal intensity increase) is of paramount

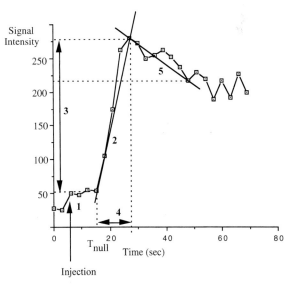

Fig. 8.6. Analysis of the signal intensity-versus-time curve. **1**, Baseline signal intensity. **2**, At T_{null} the signal intensity increases after the bolus injection of contrast media using a linear fit, **3**, The maximum signal intensity increases. **4**, The time between T_{null} and the maximum signal intensity increases. **5**, The signal intensity decreases after the peak signal intensity using an exponential fit

myocardial blood flow under hyperemic conditions to that under resting conditions. This ratio, however, may deviate from the coronary flow reserve, depending on the level of collateral blood flow (GOULD et al. 1990). The differences in regional perfusion can be quantified by defining a relative myocardial perfusion index as the ratio of the myocardial perfusion in the territory of the stenosed coronary artery to the myocardial perfusion in a remote normal zone (GOULD et al. 1990).

More fundamental parameters can also be extracted from perfusion measurements (LE BIHAN 1995). The Stewart-Hamilton equation relates the flow through an organ with the total amount of injected tracer m and the tracer concentration as measured in the draining veins cd(t):

$$F = \frac{M}{\int_0^\infty c_d(t)dt} \qquad (8.1)$$

A number of assumptions are, however, necessary:

1. the tracer is not extracted from the blood pool
2. the flow should not be affected by the tracer
3. the tracer must be thoroughly mixed with the blood
4. it must be corrected for recirculation of the tracer

Additional information is obtained from the mean transit time (MTT) of the tracer that is calculated as follows:

$$MTT = \frac{\int_0^\infty t \cdot c_d(t)d}{\int_\infty c_d(t)d} \qquad (8.2)$$

Here it is presumed that the tracer is injected as a bolus, but corrections can be made for a longer injection. Equation 8.3 further relates this MTT with the volume V occupied by the tracer and the flow:

$$MTT = \frac{V}{F} \qquad (8.3)$$

In practice, arterial input functions showing the time course of the bolus which are necessary to correct for the nonideal injection and the tracer concentration in the veins (Eq. 8.1) are not easily attained. Using blood pool agents, however, the area under the curve of the tissue concentration of the tracer is proportional to the effective tracer distribution volume. Quite often, an assessment of this parameter over a

particular organ shows regional heterogeneities that provide clinically useful information. For a thorough quantitative evaluation of perfusion from currently available MR images, the following corrections have to be considered:

1. Tracer concentrations have to be calculated from signal intensities in MR images. The relation between concentration of Gd and signal intensity is usually not known. In practice, a calibration is necessary for all sequences with their applied parameters (TR/TE/flip angle/time delays,etc.).
2. Most contrast agents used in clinical practice diffuse rapidly from the intravascular to the extravascular space. This effect can be incorporated in more difficult models that prescribe an organ as consisting of different compartments that mutually interact.
3. Correction for recirculation is usually performed using a gamma-variate fit of the arterial input function.
4. The effects of a finite contrast agent injection can be corrected using deconvolution based on the same arterial input function.

8.5
Results in Animals and Humans

A review of the perfusion studies with MR in humans and animals is given in Table 8.3. It is beyond the scope of this chapter to mention all results in detail. For the interested reader, we refer to excellent review papers in the literature (SAEED et al. 1994 ,1995). Perfusion studies have been performed in isolated hearts, animals (rats, rabbits, cats, dogs and pigs), normal volunteers, patients with coronary artery disease and patients with a history of acute myocardial infarction. Most groups have used turbo-FLASH sequences to assess myocardial perfusion, while a minority of studies have been performed with EPI techniques (both gradient-recalled-echo planar and inversion recovery EPI). This difference is very likely related to the limited availability of MR units equipped with EPI and the difficulty of acquiring satisfactory images (fat suppression, shimming, etc.). The commercially available extracellular Gd-chelates (e.g., Gd-DTPA, Gd-DOTA) have been used as contrast agents in most studies in both animals and humans (Fig. 8.7). A typical dose is 0.04–0.05 mmol/ kg body weight. The correlation between the dose of contrast agent and the effects on the myocardial signal intensity changes have been studied by

Table 8.3. Review of MR Myocardial Perfusion Studies in Animals and Humans

Author/year	Study group	MR sequence	Contrast agent	Dose (mmol/kg)	Stress	No. of Slices	Cardiac axis	Sensitivity	Specificity	Gold standard	Comments
Atkinson et al. (1990)	Rats/volunteers	t-FLASH	EC (Gd)	0.05-0.1	No	1	Ax	–	–	–	
Burstein et al (1991)	Isolated hearts	t-FLASH	EC (Gd)	Var.	No	1	Ax	–	–	–	
Manning et al. (1991)	Patients	t-FLASH	EC (Gd)	0.04	No	1	SA	–	–	CA	
van Rugge et al. (1991)	Volunteers	t-FLASH	EC (Gd)	0.05	No	1	SA	–	–	–	
Schaefer et al. (1992)	Patients	t-FLASH	EC (Gd)	0.04	DIP	1	SA	–	–	[201]Tl	
Canet et al. 1993)	Dogs	t-FLASH	IV (Fe)	0.02	No	1	SA	–	–	–	
Klein et al. (1993)	Humans	t-FLASH	EC (Gd)	0.05	DIP	1	SA	77%/81%	75%/100%	[99m]Tc/angio	
Wendland et al. (1993)	Rats	EPI	EC (Dys)	Var.	No	1	Ax	–	–	–	
Wendland et al. (1993a)	Rats	EPI	EC (Gd)	Var.	No	1	Ax	–	–	–	
Wilke et al. (1993b)	Dogs	t-FLASH	EC (Gd)	0.05	DIP	1	SA	–	–	Micro-spheres	
Artega et al. (1994)	Rabbits	t-FLASH	IV (Gd)	0.01	No	1	SA	–	–	–	
Edelman et al. (1994)	Humans	EPI	EC (Gd)	<0.2	No	1	Ax/SA	–	–	–	
Eichenberger et al. (1994)	Patients	t-FLASH	EC (Gd)	0.05	DIP	3	SA	64%	76%	[201]Tl/angio	
Hartnell et al. (1994)	Patients	t-FLASH	EC (Gd)	0.04	DIP	2	SA	92%	100%	[201]Tl/angio	+ cine MR
Kantor et al. (1994)	Dogs	EPI	EC (Gd)	0.1	DIP	1	Ax	–	–	–	
			EC (Dys)	0.1	DIP	1	Ax	–	–	–	
Wendland et al. (1994)	Rats	EPI	IV (Gd)	Var.	No	1	Ax	–	–	–	
			EC (Gd)	Var.	No	1	Ax	–	–	–	
Canet et al. (1995)	Patients	t-FLASH	EC (Gd)	Var.	No	1	SA	–	–	–	
Lima et al. (1995)	Patients	t-FLASH	EC (Gd)	0.1	No	4	SA	–	–	[201]Tl	
Walsh et al. (1995)	Patients	t-FLASH	EC (Gd)	0.05-0.1	DIP	3-4	SA	–	–	[201]Tl/[99m]Tc	
Kraitchman et al. (1996)	Dogs	t-FLASH	IV (Gd)	0.005	DOB	1	SA	–	–	Micro-spheres	+ MR tagging
Matheijssen et al. (1996)	Patients	t-FLASH	EC (Gd)	0.05	DIP	2	SA	–	–	[99m]Tc/angio	
Revel et al. (1996)	Dogs	t-FLASH	IV (Fe)	?	No	1	SA	–	–	–	
Schwitter et al. (1997)	Volunteers	EPI	EC (Gd)	Var.	No	5-7	Ax	–	–	–	
Wilke et al. (1997)	Pigs/humans	t-FLASH	EC (Gd)	0.04/0.025	AD	3-5	SA	–	–	Echo	
Cherryman et al. (1998)	Patients	t-FLASH	EC (Gd)	0.05	No	3	SA	–	–	ECG/Echo/[99m]Tc	
Chung et al. (1998)	Cats	t-FLASH	IV (Gd)	0.01	ATP	?	?	–	–	–	
Johansson et al. (1998)	Volunteers	t-FLASH	IV (Fe)	Var.	No	1	SA	–	–	–	
Panting et al. (1998)	Humans	t-FLASH/EPI	IV (Fe)	Var.	DIP	?	?	–	–	–	
Penzkofer et al. (1998)	Patients	t-FLASH	EC (Gd)	0.05	No	3	SA	83.3%	96.4%	[99m]Tc	
Wintersperger et al. (1998)	Patients	t-FLASH	EC (Gd)	0.05	No	3	SA	–	–	[99m]Tc	+ cine MR

AD, adenosine; ATP, adenosine triphosphate; Ax, axial; angio, coronary angiography; DIP, dipyridamole; DOB, low-dose dobutamine; Dys, dysprosium; EC, extracellular; Echo, Echocardiography; EPI, echo-planar; IV, intravascular contrast agent; GE, gradient-echo; Fe, ferritic particle (iron oxide); SA, short-axis; t-FLASH, turbo-FLASH; var, variable dose of contrast agent

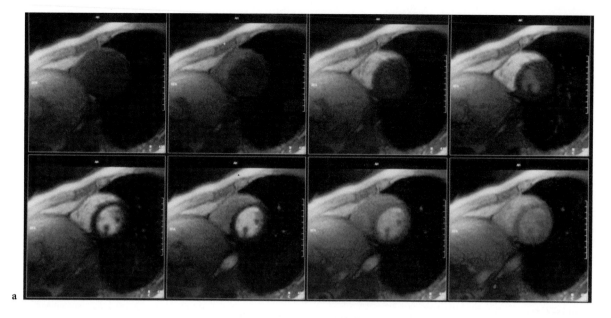

a

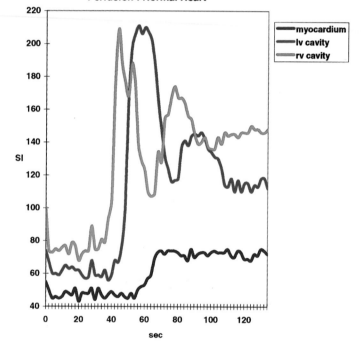

Fig. 8.7a-b. MR myocardial perfusion study in a normal volunteer. **a** First pass of Gd-DTPA (0.05 mmol/kg body-weight) through the heart following bolus injection in a cubital vein using a turbo FLASH sequence *(upper left to lower right)*. The signal of the myocardium is nulled by an inversion recovery pulse. First, the right ventricular cavity is strongly enhanced, followed by the left ventricular cavity and the myocardium. **b** Signal intensity-versus-time curve shows the changes in signal intensity in the right ventricular (RV) cavity, left ventricular (LV) cavity, and myocardium. Peak enhancement during the first pass is similar for the RV and the LV cavity. Approximately 25 s later a smaller second peak is visible, representing the second pass. The enhancement in the myocardium is much less pronounced and characterized by the absence of a sharp decline in signal intensity and of a second peak. The latter phenomena are caused by rapid extravasation of Gd-DTPA into the interstitium, which is responsible for a slow wash-out.

several groups (BURSTEIN et al. 1991; WENDLAND et al. 1993a, b,1994; CANET et al. 1995).

Other groups have investigated the role of intravascular contrast agents in assessing myocardial perfusion in animals (CANET et al. 1993, REVEL et al. 1996, KRAITCHMAN et al. 1996, CHUNG et al. 1998). As mentioned above, these contrast agents remain in the vascular space for a considerable time and thus do not require first-pass imaging. Chung and co-workers compared first-pass and steady state hemodynamics in cats with a reperfused anterior myocardial infarction, using a higher molecular weight gadolinium compound during rest and stress (Gadomer-17) (CHUNG et al. 1998). During first pass, nonviable myocardium exhibited a significant decline of the slope of the initial rise in signal intensity and a significantly lower peak signal intensity during both stress and rest. During steady state, the signal intensity increase was considerably higher for the (post)ischemic but viable regions than for the

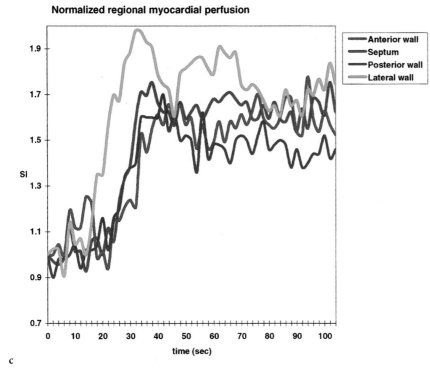

Fig. 8.7c. Signal intensity-versus-time curve in the anterior wall, septum, posterior wall, and lateral wall of the left ventricle. The y-axis shows the relative signal intensity (*SI*) rather than the absolute signal intensity. A similar enhancement pattern is shown for all myocardial regions, with a sharp rise and a slow wash-out

nonviable and normal myocardium. JOHANSSON and colleagues (1998) and PANTING and colleagues (1998) recently reported their preliminary results in humans using ultrasmall paramagnetic iron oxide (USPIO) particles. These intravascular contrast agents can be used to produce signal changes in T1- and T2*-weighted images. The role of magnetic susceptibility MR contrast agents (such as dysprosium) in the assessment of myocardial perfusion has also been evaluated (WENDLAND et al. 1993b, KANTOR et al. 1994). Stress testing has not been systematically used, but is crucial when comparisons are made with other modalities such as stress-rest radionuclide imaging. As a pharmacological stress agent, dipyridamole has been most commonly used. Other groups have used adenosine as an alternative, while Kraitchman and colleagues used dobutamine (KRAITCHMAN et al. 1996; WILKE et al. 1997).

Until now, only a relatively small number of studies have compared the ability of MR myocardial perfusion techniques to detect hypoperfused myocardial regions with clinically used imaging modalities such as ^{201}Tl and ^{99m}Tc radionuclide imaging and coronary angiography. The sensitivity of the former was found to range between 64% and 92%, and the specificity between 75% and 100% (KLEIN et al. 1993; EICHENBERGER et al. 1994; HARTNELL et al. 1994; PENZKOFER et al. 1998). HARTNELL and colleagues (1994) showed an improved accuracy (similar to scintigraphy) when combining MR myocardial perfusion with cine MR to detect associated wall motion abnormalities. WINTERSBERGER and co-workers (1998) compared myocardial perfusion with myocardial wall thickening in patients with chronic myocardial infarction. Wall thickening was significantly lower in hypoperfused areas than in normally perfused areas, and the location of hypoperfusion and restricted myocardial wall thickening correlated well. Other groups have used myocardial MR tagging for concomitant assessment of regional myocardial function and determination of the principal myocardial strains (KRAITCHMAN et al. 1996). Several studies have stressed the advantages of MR myocardial perfusion compared with radionuclide imaging for obtaining information on the heterogeneous transmural enhancement (subepi-,

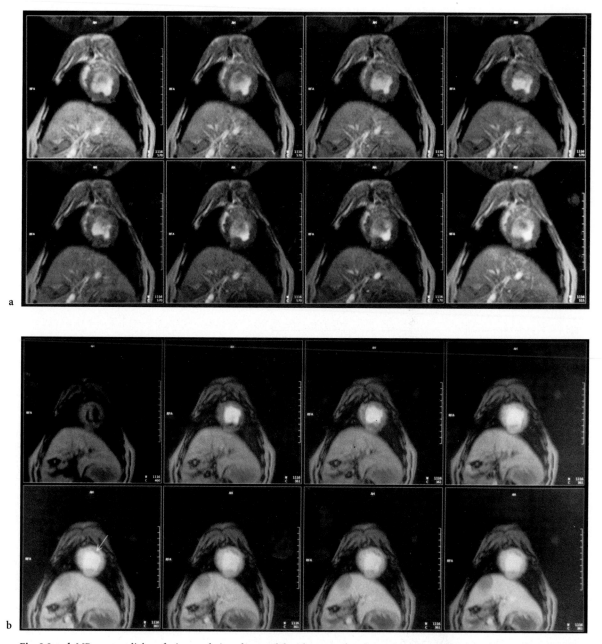

Fig. 8.8 a–d. MR myocardial perfusion study in a dog model with a reperfused anterior myocardial infarction. **a** Short-axis cine MR study. Eight time points during the cardiac cycle are shown from end-diastole *(upper left)* to mid-diastole *(lower right)*. The anterior left ventricular (LV) wall is edematously thickened (bright and inhomogeneous appearance) and is characterized by absence of wall motion (akinesis). **b** First-pass MR myocardial perfusion using 0.05 mmol/kg Gd-DTPA. While the myocardium globally shows bright enhancement, a persistent hypointense area is present in the subendocardial part of the anterior LV wall *(arrow)*. **c** Signal intensity-versus-time curve. ROI's are placed in the anterior LV wall (subendocardially in the hypointense region), the LV septum, the posterior wall, and the lateral wall. In contrast to the normal myocardium (which shows a sharp rise in signal intensity following injection of Gd-DTPA), a slow rise in signal intensity and a lower peak enhancement are found subendocardially in the anterior wall *(red line)*. **d** Corresponding post-mortem MR studies (T1-weighted spin-echo MR with Gd-DTPA administration). The hyperintense region is much larger than the small hypointense (subendocardial) region visible on the perfusion study. This discrepancy can be explained as follows: since Gd-DTPA is not specifically confined to the infarcted myocardium but also enhances the ischemic but viable myocardium perfused by open blood vessels, the hyperintense region on the morphologic study will be considerably larger than the hypointense region on the first-pass perfusion study, which depicts occluded subendocardial vessels in the infarcted region

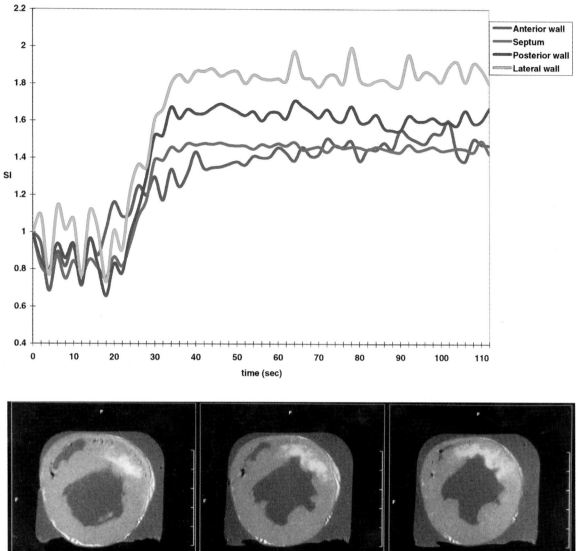

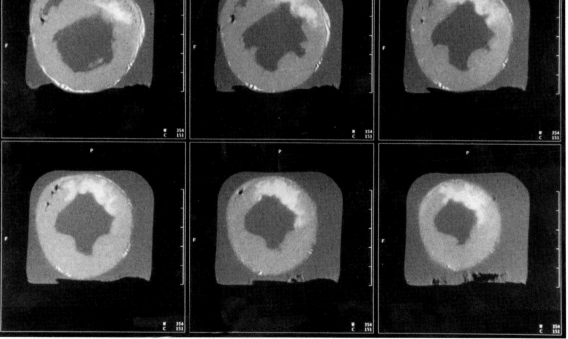

Fig. 8.8 a–d. (Continued)

mid-, and subendo cardium), which may reflect the variability in myocardial perfusion across the wall (WILKE et al. 1993; EDELMAN and LI 1994). LIMA and co-workers (1995) performed MR perfusion studies in patients with a recent acute myocardial infarction. Two different patterns of enhancement were found, which were related to the patency of the infarct-related artery. A hyperenhancement pattern in the infarct region was associated with a patent infarct artery, and with less damage on ECG and echocardiography. The second pattern consisted in a hyperenhanced region surrounding a subendo-cardial area of decreased signal at the center of the infarcted region (Fig. 8.8). This pattern was associated with coronary occlusion at angiography, Q-waves on ECG, and greater regional dysfunction on echocardiography. Moreover, the extent and location of the abnormalities on MR corresponded well with the extent and location of the fixed SPECT abnormalities. In a recent study by CHERRYMAN and co-workers (1998), 103 patients with a first acute myocardial infarction underwent ECG, echo-cardiography, ^{201}Tl SPECT and MR perfusion study. The authors concluded that dynamic contrast-enhanced MRI is consistently better than thallium SPECT in infarct detection, being the most effective test for infarcts in the anterior septal and inferior posterior regions.

8.6 Conclusions

The advent of rapid MR imaging techniques has made it possible to study physiological events such as myocardial perfusion in real-time. Comparisons with other established techniques, such as radiola-beled microspheres, are still proceeding. Preliminary experience shows that accurate information on myocardial perfusion can be obtained in a totally noninvasive manner without the need for radioactive tracers and with a spatial and temporal resolution not matched by any other modality. Due to improvements in sequence design, the perfusion in the entire ventricle can be evaluated following a single bolus injection of contrast agent.

The interpretation of MR perfusion studies with a large number of images will be simplified by the development of automated pixel-based analysis programs (PENZKOFER et al. 1998), and the creation of myocardial perfusion maps (BOUDRAA et al. 1998). Furthermore, the wider availability of intra-vascular contrast agents for clinical studies in the near future will improve our understanding of the myocardial perfusion behavior in normal and patho-logical conditions. Together with other applications of MR in the heart, MR may become a preferential technique in the evaluation of patients with CAD.

Acknowledgements

The authors would like to thank N. Wilke, MD from the University of Minneapolis, USA for and Y. Ni, MD, PhD, A. Maes, MD, PhD, and J. Nuyts, PhD from the University of Leuven, Belgium for their cooperation and helpful comments in the preparation of this chapter.

References

Anderson CM, Brown JJ (1993) Cardiovascular magnetic resonance imaging: evaluation of myocardial perfusion. Coron Artery Dis 4:354–360

Arteaga C, Canet E, Ovize M, Janier M, Revel D (1994) Myocardial perfusion assessed by subsecond magnetic resonance imaging with a paramagnetic macromolecular contrast agent. Invest Radiol 29:S54–S57

Atalay MK, Forder JR, Chacko VP, Kawamoto S, Zerhouni EA (1993) Oxygenation in the rabbit myocardium: assessment with susceptibility- dependent MR imaging. Radiology 189:759–764

Atkinson DJ, Burstein D, Edelman RR (1990) First-pass cardiac perfusion: evaluation with ultrafast MR imaging. Radiology 174:757–762

Berr SS, Mai VM (1998) Cardiac extraslice spin tagging - CEST perfusion. Proceedings of International Society for Magnetic Resonance in Medicine, sixth scientific meeting and exhibition, Sydney, Australia, April 18–24, 1998:923

Boudraa A, Canet E, Janier M, et al. (1998) A fast method for mapping first pass myocardial MR images. Proceedings of International Society for Magnetic Resonance in Medicine, sixth scientific meeting and exhibition, Sydney, Australia, April 18–24, 1998:898

Brasch RC (1992) New directions in the development of MR imaging contrast media. Radiology 183:1–11

Burstein D, Taratuta E, Manning WJ (1991) Factors in myocardial "perfusion" imaging with ultrafast MRI and Gd-DTPA administration. Magn Reson Med 20:299–305

Canet E, Revel D, Forrat R, et al. (1993) Superparamagnetic iron oxide particles and positive enhancement for myocardial perfusion studies assessed by subsecond T-1-weighted MRI. Magn Reson Imaging 11:1139–1145

Canet E, Doulk P, Janier M, et al. (1995) Influence of bolus volume and dose of gadolinium chelate for first-pass myocardial perfusion MR imaging studies. J Magn Reson Imaging 5:411–415

Cherryman GR, Tranter J, Keal R, et al. (1998) Prospective comparison of contrast-enhanced MRI with thallium 201 SPECT and 2D echocardiography in the localization of acute myocardial infarction. Proceedings of International Society for Magnetic Resonance in Medicine, sixth scientific meeting and exhibition, Sydney, Australia, April 18–24, 1998;923

Chung KI, Chung TS, Weinmann HJ, Lim TH (1998) Viable myocardium in acute myocardial infarction: assessment with steady-state and first-pass MR imaging during ATP-induced hyperemia and at rest after Gadomer-17 enhancement. Proceedings of International Society for Magnetic Resonance in Medicine, sixth scientific meeting and exhibition, Sydney, Australia, April 18–24, 1998; 890

Diesbourg LD, Prato FS, Wisenberg G, et al. (1992) Quantification of myocardial blood flow and extracellular volumes using a bolus injection of Gd-DTPA: kinetic modeling in canine ischemic disease. Magn Reson Med 23:239–253

Donahue K, Burstein D, Manning W, Gary M (1994) Studies of Gd-DTPA relaxivity and proton exchange rates in tissue. Magn Reson Med 32:66–76

Edelman RR, Li W (1994) Contrast-enhanced echo-planar MR imaging of myocardial perfusion: preliminary study in humans. Radiology 190:771–777

Eichenberger AC, Schuiki E, Kochli VD, Amann FW, McKinnon GC, von Schulthess GK (1994) Ischemic heart disease: assessment with gadolinium-enhanced ultrafast MR imaging and dipyridamole stress [see comments]. J Magn Reson Imaging 4:425–431

Gould K (1978) Noninvasive assessment of coronary stenosis by myocardial perfusion imaging during pharmacologic coronary vasodilatation. I. Physiologic basis and experimental validation. Am J Cardiol 41:267–278

Gould KL (1990) Positron emission tomography and interventional cardiology. Am J Cardiol 66: 51F–58F

Gould KL, Kirkeeide RL, Buchi M (1990) Coronary flow reserve as a physiologic measure of stenosis severity. J Am Coll Cardiol 15: 459–474

Hadjimiltiades S, Watson R, Hakki AH, Heo J, Iskandrian AS (1989) Relation between myocardial thallium-201 kinetics during exercise and quantitative coronary angiography in patients with one vessel coronary artery disease. J Am Coll Cardiol 13: 1301–1308

Hartnell G, Cerel A, Kamalesh M, et al. (1994) Detection of myocardial ischemia: value of combined myocardial perfusion and cineangiographic MR imaging. Am J Roentgenol 163:1061–1067

Henkin RE, Kalousdian S, Kikkawa RM, Kemel A (1994) 201-Thallium myocardial perfusion imaging utilizing single-photon emission computed tomography (SPECT). American Medical Association

Johansson LO, Akenson P, Ragnarsson A, Ahlström H (1998) Myocardial perfusion using a new ultra small paramagnetic iron oxide, enabling T2* perfusion with very short echo-times: first trials in humans. Proceedings of International Society for Magnetic Resonance in Medicine, sixth scientific meeting and exhibition, Sydney, Australia, April 18–24, 1998:903

Judd RM, Ataly, MK, Rottman GA, Zerhouni EA (1995a) Effects of myocardial water exchange on T1 enhancement during bolus administration of MR contrast agents. Magn Reson Med 33:215–223

Judd RM, Reeder SB, Atalar E, McVeigh ER, Zerhouni EA (1995b) A magnetization-driven gradient echo pulse sequence for the study of myocardial perfusion. Magn Reson Med 34:276–282

Kannel WB, Doyle JT, McMamara PM, et al (1976) Precursors of sudden coronary death: factors related to the incidence of sudden death. Circulation 51:606–613

Kantor HL, Rzedzian RR, Buxton R, et al. (1994) Contrast induced myocardial signal reduction: effect of lanthanide chelates on ultra high speed MR images. Magn Reson Imaging 12:51–59

Kaul S, Senior R, Dittrich H, Raval U, Khattar R, Lahiri A (1997) Detection of coronary artery disease with myocardial contrast echocardiography: comparison with

^{99m}Tc-sestamibi single-photon emission tomography. Circulation 96:785–792

Kivelitz DE, Bis KG, Wilke NM, Jerosch-Herold M, Juni JE, Hamm BK (1997a) Quantitative MR first pass perfusion imaging demonstrates coronary artery patency post interventions, Radiology 205 (Suppl): 254

Kivelitz DE, Wilke NM, Bis KG, Jerosch-Herold M, Juni JE, Hamm BK(1997b) Quantitative MR first pass versus N13-ammonia PET perfusion imaging in coronary artery disease. Radiology 205 (Suppl): 253

Klein MA, Collier BD, Hellman RS, Bamrah VS (1993) Detection of chronic coronary artery disease: value of pharmacologically stressed, dynamically enhanced turbo-fast low-angle shot MR images. Am J Roentgenol 161:257–263

Klocke F (1983) Measurements of coronary blood flow and degree of stenosis: current clinical implications and continuing uncertainties. J Am Coll Cardiol 1: 31–36

Klocke FJ (1990) Cognition in the era of technology: "seeing the shades of gray". J Am Coll Cardiol 16:763–769

Kloner RA, Przyklenk K, Rahimtoola SH, Braunwald E (1992) In: Opie LH (ed) Stunning, hibernation and calcium in myocardial ischemia and reperfusion. Kluwer, Dordrecht, pp 251–280

Kraitchman DL, Wilke N, Hexeberg E, et al. (1996) Myocardial perfusion and function in dogs with moderate coronary stenosis. Mag Reson Med 35:771–780

Kroll K, Wilke N, Jerosch-Herold M, et al. (1996) Accuracy of modeling of regional myocardial flows from residue functions of an intravascular indicator, Am J Physiol (Heart Circ Physiol) 40: H1643–H1655

Laub G, Simonetti O (1996) Assessment of myocardial perfusion with saturation-recovery Turbo FLASH sequences. ISMR, 4th Scientific Meeting, New York, p 179

Le Bihan D (1995) Diffusion and perfusion magnetic resonance imaging. Applications to functional MRI. Raven Press, New York

Lima JAC, Judd RM, Bazille A, Schulman SP, Atalar E, Zerhouni EA (1995) Regional heterogeneity of human myocardial infarcts demonstrated by contrast-enhanced MRI. Potential mechanisms. Circulation 92:1117–1125

Manning WJ, Atkinson DJ, Grossman W, Paulin S, Edelman RR (1991) First-pass nuclear magnetic resonance imaging studies using gadolinium-DTPA in patients with coronary artery disease. J Am Coll Cardiol 18:959–965

Mansfield P (1977) Multiplanar image formation using NMR spin echoes. J Physiol (Lond) 10:L55–L58

Matheijssen NA, Louwerenburg HW, van Rugge FP, et al. (1996) Comparison of ultrafast dipyridamole magnetic resonance imaging with dipyridamole SestaMIBI SPECT for detection of perfusion abnormalities in patients with one-vessel coronary artery disease: assessment by quantitative model fitting. Magn Reson Med 35:221–228

Mauss Y, Grucker D, Fornasiero D, Chambron J (1985) NMR compartmentalization of free water in the perfused rat heart. Magn Reson Med 2:187–194

Meza MF, Mobarek S, Sonnemaker R, et al. (1996) Myocardial contrast echocardiography in human beings: correlation of resting defects to sestamibi single photon emission computed tomography. Am Heart J 132:528–535

Mitchell MD, Osbakken M (1991) Estimation of myocardial perfusion using deuterium nuclear magnetic resonance. Magn Reson Imaging 9:545–552

National Heart Lung and Blood Institute: Morbidity from coronary heart disease in the United States. (1990) National Heart, Lung, and Blood Institute Data Fact Sheet, Bethesda, MD

Nienaber CA, Spielmann RP, Salge D, Clausen A, Montz R, Bleifeld W (1987) Noninvasive identification of collateralized myocardium by 201 thallium tomography in vasodilation and redistribution. Z Kardio 76: 612–620

Panting JR, Taylor AM, Gatehouse PD, et al. (1998) Equilibrium myocardial signal changes with an intravascular contrast agent NC100150: possible utility for steady state myocardial perfusion assessment. Proceedings of International Society for Magnetic Resonance in Medicine, sixth scientific meeting and exhibition, Sydney, Australia, April 18–24, 1998: 896

Patterson RE, Horowitz SF, Eisner RL (1994) Comparison of modalities to diagnose coronary artery disease. Semin Nucl Med 24:286–310

Pennell DJ (1994) Pharmacological cardiac stress: when and how? Nucl Med Commun 15:578–585

Penzkofer H, Wintersperger BJ, Knez A, Weber J, Reiser M (1998) Proceedings of International Society for Magnetic Resonance in Medicine, sixth scientific meeting and exhibition, Sydney, Australia, April 18-24, 1998: 901

Reimer KA, Jennings RB (1979) The wavefront progression of myocardial ischemic cell death. II. Transmural progression of necrosis within the framework of ischemic bed size (myocardium at risk) and collateral flow. Lab Invest 40:633–644

Revel D, Canet E, Sebbag L, et al. (1996) First-pass and delayed magnetic resonance imaging studies of reperfused myocardial infarction with iron oxide particles. Acad Radiol 3:S398–S401

Rosen BR, Belliveau JW, Vevea JM, Brady TJ (1990) Perfusion with NMR contrast agents. Magn Reson Med 14:249–265

Saeed M, Wendland MF, Higgins CB (1994) Contrast media for MR imaging of the heart. J Magn Reson Imaging 4:269–279

Saeed M, Wendland MF, Higgins CB (1995) The developing role of magnetic resonance contrast media in the detection of ischemic heart disease. Proc Soc Exp Biol Med 208:238–254

Schaefer S, Lange RA, Kulkarni PV, et al. (1989) In vivo nuclear magnetic resonance imaging of myocardial perfusion using the paramagnetic contrast agent manganese gluconate. J Am Coll Cardiol 14:472–480

Schaefer S, van Tyen R, Saloner D (1992) Evaluation of myocardial perfusion abnormalities with gadolinium-enhanced snapshot MR imaging in humans. Work in progress. Radiology 185:795–801

Schwitter J, Debatin JF, von Schulthess GK, McKinnon GC (1997) Normal myocardial perfusion assessed with multishot echo-planar imaging. Magn Reson Med 37:140–147

Siebert, JE, Eisenberg, JD, Pernicone, JR, Cooper TG (1998) Practical myocardial perfusion studies via adenosine pharmacologic stress. Proceedings of International Society for Magnetic Resonance in Medicine, sixth scientific meeting and exhibition, Sydney, Australia, April 18–24, 1998:902

Sigal SL, Soufer R, Fetterman RC, Mattera JA, Wackers FJ (1991) Reproducibility of quantitative planar thallium-201 scintigraphy: quantitative criteria for reversibility of myocardial perfusion defects. J Nucl Med 32: 759–765

Taylor AM, Pennell DJ (1996) Recent advances in cardiac magnetic resonance imaging [see comments]. Curr Opin Cardiol 11:635–642

Tong CY, Prato FS, Wisenberg G, et al. (1993) Techniques for the measurement of the local myocardial extraction efficiency for inert diffusible contrast agents such as gadopentate dimeglumine. Magn Reson Med 30:332–336

Tsekos NV, Zhang Y, Merkle H, et al. (1995) Fast anatomical imaging of the heart and assessment of myocardial perfusion with arrhythmia insensitive magnetization preparation. Magn Reson Med 34:530–536

Unger EF, Banai S, Shou M, et al. (1994) Basic fibroblast growth factor enhances myocardial collateral flow in a canine model. Am J Physiol 266: H1588–H1595

van Rugge FP, Boceel JJ, van der Wall EE et al. (1991) Cardiac first-pass and myocardial perfusion in normal subjects assessed by sub-second Gd-DTPA enhanced MR Imaging. J Comput Assist Tomogr 15: 959–965

Vatner SF (1980) Correlation between acute reductions in myocardial blood flow and function in conscious dogs. Circulation Research 47, 201

Vernon SM, Camarano G, Kaul S, Sarembock IJ, Gimple LW, Powers ER, Ragosta M (1996) Myocardial contrast echocardiography demonstrates that collateral flow can preserve myocardial function beyond a chronically occluded coronary artery. Am J Cardiol 78:958–960

Walsh EG, Doyle M, Lawson MA, Blackwell GG, Pohost GM (1995) Multislice first-pass myocardial perfusion imaging on a conventional clinical scanner. Magn Reson Med 34:39–47

Wedeking P, Sotak CH, Telser J, Kumar K, Chang CA, Tweedle MF (1992) Quantitative dependence of MR signal intensity on tissue concentration of Gd(HP-DO3A) in the nephrectomized rat. Magn Reson Imaging 10:97–108

Weinmann HJ, Brasch RC, Press WR, Wesbey GE (1983) Characteristics of gadolinium-DTPA complex: a potential NMR contrast agent. AJR 142:619–624

Weiskoff RM, Chesler D, Boxerman JL, Rosen BR (1993) Pitfalls in MR measurement of tissue blood flow with intravascular tracers: which mean transit time? Magn Reson Med 29:553–558

Wendland MF, Saeed M, Masui T, Derugin N, Moseley ME, Higgins CB (1993a) Echo-planar MR imaging of normal and ischemic myocardium with gadodiamide injection. Radiology 186:535–542

Wendland MF, Saeed M, Masui T, Derugin N, Higgins CB (1993b) First pass of an MR susceptibility contrast agent through normal and ischemic heart: gradient-recalled echo-planar imaging. J Magn Reson Imaging 3:755–760

Wendland MF, Saeed M, Yu KK, et al. (1994) Inversion recovery EPI of bolus transit in rat myocardium using intravascular and extravascular gadolinium-based MR contrast media: dose effects on peak signal enhancement. Magn Reson Med 32:319–329

Wetter DR, McKinnon GC, Debatin JF, von Schulthess G (1995) Cardiac echo-planar MR imaging: comparison of single- and multiple-shot techniques. Radiology 194:765–770

Wilke N, Simm C, Zhang J, et al. (1993) Contrast-enhanced first pass myocardial perfusion imaging: correlation between myocardial blood flow in dogs at rest and during hyperemia. Magn Reson Med 29:485–497

Wilke N, Jerosch-Herold M, Wang Y, et al. (1997) Myocardial perfusion reserve: assessment with multisection, quantitative, first-pass MR imaging. Radiology 204:373–384

Williams DS, Grandis DJ, Zhang W, Koretsky AP (1993) Magnetic resonance imaging of perfusion in the isolated rat heart using spin inversion of arterial water. Magn Reson Med 30:361–365

Wilson RF, Wyche K, Christensen BV, Zimmer S, Laxson DD (1990) Effects of adenosine on human coronary arterial circulation. Circulation 82:1595–1606

9 Myocardial Metabolism

S. Neubauer

9.1 Introduction

The signal source for magnetic resonance imaging (MRI) is exclusively the ^{1}H nucleus, more specifically the highly abundant ^{1}H nuclei in water (H_2O) and fat (CH_2 and CH_3 groups). ^{1}H-MRI is a superb method for obtaining anatomical information, but offers little biochemical insight into the state of the observed tissue. In contrast, magnetic resonance spectroscopy (MRS) allows the study of a number of additional nuclei with a nuclear spin, i.e., an uneven number of protons, neutrons, or both. MRS is the only available method for the noninvasive study of cardiac metabolism without a need for the application of external radioactive tracers, such as in positron emission tomography (PET). Nuclei of interest for metabolic MRS are shown in Table 9.1 and include, most importantly, ^{1}H (protons from metabolites other than water and fat), ^{13}C, ^{19}F, ^{23}Na, ^{31}P (the most widely studied nucleus), ^{39}K, and ^{87}Rb. In principle, many clinical questions could be addressed with cardiac MRS, if it were not for its main

limitation: restricted sensitivity of signal detection. Nuclei studied with MRS have a substantially lower MR sensitivity than ^{1}H and are present in concentrations several orders of magnitude lower than those of ^{1}H from water (Table 9.1).

Since the first ^{31}P-MR spectrum was obtained from an isolated heart (Garlick et al. 1977), MRS has become a standard method for experimental cardiology and has been used for the study of many aspects of cardiac metabolism (for reviews, see Gadian 1995; Ingwall 1982; Neubauer et al. 1991). In the 1970s, this field was pioneered by research groups led by G. Radda (Garlick et al. 1977), J. Ingwall (Ingwall 1982), and W. Jacobus (Jacobus et al. 1977). A large body of literature exists on experimental applications of MRS to the heart, and more than 90% of publications on cardiac MRS report on experimental animal work. Although this is a clinical textbook, full appreciation of MRS would be impossible without an introduction (a comprehensive overview is beyond the scope of this chapter) on the experimental applications of MRS. Thereby, we can explain the principles of MRS in well-defined experimental settings, which then point to clinical applications that might become possible in the future if we succeed in overcoming the technical challenges that presently limit the clinical utility of MRS. This chapter is not intended as a complete review of all published work on clinical MRS of the heart, which is available elsewhere (Beyerbracht et al. 1996; Bottomley 1994); rather, its purpose is to introduce the technical and physiological background of MRS studies and to provide a perspective on its clinical potential in patients with heart disease.

9.2 Basic Principles

The most widely used model for cardiac MRS is the isolated rodent heart perfused with crystalloid solutions ("Krebs-Henseleit" perfusate, etc.), and the

S. Neubauer, MD, Medizinische Universitätsklinik Würzburg, Josef Schneider-Straße 2, D-97080 Würzburg, Germany

Table 9.1. Details regarding nuclei of interest for metabolic MRS

Nucleus	Natural abundance (%)	Relative MR sensitivity	Myocardial tissue concentrations
^1H	99.98	100	H_2O 110 M; up to ~90 mM (CH_3-^1H of creatine)
^{13}C	1.1	1.6×10^{-2}	Labelled compounds, several mM
^{19}F	100	83	Trace
^{23}Na	100	9.3	10 mM (intracellular); 140 mM (extracellular)
^{31}P	100	6.6	Up to ~18 mM (PCr)
^{39}K	9.1	4.6×10^{-2}	140 mM (intracellular); 4 mM (extracellular)
^{87}Rb	27.85	17	Trace

most widely studied nucleus is ^{31}P. Therefore, the basic principles of MRS [see GADIAN (1995) for a textbook on the basics of MRS] shall be derived from an example describing ^{31}P-MRS in an isolated heart; the principles, however, apply to MRS of all nuclei. An MR spectrometer consists of a high-field vertical or horizontal superconducting magnet (up to 12 T) with a bore size ranging from ca. 5 cm up to clinical dimensions. The magnet bore holds the nucleus-specific probe head with the radiofrequency (RF) coils used for MR excitation and signal reception. The magnet is interfaced with a computer console, the RF transmitter, and receiver. In an MRS experiment, after homogenizing the magnetic field with shim gradients, an RF impulse is sent into the RF coils for spin excitation. Thereafter, the resulting MR signal, the free induction decay (FID) is recorded and stored. Next, the FID, which relates time and signal intensity and represents an exponential decrease of signal with time, is subjected to a mathematical manipulation termed "Fourier transformation," resulting in an MR spectrum, which relates resonance frequency and signal intensity. Since MRS is an intrinsically insensitive technique, many RF impulses have to be applied (e.g., 100–200 for ^{31}P-MRS of isolated hearts) and the resulting FIDs have to be signal-averaged in order to obtain MR spectra with a sufficient "signal-to-noise ratio" (SNR) (signal amplitude divided by the standard deviation of background noise). The required number of "iterations" depends, among other factors, on the metabolite concentration of the sample, the filling factor, i.e., the mass of the observed object relative to the coil size, the natural abundance of the nucleus under study, its relative MR sensitivity (Table 9.1), the pulse angle, and the TR. When selecting pulse angles and TR for an MRS experiment, one has to be aware of the effects of "saturation." In analogy to principles inherent to MRI, a full MR signal from a given nucleus can only be obtained when the nucleus is excited from a fully relaxed spin state, i.e., when a time of at least ~5 × T1 has passed since the previous

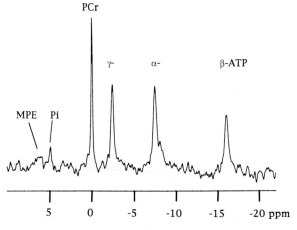

Fig. 9.1. ^{31}P-MR spectrum of an isolated, buffer-perfused rat heart obtained within 5 min at 7 T

excitation [for example T1 of phosphocreatine (PCr) at 7 T ~ 3 s, at 1.5 T ~ 6 s]; i.e., "fully relaxed" spectra can only be obtained with long TRs necessitating extensive measuring times. Since the initial part of the FID contains most of the information on the signal, use of faster TRs yields spectra with higher SNR for a given acquisition time. On the other hand, with TRs , < 5 × T1, part of the signal is lost due to saturation effects. Since the T1s of ^{31}P-metabolites such as PCr and adenosine triphosphate (ATP) differ, the extent of saturation is also different. When quantitating partially saturated spectra, one therefore has to apply "saturation factors" for defined experimental conditions. Such factors are determined individually for each metabolite by comparing fully relaxed and saturated spectra obtained sequentially. In practice, TRs and pulse angles for MRS are chosen to yield acceptable measurement times at a ~20%–50% degree of saturation. Larger degrees of saturation (i.e., very short TRs) make the quantification of spectra unreliable.

Figure 9.1 shows a ^{31}P-MR spectrum from an isolated, beating rat heart, obtained in 5 min at 7 T with a TR of 1.93 s and a pulse angle of 45°. Six resonances are identified (three ^{31}P atoms of ATP (γ–, α–, β–), PCr, inorganic phosphate, and monophosphate esters), which meet the following requirements: present in sufficient concentration (for ^{31}P > ca. 0.6 mM) and free in solution (immobilized metabolites such as plasma membrane phosphates give no quantifiable MR signal due to very short T2 values but rather contribute to a broad "baseline hump"). The phenomenon that different metabolites resonate at distinct frequencies, allowing their discrimination from each other, is termed "chemical shift" (expressed relative to the B1 field in ppm = parts per million): different positions in the molecule lead to subtle differences in the strength of the local magnetic field, thus spreading the resonance frequencies of ^{31}P metabolites over a range of ca. 30 ppm. The area under each resonance is proportional to the amount of each ^{31}P nucleus in the sample. Metabolite resonances are therefore quantified by integrating the peak area. For all but spectra with very high SNR, this is aided by using Lorentzian line curve fit routines. Relative metabolite levels can be calculated directly (e.g., the PCr/ATP ratio), but absolute metabolite concentrations can only be evaluated by comparing tissue resonance areas with those from an external ^{31}P reference standard (e.g., phenylphosphonate) (CLARKE et al. 1993; INGWALL 1982; NEUBAUER et al. 1991). Since the MRS measurement is noninvasive, sequential spectra can be obtained during any given protocol, and the dynamic response of metabolites in response to ischemia, inotropic stimulation, etc. can then be followed. This is in contrast to traditional biochemical methods where the tissue has to be frozen and extracted, allowing the study of only one time point.

9.3
Experimental Applications

9.3.1
^{31}P

^{31}P-MR allows the study of cardiac high-energy phosphate metabolism to noninvasively estimate the energetic state of the heart. Metabolites identified in the ^{31}P-MR spectrum from Fig. 9.1 were described above, i.e., ATP (γ–, α–, and β– atoms of ^{31}P; the resonance at the right shoulder of the α-P-ATP peak represents the P atom of NAD+), PCr, inorganic phosphate (Pi) and monophosphate esters [MPE; comprising mostly adenosine monophosphate (AMP) and glycolytic intermediates]. ATP is the main substrate

Creatine Kinase - Phosphocreatine Energy Shuttle

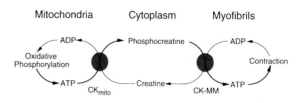

Fig. 9.2. Creatine kinase – phosphocreatine energy shuttle. For details, see text

for all energy-consuming reactions in the cell (LEHNINGER 1982). PCr, the other major high-energy phosphate compound, acts as an energy reservoir and probably has additional roles: First, PCr may serve as an energy transport molecule in the "creatine kinase/PCr energy shuttle" (INGWALL et al. 1985; WALLIMANN et al. 1992) (Fig. 9.2). It is believed that the high-energy phosphate bond is transferred from ATP to creatine at the site of ATP production, the mitochondria, yielding PCr and adenosine diphosphate (ADP). This reaction is catalyzed by the mitochondrial isoenzyme of creatine kinase. PCr, a much smaller molecule than ATP, then diffuses through the cytoplasm to the site of ATP utilization, the myofibrils, where the back reaction occurs, ATP is reformed and is used for contraction. This reaction is catalyzed by the myofibrillar-bound MM creatine kinase isoenzyme. Free creatine then diffuses back to the mitochondria. The existence of this "energy shuttle" is likely because the very low free cytosolic ADP concentration (40–80 µM) does not provide sufficient capacity for the back diffusion to the mitochondria (JACOBUS 1985; WALLIMANN et al. 1992). This function is therefore assigned to free creatine, which is present at concentrations that are at least two orders of magnitude higher than those of ADP. Second, PCr and creatine kinase serve to maintain free cytosolic ADP at its low concentration of 40–80 µM. Free ADP cannot be measured by any method but is calculated from the creatine kinase equilibrium assumption:

$$\text{ADP} = (\text{ATP} \times \text{creatine}) : (\text{PCr} \times \text{H}^+ \times K_{eq}),$$

where H$^+$ is the intracellular hydrogen ion concentration, and K_{eq} is the equilibrium constant of the creatine kinase reaction (LAWSON and VEECH 1979).

Maintenance of a low free cytosolic ADP concentration is crucial for normal cardiac function because ADP determines the free energy change of ATP hydrolysis (ΔG; KJ/mol), a measure of the amount of energy released from ATP hydrolysis:

$$\Delta G = \Delta G_0 + RT\ln(\text{ADP} \times \text{inorganic}$$
$$\text{phosphate}) : \text{ATP},$$

where ΔG_0 is the standard free energy change at 37°C, $Mg^{2+} = 1\,mM$; R = gas constant; T = temperature (K).

In normal cardiomyocytes, ΔG is in the order of $-58\,KJ/mol$. Below a threshold value for ΔG of about $-52\,KJ/mol$ many intracellular enzymes such as SR-Ca^{2+}-ATPase and others will not function properly (KAMMERMEIER et al. 1982). Thus, PCr has multiple important functions in cellular energy metabolism [see JACOBUS and INGWALL (1980) for further reading].

Inorganic phosphate is formed when ATP is hydrolyzed: ATP $\Leftrightarrow$ ADP + Pi, and increases when ATP utilization exceeds ATP production, such as in ischemia. In addition, intracellular pH (pHi) can be quantified from the chemical shift difference between PCr and inorganic phosphate, which is pH-sensitive (MOON and RICHARDS 1973), and similarly, the free cytosolic magnesium concentration (0.2–$0.6\,mM$) can be calculated from the chemical shift difference or peak height of α- and β-P-ATP (CLARKE et al. 1996; GUPTA et al. 1983; WU et al. 1981).

^{31}P-MRS can be used to study the dynamic changes of cardiac energy metabolism under various experimental conditions. An isolated perfused rat heart model is functionally and metabolically stable for ~ 90 min. The simplest application of this model is to study the effects of various substrates: PCr concentrations are, for example, higher for pyruvate and/or fatty acid substrates and for perfusion with blood (PCr/ATP ratio ~ 1.5–2.0) than when glucose is the only substrate (PCr/ATP ratio ~ 1.3) (INGWALL 1982). When cardiac workload is increased substantially, PCr levels also decrease (BITTL and INGWALL 1985; ZHANG et al. 1995). ATP content remains constant under all these conditions: due to the creatine kinase equilibrium favoring ATP synthesis over PCr synthesis by a factor of ~ 100, for any stress situation, ATP will only decrease when PCr is substantially depleted, as long as creatine kinase is not inhibited. This is the reason why the PCr/ATP ratio can be considered a measure of the energetic state of the heart. ^{31}P-MRS is ideally suited to study the changes of myocardial energy metabolism simultaneous to the alterations of cardiac function in ischemia and reperfusion (as a model for acute myocardial infarction and reperfusion due to thrombolysis). A related injury model is hypoxia/reoxygenation; hypoxia differs from ischemia in that only oxygen supply is stopped while reperfusion and

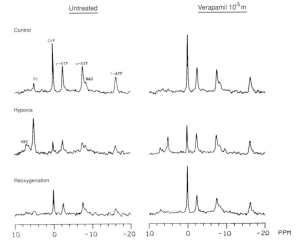

Fig. 9.3. ^{31}P-NMR spectra from an untreated perfused rat heart and a heart treated with verapamil during control, at the end of 30 min of hypoxia and at the end of 30 min of reperfusion. *NAD*, Nicotine adenine dinucleotide. For details, see text. *CP* or *CrP* = creatine phosphate, a term synonymous with phosphocreatine. [From NEUBAUER S and INGWALL JS (1989) J Mol Cell Cardiol 21:1163–1178. Reproduced with permission from Academic Press Limited]

substrate supply are maintained. As an example, Fig. 9.3 illustrates the changes of energy metabolism in a protocol of control perfusion, hypoxia, and reoxygenation: after 30 min of hypoxia, ATP resonances are reduced by $\sim 50\%$, PCr by $\sim 80\%$, and the resonances for inorganic phosphate and monophosphate esters have increased. With reoxygenation, inorganic phosphate shows full, PCr partial, and ATP no recovery. When hearts are pretreated with a Ca^{2+} antagonist (verapamil), changes in energetics are attenuated, i.e., verapamil protects hearts from the effects of hypoxic injury (NEUBAUER and INGWALL 1989). Using ^{31}P-MRS with a 12 s temporal resolution by summing spectra from multiple experiments, CLARKE et al. (1987) showed that the decrease in PCr and the increase in inorganic phosphate are among the very earliest metabolic responses in myocardial ischemia, changing only seconds after the onset of flow reduction; decreases in ATP and in pHi occur later, i.e., within minutes. For further details on energy metabolism in ischemia, the reader is referred to the literature (e.g., BAK and INGWALL 1994; NEUBAUER et al. 1988, 1994; NUNNALLY and HOLLIS 1979).

^{31}P-MRS has been used to examine the question of whether high-energy phosphate concentrations show oscillations as a function of the cardiac cycle (systole vs diastole). While some experiments in isolated hearts have detected such cyclic oscillations (FOSSEL et al. 1980; TOYO OKA et al. 1986), studies in large animals (KANTOR et al. 1986) and in man (GRIST et al. 1989) have not detected cyclical changes in ATP, PCr, or inorganic phosphate. A unique aspect of ^{31}P-MRS is that it can be used not only to quantitate steady state metabolite levels but also to measure the rate and velocity of chemical reactions in vivo (in mM/s), using *magnetization (saturation) transfer* methods (for further reading see FORSEN and HOFMAN 1963; SPENCER et al. 1988). In heart, the creatine kinase and ATP synthesis reactions are most suitable. It was shown, for example, that creatine kinase reaction velocity correlates with cardiac workload (BITTL and INGWALL 1985). During recovery after ischemia, creatine kinase reaction velocity is closely correlated with the recovery of mechanical function (NEUBAUER et al. 1988). It is important to apply this method to the human heart (BOTTOMLEY and HARDY 1992), which has yet to be done in patients with heart disease.

Experimental ^{31}P-MRS studies have contributed to our understanding of the pathophysiology of heart failure. A number of heart failure models have been examined, including the spontaneously hypertensive rat (BITTL and INGWALL 1987), the Syrian cardiomyopathic hamster (BUSER et al. 1989; NASCIMBEN et al. 1995), furazolidone-induced cardiomyopathy in the turkey (LIAO et al. 1996), and, as the clinically most relevant model, chronic coronary artery ligation in rat (NEUBAUER et al. 1995a) and pig (ZHANG et al. 1996). Uniformly, the failing myocardium is characterized by reduced PCr, unchanged or moderately reduced ATP, unchanged or increased inorganic phosphate, substantially reduced creatine kinase reaction velocity (parameters measured with ^{31}P-MRS) and also by reduced total creatine content, total and mitochondrial creatine kinase activity and increased fetal BB- and MB-creatine kinase isoenzymes (parameters measured with traditional biochemical techniques). These changes are likely to contribute to the impairment of the contractile reserve of the failing myocardium, probably due to the failure to maintain high ΔG values (see above) during inotropic stimulation (INGWALL 1993). These experimental reports have set the stage for the clinical studies of human heart failure described later. Recently, using molecular gene ablation methods, mice with a null mutant (i.e., total lack) of both MM- (VAN DEUSSEN et al. 1993) and "double" (MM- and mitochondrial-) creatine kinase isoenzymes (STEEGHS et al. 1997) have been created. These new "knockout" models will undoubtedly provide unique information on the role of energetics in heart failure.

Most experimental ^{31}P-MRS studies have been performed without spatial localization or with the crude localization achieved with surface coils. More recently, spectroscopic imaging in one (FRIEDRICH et al. 1995) or three (VON KIENLIN et al. 1998) dimensions has been reported, allowing the analysis of regional heterogeneity of cardiac energy metabolism. In large animals such as dog and pig, ROBITAILLE et al. (1989) and ZHANG et al. (1993) were able to obtain ^{31}P spectra from five distinct voxels spanning the LV wall, thereby examining transmural heterogeneity of energy metabolism. These studies suggest that during cardiac stress energetic changes are more pronounced in the subendocardium than in the subepicardium.

9.3.2
^{1}H, ^{13}C, ^{19}F, ^{23}Na, ^{39}K, and ^{87}Rb

^{1}H shows high natural abundance and the highest MR sensitivity of all MR-detectable nuclei (Table 9.1). Since ^{1}H is contained in the largest number of metabolites, in principle, many metabolites can be detected such as creatine, lactate, carnitine, taurine, -CH$_3$ and -CH$_2$ resonances of lipids, and so on (BALSCHI et al. 1995; UGURBIL et al. 1984). Most promising may be the measurement of total creatine (in conjunction with ^{31}P-MRS, this allows quantification of total, free, and phosphorylated creatine) (BOTTOMLEY et al. 1996a) and of the deoxymyoglobin resonances (KREUTZER and JUE 1991). On the downside, ^{1}H-MRS is technically demanding, requiring pulse sequences for suppression of the large ^{1}H signal from water. ^{1}H spectra are complex and show overlapping resonances, many of which still have to be identified. However, next to ^{31}P, ^{1}H-MRS has the greatest potential for clinical application.

The ^{13}C nucleus has a low natural abundance (1.1%); for this reason, one has to supply the heart with nontracer amounts of ^{13}C-labelled compounds such as, for example, 99% enriched 1-^{13}C-glucose, which are typically added to perfusion media or infused into the coronary arteries for a defined length of time. We can then study substrate selection by the heart for fueling energy metabolism (MALLOY et al. 1996; SOLOMON et al. 1996) or use a specifically selected substrate to probe the activities of key enzymes or entire metabolic pathways, most prominently, citric acid cycle kinetics, pyruvate dehydrogenase flux, and beta-oxidation of fatty acids (LEWANDOWSKI et al. 1996; LEWANDOWSKI and

WHITE 1995; ROBITAILLE et al. 1993; WEISS et al. 1992). Experimentally, these methods have been of tremendous use for the analysis of intermediary metabolism and mitochondrial function in animal models of heart disease. Clinical applications, however, have not yet been reported for the heart, if only for methological reasons: (1) the ^{13}C nucleus does not provide the required sensitivity for spatially resolved detection in a reasonable measuring time; (2) the high concentrations of exogenous, ^{13}C-labeled precursors are generally unphysiological; and (3) for in vivo studies it is necessary to infuse the ^{13}C-labeled compounds into coronary arteries to avoid confounding effects of intravenous infusion, which has the problem of systemic delivery to other organs and global metabolic effects of the precursor.

^{19}F-MRS has been used to follow the fate of ^{19}F-labeled pharmacological agents, particularly in tumor therapy (PRESANT et al. 1994). In experimental cardiology, ^{19}F-labeled Ca^{2+}-indicators such as 5-F-BAPTA have been used to indirectly measure intracellular Ca^{2+} concentrations (MURPHY et al. 1994), since the naturally abundant ^{40}Ca escapes MR detection due to the absence of a nuclear spin. Clinical cardiac applications of ^{19}F-MRS cannot be foreseen at present.

Maintenance and control of the extra- /intracellular Na^+ gradient ($\sim 140\,mM$ vs $\sim 10\,mM$) is one characteristic of normal functioning heart cells (EISNER et al. 1984; KIM et al. 1987). This gradient is largely responsible for setting the membrane potential. During excitation, Na^+ enters the cardiomyocyte through the "fast" Na^+ channel; Na^+ is removed from the cell by the action of the ouabain-sensitive Na^+/K^+-ATPase. In addition, Na^+ movements involve Na^+–Ca^{2+} and Na^+–H^+ exchange mechanisms. ^{23}Na-MRS, therefore, has become a valuable, in fact the only, noninvasive (as opposed to microelectrode techniques) method to evaluate changes in intra- and extracellular Na^+ during cardiac injury (KOHLER et al. 1991; PIKE et al. 1985; SPRINGER et al. 1985). A ^{23}Na spectrum from the heart shows one single peak representing the total Na^+ signal. In order to discriminate intra- and extracellular Na^+ pools, paramagnetic shift reagents, such as $[DyTTHA]^{3-}$ or $[TmDOTP]^{5-}$, are added to the perfusate. These chelate complexes are distributed in the extracellular (i.e., intravascular and interstitial) compartments but do not enter the intracellular space. Na^+ in the immediate vicinity of shift reagent experiences a downfield chemical shift of its resonance frequency, the extent of the shift being proportional to the shift reagent concentration. Experimentally, this method

has been used to examine the mechanisms of Na^+ accumulation in ischemia (INGWALL 1995; MALLOY et al. 1990; VAN ECHTELD et al. 1991) (Fig. 9.4) or the mechanisms of ventricular fibrillation, which is preceded by accumulation of intracellular Na^+ (NEUBAUER et al. 1992c). Currently, the author is unaware of attempts to develop ^{23}Na shift reagents for clinical use. This is regrettable, since, although no such studies have been done, ^{23}Na-MRS is promising for clinical applications, being potentially useful for detection of exercise-induced ischemia and evaluation of myocardial viability. In the meantime, experimental MRI of total ^{23}Na has been reported (DELAYRE et al. 1981), increased total Na signal being demonstrated in acutely ischemic myocardium (KIM et al. 1997). Due to the relatively high sensitivity of ^{23}Na and its short T1, allowing for rapid TRs, total Na imaging appears well feasible in humans; however, whether imaging of total Na instead of intra- vs extracellular pools has clinical value will have to be determined.

The potential of ^{39}K-MRS is, in principle, similar to that of ^{23}Na-MRS, but, due to the much lower MR sensitivity, ^{39}K-MRS studies have been much more difficult (PIKE et al. 1985). To overcome the problem of low sensitivity of the ^{39}K nucleus, ^{87}Rb-MRS (with Rb^+ as K^+ analogue) has been used with success to evaluate K^+ movements in the heart (CROSS et al. 1995; KUPRIYANOV et al. 1995).

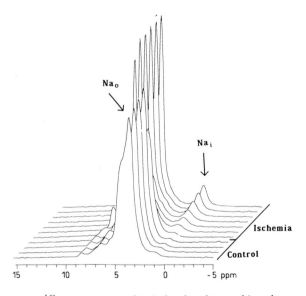

Fig. 9.4. ^{23}Na MR spectra of an isolated rat heart subjected to control and total, global ischemia. The increase in intracellular Na during ischemia is evident. Each spectrum was obtained in 4 min at 8.4 T, 960 FIDs, pulse angle 90°, and TR = 122 ms. Na_o, extracellular Na; Na_i, intracellular Na. (From NEUBAUER S, INGWALL JS, unpublished figure)

9.4
Clinical Applications

9.4.1
Technical Considerations

Almost without exception, human cardiac spectroscopy has been confined to the ^{31}P nucleus. The reasons for this include the extensive experience with the method from experimental work, the relevance of energetics for various forms of heart disease, and the relatively high concentrations of the ^{31}P metabolites ATP and PCr in heart muscle. Methodologically, clinical cardiac spectroscopy faces a number of major technical challenges. Total examination time (including imaging and spectroscopy) should not exceed 1 h, and even this may not be tolerated by patients with severe cardiac disease; thus, time for signal acquisition is limited. The heart is rapidly moving, requiring gating to the heart beat, and, possibly, to respiration as well. Cardiac muscle is situated behind a layer of chest wall skeletal muscle, giving rise to a strong ^{31}P signal that must be suppressed; unlike in experimental studies, this necessitates the use of additional localization techniques, which, in turn, are unavoidably associated with substantial signal loss. Localization techniques that have been applied to the human heart include DRESS (depth-resolved-surface-coil-spectroscopy), rotating frame, 1D-CSI (chemical shift imaging), ISIS (image-selected in vivo spectroscopy), and 3D-CSI. Some details are given in Fig. 9.5; a full review (BOTTOMLEY 1994) is beyond the scope of this chapter.

Most of the methodological work on human cardiac MRS has been pioneered by P. Bottomley (BOTTOMLEY 1995; BOTTOMLEY et al. 1990, 1996b). VON KIENLIN and MEJIA (1991) introduced a new localization method termed SLOOP (spectra localization with optimum pointspread function), which allows selection of voxel sizes of not only rectangular, but any, even curved, shape; this should aid cardiac MRS by improved matching of voxel and heart shape. Most groups have examined patients in the prone rather than the supine position, since this reduces motion artifacts as well as the distance of the heart to the surface coil. For most spectroscopic techniques, a series of ^{1}H scout images is first obtained, which is used to select the spectroscopic volume(s). Due to the relatively low sensitivity of Space ^{31}P-MRS, required voxel sizes have been quite large, usually >30 cm^3. However, improvements in coil design, localization techniques, and, possibly,

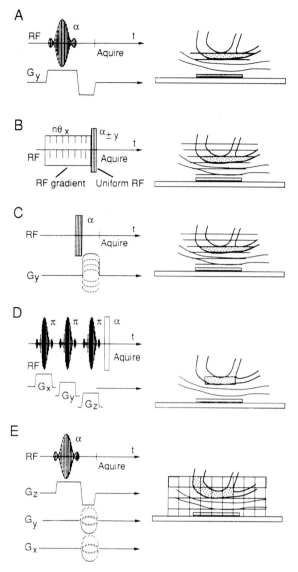

Fig. 9.5 A–E. Basic pulse sequences for localized cardiac spectroscopy with surface coils. **A** "Depth-resolved surface coil spectroscopy." A single section parallel to the plane of the surface coil is selected by applying an MRI gradient G in the presence of a modulated RF excitation pulse of flip angle α. **B** The "rotating frame" MR method uses the gradient inherent in a surface coil to simultaneously spatially encode spectra from multiple sections parallel to the surface coil by means of application of a θ flip angle pulse, which is stepped in subsequent applications of the sequence. **C** The "one-dimensional chemical shift imaging" method similarly encodes multiple sections but uses an MRI gradient whose amplitude is stepped. **D** The "image-selected in vivo spectroscopy" method localizes to a single volume with selective inversion pulses applied with G_x, G_y, and G_z MRI gradients. All eight combinations of the three pulses must be applied and the resultant signals added and subtracted. **E** A section-selective "three-dimensional chemical shift imaging" sequence employs MRI section selection in one dimension and phase encoding in two dimensions. [From BOTTOMLEY P (1994) Radiology 191:596. Figure and legend reprinted with permission from the Radiological Society of North America]

field strength (HETHERINGTON et al. 1995; MENON and HENDRICH 1992) should allow ³¹P spectroscopicimaging with voxel sizes of <10 cm³. Figure 9.6 shows a typical ³¹P-MR spectrum of a healthy volunteer acquired from a ~60 cm³ voxelusing ISIS and a TR of 15 s. Compared with the rat heart spectrum, SNR is lower, and two additional resonances appear: 2,3-diphosphoglycerate (2,3-DPG), arising from the presence of blood (erythrocytes) in the selected voxel, and phosphodiesters, a signal assigned to membrane as well as serum phospholipids. The 2,3-DPG resonances appear at a similar frequency as inorganic phosphate, which therefore cannot be detected in blood-contaminated human spectra. For the same reason, intracellular pH cannot be determined; intracellular inorganic phosphate and pH should ultimately be measurable in human myocardium when voxel sizes are small enough to avoid major blood contamination of ³¹P spectra.

Human ³¹P spectra can be directly quantified in relative terms, i.e., the PCr/ATP and phosphodiester/ATP peak area ratios are calculated. PCr/ATP is considered an index of the energetic state of the heart (see above), while the meaning of the phosphodiester/ATP ratio is poorly understood; it was suggested that an increase in phosphodiester/ATP indicates membrane damage (AUFFERMANN et al. 1991), but phosphodiester/ATP ratios do not seem to change with cardiac disease. Absolute quantification of PCr and ATP is technically demanding, but required if ³¹P-MRS is to evolve as a clinical modality. In principle, absolute ³¹P metabolite levels can be quantified by obtaining simultaneous signal from a ³¹P standard as well as estimates of myocardial mass based on MRI (BOTTOMLEY et al. 1990). Recently, an elegant method for absolute quantification has been introduced (BOTTOMLEY et al. 1996b),

which is based on simultaneous acquisition of a ¹H spectrum that is used to calibrate the ³¹P signal to the tissue water proton content. This method allows absolute quantification without estimates of myocardial mass based on MRI.

Human ³¹P spectra need to be corrected for the effects of partial saturation based on the principles described above (Sect. 9.2). After initial conflicting results on T1 values of human cardiac ³¹P metabolites (NEUBAUER et al. 1992a; van DOBBENBURGH et al. 1994), a consensus exists that at 1.5 T, the T1 of PCr is ~4.4. ± 0.5 s, and the T1 of ATP is ~2.4 ± 0.4 s (BOTTOMLEY 1994). ³¹P T1s do not seem to change with cardiac disease (BOTTOMLEY et al. 1991a), although this remains to be examined in detail. Correction for the amount of blood contamination is also required: blood contributes signal from ATP, 2,3-DPG, and phosphodiesters to the ³¹P heart spectrum. A practical approach for blood correction involves obtaining ³¹P spectra from human blood. In our hands, such spectra show an ATP/2,3-DPG area ratio of ~0.11, corresponding to a molar ratio of 0.22, and a phosphodiester/2,3-DPG area ratio of ~0.19. Thus, for blood correction, the ATP resonance area is reduced by 11% of the 2,3-DPG resonance area (NEUBAUER et al. 1992b). ³¹P-metabolite ratios in the blood may change in the presence of disease, however (HORN et al. 1993), so that measurement of individual blood ³¹P signals is advisable for correction. In the long term, hopefully, blood correction will no longer be required when voxel sizes are further reduced to obtain spectra largely uncontaminated by blood. Due to limited SNR, for area integration of resonances from human ³¹P spectra, an algorithm is required that allows for time domain or frequency domain Lorentzian line fitting. Generally, an effort should be undertaken to develop technical standards for acquisition and processing of human cardiac MR spectra. The ultimate success of this method will also depend on comparability and compatibility of MRS measurements from centers at different locations, necessitating standardized procedures that currently do not exist.

A present limitation of ³¹P-MRS is that the method can interrogate the anterior portion of the heart only. Typical parameters for ³¹P surface coils range from 8 to 15 cm, and the B1 field characteristics of these coils make detection of the more distant, posterior parts of the heart impossible. Whether novel approaches to coil design, such as phased array ³¹P coils (HARDY et al. 1992), will allow interrogation of the posterior wall remains to be seen.

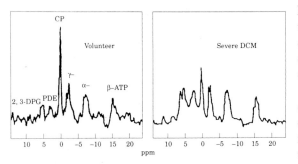

Fig. 9.6. ³¹P-MR spectrum from the human heart of a volunteer and a patient with dilated cardiomyopathy. The reduction of the PCr resonance in the patient is apparent. [From NEUBAUER S et al. (1995b) Eur Heart J 16 (Suppl O):115–118. Reproduced with permission from W.B. Saunders Company Ltd.]

9.4.2
Normal Values for Human Cardiac High-Energy Phosphates

The available literature suggests that in normal human heart the PCr/ATP ratio is ~1.8 (BOTTOMLEY 1994); for our own volunteer group we obtained a value of ~2.0 (NEUBAUER et al. 1992b). The normal myocardial ATP concentration is ~10 mM, and thus, the PCr concentration is ~18 mM (INGWALL 1993). These numbers agree with measurements in animal hearts in vivo (LANGE et al. 1984; NEUBAUER and INGWALL 1989). It is likely, and our own experience indicates, that PCr/ATP ratios do no change with age in the absence of cardiac disease, although no systematic studies on this subject are available.

9.4.3
Heart Failure and Cardiac Transplantation

As described above, experimental studies have shown reduced PCr, total creatine and creatine kinase reaction velocity in chronically failing myocardium (NASCIMBEN et al. 1995; NEUBAUER et al. 1995a). For human ^{31}P-MRS in heart failure, these results would predict a decrease in the PCr/ATP ratio. Initial studies, however, failed to detect significant reductions in the PCr/ATP ratio (AUFFERMANN et al. 1991; DE ROOS et al. 1992; MASUDA et al. 1992; SCHAEFER et al. 1990). These early reports did not grade patients for the severity of heart failure and included all stages of disease severity. Hardy et al. were the first to show that the myocardial PCr/ATP ratio was significantly reduced (from 1.80 ± 0.06 to 1.46 ± 0.07) in symptomatic patients with heart failure of ischemic or nonischemic origin (HARDY et al. 1991). We reported that the decrease in PCr/ATP ratios in dilated cardiomyopathy (DCM) correlated with the clinical severity of heart failure according to the New York Heart Association (NYHA) class (NEUBAUER et al. 1992b) (Fig. 9.7) and also with LV ejection fraction (NEUBAUER et al. 1995b). Thus, the PCr/ATP ratio decreases for the highly symptomatic stages of heart failure but remains normal during initial stages. This observation suggests that changes in cardiac energetics are unlikely to be primary causal events leading to the development of failure, but rather that altered energetics are a contributing factor worsening heart failure during the more advanced stages.

Given that the PCr/ATP ratio changes only in advanced heart failure, what clinical information could

^{31}P-MRS provide in these patients? First, as the only noninvasive method to probe high-energy phosphate metabolism in humans, ^{31}P-MRS may be applied to study the changes in cardiac energetics in response to medical therapy in heart failure. Our initial observations showed that in six patients with DCM treated with standard medical therapy including ACE inhibitors, digitalis, diuretics, and, in four patients, beta-blockers, clinical recompensation occurred over a 3-month period. During this time, the PCr/ATP ratio of the patients improved significantly from 1.51 ± 0.32 to 2.15 ± 0.27 (NEUBAUER et al. 1992b). Currently, we are performing a larger, blinded, placebo-controlled trial of the effects of chronic beta-blocker therapy on symptoms, cardiac hemodynamics and energetics in patients with heart failure due to DCM. Evaluation of energetic effects of various forms of medical therapy in heart failure may become clinically important. Second, the PCr/ATP ratio may provide prognostic information on survival of patients with heart failure that extends beyond the prognostic relevance of clinical and hemodynamic variables. We recently showed that in DCM, the myocardial PCr/ATP ratio was a better predictor of long-term survival than LV ejection fraction or NYHA class (NEUBAUER et al. 1997a) (Fig. 9.8). Thus, ^{31}P-MRS may become established as a tool for prognostic evaluation in heart failure. It is possible that determination of creatine kinase reaction velocity in heart failure will provide an even more relevant energetic index, but presently, this parameter has been measured in volunteers only (BOTTOMLEY and HARDY 1992), and studies in heart

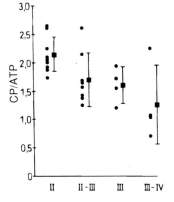

Fig. 9.7. Phosphocreatine (CP)/ATP ratios in patients with dilated cardiomyopathy graded according to the NYHA classification for heart failure. For each NYHA grade, raw and mean data are shown. Correlation between the NYHA grade and CP/ATP was highly significant ($r = 0.60$; $P < 0.005$). [From NEUBAUER S et al. (1992) Circulation 86:1810–1818. Reproduced with permission from the American Heart Assocation]

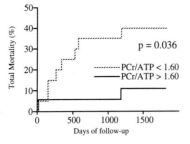

Fig. 9.8. Kaplan-Meier life table analysis for total mortality of dilated cardiomyopathy patients divided into two groups split by the myocardial PCr/ATP ratio (<1.60 vs >1.60). Patients with an initially low PCr/ATP ratio showed increased mortality over the study period of, on average, 2.5 years. [From NEUBAUER S et al. (1997) Circulation 96:2190–2196. Reproduced with permission from the American Heart Association]

failure are eagerly awaited, although technically demanding.

With regard to cardiac transplantation, experimental reports had raised the hope that ^{31}P-MRS might be used to detect transplant rejection and possibly, at least in part, substitute for repetitive biopsies (FRASER et al. 1990; HAUG et al. 1987). However, clinical studies have been less promising. In the only published full paper on this subject, the PCr/ATP ratio was reduced in transplanted hearts with rejection, but there was no correlation with histological scores estimated from myocardial biopsies (BOTTOMLEY et al. 1991b). To complicate matters further, the PCr/ATP ratio seems to decrease during the first few weeks after transplantation as a result of myocardial ischemia during the acute operative procedure (VAN DOBBENBURGH et al. 1993), slowly recovering thereafter. Thus, PCr/ATP ratios presently do not appear suitable for the detection of acute cardiac transplant rejection. However, it is conceivable that measurement of absolute concentrations of ATP and PCr may prove more useful in this context: if myocyte mass is reduced during rejection, the PCr/ATP ratio may be unaltered because ATP and PCr decrease in parallel. Such studies remain to be done.

9.4.4
Valvular Heart Disease and Other Forms of Cardiac Hypertrophy

As in the case of heart failure, experimental work indicates alterations in myocardial energy metabolism at least for higher grades of LV hypertrophy (WEXLER et al. 1988; ZHANG et al. 1993). Only two

complete studies have been reported on changes of cardiac energy metabolism in human valvular heart disease. In patients with aortic stenosis or incompetence, CONWAY et al. (1991) found a reduced PCr/ATP ratio (1.10 ± 0.32 vs 1.50 ± 0.20 in volunteers; mean $\pm$ SD) only when clinical signs of heart failure were present, while the PCr/ATP ratio remained unchanged (1.56 ± 0.15) for clinically asymptomatic stages, in analogy to our findings in DCM. Our own work on patients with aortic valve disease, similarly, indicates a reduction in PCr/ATP ratios for patients with NYHA class III or more but not for those with NYHA class I or II. Also, for the same degree of heart failure, energy metabolism may be more affected in aortic stenosis (pressure overload) than in aortic incompetence. Finally, we showed that in aortic stenosis, reductions in the PCr/ATP ratio correlate with LV end-diastolic pressures and also with end-diastolic wall stress (NEUBAUER et al. 1997b). The challenge for ^{31}P-MRS is to provide additional clinical information that might contribute to the optimum timing for valve replacement in these patients. For aortic stenosis, the consensus is that symptomatic patients should be operated on, but how to proceed with asymptomatic or marginally symptomatic cases remains a matter of debate. In aortic incompetence, available grading methods, such as echocardiography or radionuclide ventriculography, often leave cardiologists with the difficult decision at what time valve replacement would be of greatest benefit for the patient. Long-term prospective clinical studies will have to answer the question whether ^{31}P-MRS measurements of the myocardial PCr/ATP ratio and, in the future, also of absolute levels of ATP and PCr, provide clinically relevant independent information on the optimum timing for valve replacement. Furthermore, future studies should examine the question whether and/or when alterations in energy metabolism are reversible following valve replacement, and how energetic changes relate to the recovery of LV function, volumes and mass.

Although reports based on small patient numbers have appeared (MASUDA et al. 1992; SCHAEFFER et al. 1990), systematic clinical studies of cardiac energy metabolism in patients with LV hypertrophy due to long-term hypertensive heart disease in relation to LV function, volumes, and mass remain to be reported. ^{31}P-MRS would allow one to follow the energetic correlates of hypertrophy regression during various forms of antihypertensive therapy. An interesting recent study by PLUIM et al. (1996) showed that "physiological" hypertrophy in the athlete's heart differs from hypertrophy due to pathological causes in that the myocardial PCr/ATP ratio remains normal (2.2 ± 0.3 vs 2.2 ± 0.2 in volunteers; mean ± SD); experimental work in rats subjected to swim exercise had predicted this finding (SPENCER et al. 1997). The molecular reasons for these differences in energy metabolism between physiological and pathological myocardial hypertrophy are an important area for future basic and clinical research.

Hypertrophic cardiomyopathy (HCM) is, in most cases, due to well-characterized genetic mutations associated with substantial increases in LV wall thickness and structural disarray of myofibrils (SPIRITO et al. 1997). HCM can, but does not have to, be associated with an LV outflow gradient (obstructive or nonobstructive HCM). Recent experimental studies of a gene-targeted mouse model of HCM suggest an alteration of cardiac energetics (SPINDLER et al. 1996). Similarly, human studies in HCM (DE ROOS et al. 1992; MASUDA et al. 1992; RAJAGOPALAN et al. 1987; SAKUMA et al. 1993; SIEVERDING et al. 1997; WEISS et al. 1990) have mostly shown reduced PCr/ATP ratios in myocardial tissue affected by hypertrophy. While these studies are promising, many questions remain: Problems to be solved in MRS of HCM patients include spatial localization exclusively to affected in contrast to neighbouring nonhypertrophied myocardium, exact definition of the subtype of HCM including underlying genetic mutations in relation to the energetic imbalance (HCM comprises a whole family of distinct gene mutations), and absolute quantification of ATP and phosphocreatine, since myocyte loss may not be detectable from metabolite ratio measurements.

9.4.5
Coronary Artery Disease

The largest field for potential clinical applications of ^{31}P-MRS is coronary artery disease leading to acute or chronic myocardial ischemia, i.e., an imbalance between myocardial oxygen supply and demand. Two applications are conceivable: (1) "biochemical ergometry" and (2) evaluation of myocardial viability. As described above (Sect. 9.3.1), a decrease in PCr and an increase in inorganic phosphate are among the very earliest metabolic responses in myocardial ischemia, changing within seconds after reduction of oxygen supply. One can therefore envision a "biochemical stress test" that allows for the detection of the regional biochemical consequences of myocardial ischemia at rest, during

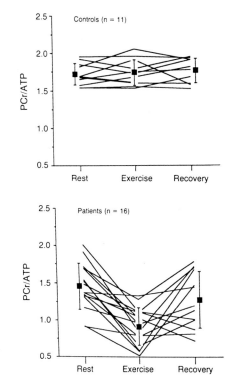

Fig. 9.9. PCr/ATP ratios at rest, during handgrip exercise, and after recovery in controls and in patients with stenosis of the LAD. PCr/ATP decreased in patients but not in healthy volunteers. [From WEISS RG et al. (1992) N Engl J Med 323:1593–1600. Reproduced with permission of the New England Journal of Medicine]

exercise and after recovery. WEISS et al. were first to report this application (Fig. 9.9). In patients with high-grade stenosis of the left anterior descending coronary artery (LAD), they found a normal PCr/ATP ratio at rest; PCr/ATP decreased during hand grip exercise, leading to a 30%–35% increase in cardiac work, from 1.5 ± 0.3 to 0.9 ± 0.2, and returned towards normal after recovery from exercise (WEISS et al. 1990). After revascularization, the PCr/ATP ratio no longer changed with exercise. These results were reproduced by YABE et al. (1994); these authors also demonstrated that a decrease in PCr/ATP ratios could be detected in patients with reversible defects on thallium scintigraphy (presumably viable myocardium capable of becoming acutely ischemic) but not in those with fixed thallium defects (presumably scar), where PCr/ATP was already reduced at rest (YABE et al. 1995). It is clear that such a biochemical stress test would find its way into routine cardiological practice as a way to noninvasively study the direct biochemical consequences of exercise on the heart, if technical advances could achieve a sufficient spatial (i.e., 5 cm^3 and less) and temporal (i.e., 10 min and less) resolution. Such a method would, for example, allow the noninvasive study of the effectiveness of revascularization procedures or of various antianginal therapies. One can envision that a "PCr threshold" may emerge as a clinically relevant parameter, representing the level of exercise achievable without a decrease in myocardial PCr concentrations.

The second potential area for application of ^{31}P-MRS in coronary artery disease is the evaluation of myocardial viability (see Chap. 7). Akinetic, i.e., noncontracting myocardium, that is supplied by a stenotic coronary artery may be nonviable (scarred), in which case revascularization by percutaneous transluminal coronary angioplasty or bypass grafting will not restore contractility and is probably of litte clinical benefit. Alternatively, such myocardium may be viable, i.e., biochemically and morphologically largely intact, but has downregulated contractility in order to reduce its energetic needs, thereby adjusting the balance between oxygen supply and demand ("hibernating myocardium"; VANOVERSCHELDE et al. 1997). Experimentally, both biochemical (NEUBAUER et al. 1995a) and ^{31}P-MRS measurements (FRIEDRICH et al. 1995; VON KIENLIN et al., 1998) have shown that myocardial scar tissue contains negligible amounts of ATP (<1% of control levels), while in hibernating myocardium, ATP levels remain close to normal (FLAMENG et al. 1987). Therefore, a method that allows evaluation of myocardial ATP content levels with high spatial (5 cm^3 or less) and acceptable temporal resolution (30 min or less) should be ideally suited for detection of myocardial viability, especially since current clinical methods for viability assessment (see below) are problematic. So far, only one clinical study has addressed this; YABE et al. (1995) reported that the absolute myocardial ATP content was significantly reduced in patients with fixed thallium defects (nonviable) but unchanged in those with reversible thallium defects (viable myocardium). While these initial results are promising, technical advances are required to achieve the necessary resolution, and systematic clinical studies comparing ^{31}P-MRS evaluation of ATP content with traditional viability measures such as ^{201}Tl uptake (scintigraphy), ^{18}F-deoxyglucose uptake (PET), or recruitment of inotropic reserve with dobutamine (echocardiography or MRI) are needed to establish the clinical value of the technique. It is conceivable that ^{31}P-MRS may evolve as a superior method with highest sensitivity and specificity, since it relies on quantification of an intrinsic marker (ATP) and is thus independent from myocardial perfusion, tracer uptake or inotropic response (severely ischemic myocardium may not increase but rather decrease its contractility upon dobutamine stimulation).

A promising new technique that may prove valuable for viability detection is determination of the absolute content of total creatine (i.e., free and phosphorylated creatine) by means of localized ^{1}H-MRS (BOTTOMLEY et al. 1996a). Scar tissue is not only characterized by reduced ATP content but also by an almost complete loss of total creatine. The resolution of this method is superior to that of ^{31}P-MRS, due to higher MR sensitivity of ^{1}H compared to ^{31}P and also because the concentration of CH$_3$-creatine protons is ca. tenfold higher than the ^{31}P concentration of ATP. Voxel sizes of ~1 cm^3 are achievable, and, in addition, the posterior wall can be interrogated. On the other hand, several methodological problems associated with ^{1}H-MRS (see Sect. 9.3.2) remain to be solved prior to more widespread clinical application. It is conceivable, however, that measurement of total creatine content by ^{1}H-MRS for viability assessment will become a practical, accepted, and clinically relevant diagnostic procedure (BOTTOMLEY and WEISS 1998).

9.5
Conclusions and Future Perspective

This chapter has described the technical principles and pathophysiological background for MRS of the heart, as well as the potential clinical applications, which are manifold. If cardiac MRS is as attractive as is claimed, why, then, has it not yet found its way into clinical practice, and why has development of the method been relatively slow? Several factors are responsible: For researchers potentially interested in clinical cardiac MRS, the technical challenges are substantial. At the same time, interpretation of MRS results requires a thorough knowledge of cardiac physiology and biochemistry. These factors necessitate a multidisciplinary collaboration involving cardiologists, radiologists, physicists and biochemists, and only a small number of institutions have been able to assemble such a broad team of scientists. Finally, the lack of industry support has slowed progress substantially. While, presently, development of imaging methods promises financial returns within a foreseeable time, development of cardiac MRS requires a long-term perspective, and the motivation of manufacturers is currently low.

What are the necessary developments for clinical cardiac MRS? Most importantly, there is a need to substantially improve temporal and spatial resolution. Using nuclear Overhauser enhancement, higher field strengths, and other improvements in hardware and software design, true 3D metabolic imaging with voxel sizes of $5\,cm^3$ for ^{31}P and $1\,cm^3$ for ^1H may be achievable (HETHERINGTON et al. 1995). Stratification of technical design for MRS protocols will be required in order to render measurements taken on different MR systems comparable. For this purpose, research groups using this method will have to agree on standards for localization procedures, pulse sequences, spectral processing, curve fit routines, etc. Absolute quantification of ^{31}P metabolites (as opposed to metabolite ratio measurements) must become a routine approach, and many of the clinical questions described in this chapter will have to be readdressed with measurements of absolute contents of ATP and PCr. Combination of ^1H- and ^{31}P-MRS in one examination is highly desirable and will allow estimation of energetic parameters such as free ADP and free energy change of ATP hydrolysis, which are probably more powerful indicators of cardiac disease states than steady state levels of ATP and PCr. In the long term, success of MRS will also depend on development of an "integrated cardiac MR examination" that allows the evaluation of morphology, global and regional function, perfusion, coronary anatomy, and metabolism within one diagnostic test (POHOST 1995). Human cardiac MRS of nuclei other than ^{31}P and ^1H, such as ^{13}C or ^{23}Na, may also offer unique insights into human cardiac metabolism in heart disease; these techniques should be established, although many methodological problems remain to be solved.

In summary, at the present time no routine clinical applications exist for human cardiac spectroscopy in patients with cardiac disease. However, if the technical advances indicated above can be made, this noninvasive method for the study of cardiac metabolism in human heart disease without the need for external radioactive tracers could well find its way into routine clinical cardiological practice.

Acknowledgements. The author would like to thank the following colleagues (listed in alphabetic order) for their contributions over many years of collaboration: GERALD BERTSCH, MEINRAD BEER, CHARLOTTE DIENESCH, GEORG ERTL, MARK DE GROOT, AXEL HAASE, DIETBERT HAHN, MICHAEL HORN, STEPHANIE HÜGEL, KAI HU, JOANNE S. INGWALL, MARKUS VON KIENLIN, KURT KOCHSIEK, THOMAS KRAHE, KLAUS LACKNER, WILFRIED LANDSCHÜTZ, ANDREA LEUPOLD, MARTIN MEININGER, THOMAS PABST, HELGA REMKES, JÖRN SANDSTEDE, KLAUS SCHNACKERZ, MATTHIAS SPINDLER, HINRIK STRÖMER, RONG TIAN, FRANK WIESMANN. The author also thanks Paul Bottomley for contributing Fig. 9.5, and Douglas Lewandowski for discussion on the paragraph on ^{13}C-MRS.

References

Auffermann W, Chew WM, Wolfe CL, et al. (1991) Normal and diffusely abnormal myocardium in humans: functional and metabolic characterization with P-31 MR spectroscopy and cine MR imaging. Radiology 179:253–259

Bak MI, Ingwall JS (1994) Acidosis during ischemia promotes adenosine triphosphate resynthesis in postischemic rat heart. In vivo regulation of 5′-nucleotidase. J Clin Invest 93:40–49

Balschi JA, Hetherington HP, Bradley EL Jr, Pohost GM (1995) Water-suppressed one-dimensional ^1H NMR chemical shift imaging of the heart before and after regional ischemia. NMR Biomed 8:79–86

Beyerbacht HP, Vliegen HW, Lamb HJ, Doornbos J, de Roos A, van der Laarse A, van der Wall EE (1996) Phosphorus magnetic resonance spectroscopy of the human heart: current status and clinical implications. Eur Heart J 17:1158–1166

Bittl JA, Ingwall JS (1985) Reaction rates of creatine kinase and ATP synthesis in the isolated rat heart. A ^{31}P NMR magnetization transfer study. J Biol Chem 260:3512–3517

Bittl JA, Ingwall JS (1987) Intracellular high-energy phosphate transfer in normal and hypertrophied myocardium. Circulation 75:196–201

Bottomley PA (1985) Noninvasive study of high-energy phosphate metabolism in human heart by depth-resolved ^{31}P NMR spectroscopy. Science 229:769–772

Bottomley PA (1994) MR spectroscopy of the human heart: the status and the challenges. Radiology 191:593–612

Bottomley PA, Hardy CJ (1992) Mapping creatine kinase reaction rates in human brain and heart with 4 Tesla saturation transfer ^{31}P NMR. J Magn Reson 99:443–448

Bottomley PA, Weiss RG (1998) Non-invasive magnetic resonance detection of creatine depletion in non-viable infarcted myocardium. Lancet 351:714–718

Bottomley PA, Hardy CJ, Roemer PB (1990) Phosphate metabolite imaging and concentration measurements in human heart by nuclear magnetic resonance. Magn Reson Med 14:425–434

Bottomley PA, Hardy CJ, Weiss RG (1991a) Correcting human heart ^{31}P NMR spectra for partial saturation: evidence that saturation factors for PCr/ATP are homogeneous in normal and disease states. J Magn Reson 95:341–355

Bottomley PA, Weiss RG, Hardy CJ, Baumgartner WA (1991b) Myocardial high-energy phosphate metabolism and allograft rejection in patients with heart transplants. Radiology 181:67–75

Bottomley PA, Lee SYH, Weiss RG (1996a) Proton MR spectroscopy of creatine in myocardial infarction. In "ISMRM 4th scientific meeting," p 426

Bottomley PA, Atalar E, Weiss RG (1996b) Human cardiac high-energy phosphate metabolite concentrations by 1D-resolved NMR spectroscopy. Magn Reson Med 35:664–670

Buser PT, Camacho SA, Wu ST, Higgins CB, Jasmin G, Parmley WW, Wikman-Coffelt J (1989) The effect of dobutamine on myocardial performance and high-energy phosphate metabolism at different stages of heart failure in cardiomyopathic hamsters: a ^{31}P MRS study. Am Heart J 118:86–91

Clarke K, O'Connor AJ, Willis RJ (1987) Temporal relation between energy metabolism and myocardial function during ischemia and reperfusion. Am J Physiol 253:H412–H421

Clarke K, Stewart LC, Neubauer S, et al. (1993) Extracellular volume and transsarcolemmal proton movement during ischemia and reperfusion: a ^{31}P NMR spectroscopic study of the isovolumic rat heart. NMR Biomed 6:278–286

Clarke K, Kashiwaya Y, King MT, et al. (1996) The beta/alpha peak height ratio of ATP. A measure of free $[Mg^{2+}]$ using ^{31}P NMR. J Biol Chem 271:21142–21150

Conway MA, Allis J, Ouwerkerk R, Niioka T, Rajagopalan B, Radda GK (1991) Detection of low phosphocreatine to ATP ratio in failing hypertrophied human myocardium by ^{31}P magnetic resonance spectroscopy. Lancet 338:973–976

Cross HR, Radda GK, Clarke K (1995) The role of Na$^+$/K$^+$ ATPase activity during low-flow ischemia in preventing myocardial injury: a ^{31}P, ^{23}Na and [87]Rb NMR spectroscopic study. Magn Reson Med 34:673–685

de Roos A, Doornbos J, Luyten PR, Oosterwaal LJ, van der Wall EE, den Hollander JA (1992) Cardiac metabolism in patients with dilated and hypertrophic cardiomyopathy: assessment with proton-decoupled P-31 MR spectroscopy. J Magn Reson Imaging 2:711–719

DeLayre JL, Ingwall JS, Malloy C, Fossel ET (1981) Gated sodium-23 nuclear magnetic resonance images of an isolated perfused working rat heart. Science 212:935–936

Eisner DA, Lederer WJ, Vaughan-Jones RD (1984) The quantitative relationship between twitch tension and intracellular sodium activity in sheep cardiac Purkinje fibres. J Physiol 355:251–266

Flameng W, Vanhaecke J, Van Belle H, Borgers M, De Beer L, Minten J (1987) Relation between coronary artery stenosis and myocardial purine metabolism, histology and regional function in humans. J Am Coll Cardiol 9:1235–1242

Forsen S, Hofman RA (1963) Study of moderately rapid chemical exchange reactions by means of nuclear magnetic double resonance. J Chem Phys 39:2892–2901

Fossel ET, Morgan HE, Ingwall JS (1980) Measurement of changes in high-energy phosphates in the cardiac cycle using gated ^{31}P nuclear magnetic resonance. Proc Natl Acad Sci USA 77:3654–3658

Fraser CJ, Chacko VP, Jacobus WE, et al. (1990) Early phosphorus 31 nuclear magnetic resonance bioenergetic changes potentially predict rejection in heterotopic cardiac allografts. J Heart Transplant 9:197–204

Friedrich J, Apstein CS, Ingwall JS (1995) ^{31}P nuclear magnetic resonance spectroscopic imaging of regions of remodeled myocardium in the infarcted rat heart. Circulation 92:3527–3538

Gadian DG (1995) NMR and its applications to living systems. Oxford University Press, New York

Garlick PB, Radda GK, Seeley PJ (1977) Phosphorus NMR studies on perfused heart. Biochem Biophys Res Commun 74:1256–1262

Grist TM, Kneeland JB, Rilling WR, Jesmanowicz A, Froncisz W, Hyde JS (1989) Gated cardiac MR imaging and P-31 MR spectroscopy in humans at 1.5 T. Work in progress. Radiology 170:357–361

Gupta RK, Gupta P, Yushok WD, Rose ZB (1983) On the noninvasive measurement of intracellular free magnesium by ^{31}P NMR spectroscopy. Physiol Chem Phys Med NMR 15:265–280

Hardy CJ, Weiss RG, Bottomley PA, Gerstenblith G (1991) Altered myocardial high-energy phosphate metabolites in patients with dilated cardiomyopathy. Am Heart J 122:795–801

Hardy CJ, Bottomley PA, Rohling KW, Roemer PB (1992) An NMR phased array for human cardiac ^{31}P spectroscopy. Magn Reson Med 28:54–64

Haug CE, Shapiro JI, Chan L, Weil RD (1987) P-31 nuclear magnetic resonance spectroscopic evaluation of heterotopic cardiac allograft rejection in the rat. Transplantation 44:175–178

Hetherington HP, Luney DJ, Vaughan JT, et al. (1995) 3D ^{31}P spectroscopic imaging of the human heart at 4.1 T. Magn Reson Med 33:427–431

Horn M, Neubauer S, Bomhard M, Kadgien M, Schnackerz K, Ertl G (1993) ^{31}P-NMR spectroscopy of human blood and serum: results from volunteers and patients with congestive heart failure, diabetes mellitus and hyperlipidemia. MAGMA 1:55–60

Ingwall JS (1982) Phosphorus nuclear magnetic resonance spectroscopy of cardiac and skeletal muscles. Am J Physiol 242:H729–H744

Ingwall JS (1993) Is cardiac failure a consequence of decreased energy reserve? Circulation 87 Suppl VII:58–62

Ingwall JS (1995) How high does intracellular sodium rise during acute myocardial ischaemia? A view from NMR spectroscopy. Cardiovasc Res 29:2

Ingwall JS, Kramer MF, Fifer MA, Lorell BH, Shemin R, Grossman W, Allen PD (1985) The creatine kinase system in normal and diseased human myocardium. N Engl J Med 313:1050–1054

Jacobus WE (1985) Respiratory control and the integration of heart high-energy phosphate metabolism by mitochondrial creatine kinase. Annu Rev Physiol 47:707–725

Jacobus WE, Ingwall JS (1980) "Heart creatine kinase". Williams & Wilkins, Baltimore, London

Jacobus WE, Taylor GJ, Hollis DP, Nunnally RL (1977) Phosphorus nuclear magnetic resonance of perfused working rat hearts. Nature 265:756–758

Kammermeier H, Schmidt P, Jüngling E (1982) Free energy change of ATP-hydrolysis: a causal factor of early hypoxic failure of the myocardium? J Mol Cell Cardiol 14:267–277

Kantor HL, Briggs RW, Metz KR, Balaban RS (1986) Gated in vivo examination of cardiac metabolites with ^{31}P nuclear magnetic resonance. Am J Physiol 251:H171–H175

Kim D, Cragoe EJ, Smith TW (1987) Relations among sodium pump inhibition. Na$^+$-Ca$^+$ and Na$^+$-H$^+$ exchange activities, and Ca-H interaction in cultured chick heart cells. Circ Res 60:185–193

Kim RJ, Lima JAC, Chen EL, Reeder SB, Klocke FJ, Zerhouni EA, Judd RM (1997) Fast [23]Na magnetic resonance imaging of acute reperfused myocardial infarction. Potential to assess myocardial viability. Circulation 95:1877–1885

Kohler SJ, Perry SB, Stewart LC, Atkinson DE, Clarke K, Ingwall JS (1991) Analysis of [23]Na spectra from isolated perfused hearts. Magn Reson Med 18:15–27

Kreutzer U, Jue T (1991) [1]H-nuclear magnetic resonance deoxyhemoglobin signal as indicator of intracellular oxygenation in myocardium. Am J Physiol 261:H2091–H2097

Kupriyanov VV, Stewart LC, Xiang B, Kwak J, Deslauriers R (1995) Pathways of Rb$^+$ influx and their relation to intracellular [Na$^+$] in the perfused rat heart. A [87]Rb and ^{23}Na NMR study. Circ Res 76:839–851

Lange R, Ingwall JS, Hale SL, Alker KJ, Braunwald E, Kloner RA (1984) Preservation of high-energy phosphates by verapamil in reperfused myocardium. Circulation 70:734–741

Lawson JWR, Veech RL (1979) Effects of pH and free Mg^{2+} on the Keq of the creatine kinase reaction and other phosphate hydrolyses and phosphate transfer reactions. J Biol Chem 254:6528–6537

Lehninger AL (1982) In: Anderson S, Fox J (eds) Principles of biochemistry. Worth, New York, pp 467–510

Lewandowski ED, White LT (1995) Pyruvate dehydrogenase influences postischemic heart function. Circulation 91:2071–2079

Lewandowski ED, Doumen C, White LT, LaNoue KF, Damico LA, Yu X (1996) Multiplet structure of ^{13}C NMR signal from glutamate and direct detection of tricarboxylic acid (TCA) cycle intermediates. Magn Reson Med 35:149–154

Liao R, Nascimben L, Friedrich J, Gwathmey JK, Ingwall JS (1996) Decreased energy reserve in an animal model of dilated cardiomyopathy. Relationship to contractile performance. Circ Res 78:893–902

Malloy CR, Buster DC, Castro MM, Geraldes CF, Jeffrey FM, Sherry AD (1990) Influence of global ischemia on intracellular sodium in the perfused rat heart. Mag Reson Med 15:33–44

Malloy CR, Jones JG, Jeffrey FM, Jessen ME, Sherry AD (1996) Contribution of various substrates to total citric acid cycle flux and anaplerosis as determined by ^{13}C isotopomer analysis and O_2 consumption in the heart. Magma 4:35–46

Masuda Y, Tateno Y, Ikehira H, et al. (1992) High-energy phosphate metabolism of the myocardium in normal subjects and patients with various cardiomyopathies. The study using ECG gated MR spectroscopy with a localization technique. Jpn Circ J 56:620–626

Menon RS, Hendrich K (1992) ^{31}P NMR spectroscopy of human heart at 4T: detection of substantially uncontaminated cardiac spectra and differentiation of subepicardium and subendocardium. Magn Reson Med 26:368–376

Moon RB, Richards JH (1973) Determination of intracellular pH by ^{31}P magnetic resonance. J Biol Chem 248:7276–7278

Murphy E, Steenbergen C, Levy LA, Gabel S, London RE (1994) Measurement of cytosolic free calcium in perfused rat heart using TF-BAPTA. Am J Physiol 266:C1323–C1329

Nascimben L, Friedrich J, Liao R, Pauletto P, Pessina AC, Ingwall JS (1995) Enalapril treatment increases cardiac performance and energy reserve via the creatine kinase reaction in myocardium of Syrian myopathic hamsters with advanced heart failure. Circulation 91:1824–1833

Neubauer S, Ingwall JS (1989) Verapamil attenuates ATP depletion during hypoxia: ^{31}P NMR studies of the isolated rat heart. J Mol Cell Cardiol 21:1163–1178

Neubauer S, Hamman BL, Perry SB, Bittl JA, Ingwall JS (1988) Velocity of the creatine kinase reaction decreases in postischemic myocardium: a ^{31}P-NMR magnetization transfer study of the isolated ferret heart. Circ Res 63:1–15

Neubauer S, Ertl G, Krahe T, Schindler R, Hillenbrand H, Lackner K, Kochsiek K (1991) Experimentelle und klinische Möglichkeiten der MR-Spektroskopie des Herzens. Z Kardiol 80:25–36

Neubauer S, Krahe T, Schindler R, et al. (1992a) Direct measurement of spin-lattice relaxation times of phosphorus metabolites in human myocardium. Magn Reson Med 26:300–307

Neubauer S, Krahe T, Schindler R, et al. (1992b) (31)P magnetic resonance spectroscopy in dilated cardiomyopathy and coronary artery disease: altered cardiac high-energy phosphate metabolism in heart failure. Circulation 86:1810–1818

Neubauer S, Newell JB, Ingwall JS (1992c) Metabolic consequences and predictability of ventricular fibrillation in hypoxia. A ^{31}P- and ^{23}Na-nuclear magnetic resonance study of the isolated rat heart. Circulation 86:302–310

Neubauer S, Horn M, Ertl G (1994) The value of ^{31}P-NMR spectroscopy of the study of myocardial ischemia. Cardioscopies 20:37–43

Neubauer S, Horn M, Naumann A, et al. (1995a) Impairment of energy metabolism in intact residual myocardium of rat hearts with chronic myocardial infarction. J Clin Invest 95:1092–1100

Neubauer S, Horn M, Pabst T, et al. (1995b) Contributions of ^{31}P-magnetic resonance spectroscopy to the understanding of dilated heart muscle disease. Eur Heart J 16 (Suppl O):115–118

Neubauer S, Horn M, Cramer M, et al. (1997a) In patients with dilated cardiomyopathy the myocardial phosphocreatine-to-ATP ratio is a predictor of mortality. Circulation 96:2190–2196

Neubauer S, Horn M, Pabst T, et al. (1997b) Cardiac high-energy phosphate metabolism in patients with aortic valve disease assessed by ^{31}P-magnetic resonance spectroscopy. J Invest Med 45:453–462

Nunnally RL, Hollis DP (1979) Adenosine triphosphate compartmentation in living hearts: a phosphorus nuclear magnetic resonance saturation transfer study. Biochemistry 18:3642–3646

Pike MM, Frazer JC, Dedrick DF, Ingwall JS, Allen PD, Springer CS Jr, Smith TW (1985) ^{23}Na and ^{39}K nuclear magnetic resonance studies of perfused rat hearts. Discrimination of intra- and extracellular ions using a shift reagent. Biophys J 48:159–173

Pluim BM, Chin JC, De Roos A, et al. (1996) Cardiac anatomy, function and metabolism in elite cyclists assessed by magnetic resonance imaging and spectroscopy [see comments]. Eur Heart J 17:1271–1278

Pohost GM (1995) Is ^{31}P-NMR spectroscopic imaging a viable approach to assess myocardial viability? Circulation 92:9–10

Presant CA, Wolf W, Waluch V, Wiseman C, Kennedy P, Blayney D (1994) Association of intratumoural pharmacokinetics of fluorouracil with clinical response. Lancet 343:1184–1187

Rajagopalan B, Blackledge MJ, McKenna WJ, Bolas N, Radda GK (1987) Measurement of phosphocreatine to ATP ratio in normal and diseased human heart by ^{31}P magnetic resonance spectroscopy using the rotating frame-depth selection technique. Ann N Y Acad Sci 508:321–332

Robitaille PM, Lew B, Merkle H, et al. (1989) Transmural metabolite distribution in regional myocardial ischemia as studied with ^{31}P NMR. Magn Reson Med 10:108–118

Robitaille PM, Rath DP, Abduljalil AM, O'Donnell JM, Jiang Z, Zhang H, Hamlin RL (1993) Dynamic ^{13}C NMR analysis of oxidative metabolism in the in vivo canine myocardium. J Biol Chem 268/35:26296–26301

Sakuma H, Takeda K, Tagami T, Nakagawa T, Okamoto S, Konishi T, Nakano T (1993) ^{31}P MR spectroscopy in hypertrophic cardiomyopathy: comparison with Tl-201 myocardial perfusion imaging. Am Heart J 125:1323–1328

Schaefer S, Gober JR, Schwartz GG, Twieg DB, Weiner MW, Massie B (1990) In vivo phosphorus-31 spectroscopic imaging in patients with global myocardial disease. Am J Cardiol 65:1154–1161

Sieverding L, Jung WI, Breuer J, et al. (1997) Proton-decoupled myocardial ^{31}P NMR spectroscopy reveals decreased PCr/Pi in patients with severe hypertrophic cardiomyopathy. Am J Cardiol 80(3A):34A–40A

Solomon MA, Jeffrey FM, Storey CJ, Sherry AD, Malloy GR (1996) Substrate selection early after reperfusion of ischemic regions in the working rabbit heart. Magn Reson Med 35:820–826

Spencer RG, Balschi JA, Leigh JS Jr, Ingwall JS (1988) ATP synthesis and degradation rates in the perfused heart. ^{31}P-nuclear magnetic resonance double saturation transfer measurements [published erratum appears in Biophys J 1988 Dec;54(6): following 1186]. Biophys J 54:921–929

Spencer RG, Buttrick PM, Ingwall JS (1997) Function and bioenergetics in isolated perfused trained rat hearts. Am J Physiol 272:H409–H417

Spindler M, Saupe KW, Christe ME, Seidman CE, Seidman JG, Ingwall JS (1996) A murine model of familial hypertrophic cardiomyopathy shows a markedly impaired response to inotropic stimulation (abstract). Circulation 94 (Suppl I):I-433

Spirito P, Seidman CE, McKenna WJ, Maron BJ (1997) The management of hypertrophic cardiomyopathy. N Engl J Med 336:775–785

Springer CS Jr, Pike MM, Balschi JA, Chu SC, Frazier JC, Ingwall JS, Smith TW (1985) Use of shift reagents for nuclear magnetic resonance studies of the kinetics of ion transfer in cells and perfused hearts. Circulation 72:89–93

Steeghs K, Benders A, Oerlemans F, et al. (1997) Altered Ca^{2+} responses in muscles with combined mitochondrial and cytosolic creatine kinase deficiencies. Cell 89:93–103

Toyo Oka T, Nagayama K, Umeda M, Eguchi K, Hosoda S (1986) Rhythmic change of myocardial phosphate metabolite content in cardiac cycle observed by depth-selected and EKG gated in vivo ^{31}P-NMR spectroscopy in a whole animal. Biochem Biophys Res Commun 135:808–815

Ugurbil K, Petein M, Madian R, Michurski S, Cohn JN, From AH (1984) High resolution proton NMR studies of perfused rat hearts. FEBS Lett 167:73–78

van Deurssen J, Heerschap A, Oerlemans F, Ruitenbeek W, Jap P, ter Laak H, Wieringa B (1993) Skeletal muscles of mic deficient in muscle creatine kinase lack burst activity. Cell 74:621–631

van Dobbenburgh JO, Klopping C, Lahpor JR, Wolley SR, van Echteld CJA (1993) Altered myocardial energy metabolism in heart transplant patients: consequence of rejection or a postischemic phenomenon? In: Proceedings of the Society of Magnetic Resonance in Medicine, p 103

van Dobbenburgh JO, Lekkerkerk C, van Echteld CJ, de Beer R (1994) Saturation correction in human cardiac ^{31}P MR spectroscopy at 1.5 T. NMR Biomed 7:218–224

van Echteld CJ, Kirkels JH, Eijgelshoven MH, van der Meer P, Ruigrok TJ (1991) Intracellular sodium during ischemia and calcium-free perfusion: a ^{23}Na NMR study. J Mol Cell Cardiol 23:297–307

Vanoverschelde JLJ, Wijns W, Borgers M, Heyndrickx G, Depré C, Flameng W, Melin JA (1997) Chronic myocardial hibernation in humans. Circulation 95:1961–1971

von Kienlin M, Mejia R (1991) Spectral localization with optimal pointspread function. Magn Reson Med 94:268–287

von Kienlin M, Rösch C, Le Fur Y, et al. (1998) Three-dimensional ^{31}P magnetic resonance spectroscopic imaging of regional high-energy phosphate metabolism in injured rat heart. Magn Reson Med 39:731–741

Wallimann T, Wyss M, Brdiczka D, Nicolay K, Eppenberger HM (1992) Intracellular compartmentation, structure and function of creatine kinase isoenzymes in tissues with high and fluctuating energy demands: The "phosphocreatine circuit" for cellular energy homeostasis. Bioph J 281:21–40

Weiss RG, Bottomley PA, Hardy CJ, Gerstenblith G (1990) Regional myocardial metabolism of high-energy phosphates during isometric exercise in patients with coronary artery disease. N Engl J Med 323:1593–1600

Weiss RG, Gloth ST, Kalil Filho R, Chacko VP, Stern MD, Gerstenblith G (1992) Indexing tricarboxylic acid cycle flux in intact hearts by carbon-13 nuclear magnetic resonance. Circ Res 70:392–408

Wexler LF, Lorell BH, Momomura S, Weinberg EO, Ingwall JS, Apstein CS (1988) Enhanced sensitivity to hypoxia-induced diastolic dysfunction in pressure-overload left ventricular hypertrophy in the rat: role of high-energy phosphate depletion. Circ Res 62:766–775

Wu ST, Pieper GM, Salhany JM, Eliot RS (1981) Measurement of free magnesium in perfused and ischemic arrested heart muscle. A quantitative phosphorus-31 nuclear magnetic resonance and multiequilibria analysis. Biochemistry 20:7399–7403

Yabe T, Mitsunami K, Okada M, Morikawa S, Inubushi T, Kinoshita M (1994) Detection of myocardial ischemia by ^{31}P magnetic resonance spectroscopy during handgrip exercise. Circulation 89:1709–1716

Yabe T, Mitsunami K, Inubushi T, Kinoshita M (1995) Quantitative measurements of cardiac phosphorus metabolites in coronary artery disease by ^{31}P magnetic resonance spectroscopy [see comments]. Circulation 92:15–23

Zhang J, Merkle H, Hendrich K, Garwood M, From AH, Ugurbil K, Bache RJ (1993) Bioenergetic abnormalities associated with severe left ventricular hypertrophy. J Clin Invest 92:993–1003

Zhang J, Duncker DJ, Xu Y, et al. (1995) Transmural bioenergetic responses of normal myocardium to high workstates. Am J Physiol 268:H1891–H1905

Zhang J, Wilke N, Wang Y, et al. (1996) Functional and bioenergetic consequences of postinfarction left ventricular remodeling in a new porcine model. MRI and ^{31}P-MRS study. Circulation 94:1089–1100

10 Cardiac Masses

J. Bogaert

CONTENTS

10.1 Introduction

Before the era of modern cardiac imaging techniques, the diagnosis of cardiac tumors was extremely difficult and often not made antemortem. Nowadays, the availability of transthoracic (TTE) and transesophageal echocardiography (TEE), computed tomography (CT), and magnetic resonance imaging (MRI) has greatly facilitated their detection. However, because of their rarity and the nonspecific, often misleading, symptomatology that causes them to be placed at the bottom of the differential diagnostic list, their diagnosis may be considerably delayed. Therefore, a great deal of suspicion is required to direct the clinician toward the proper diagnosis.

As the title to this chapter, "Cardiac Masses" was preferred to "Cardiac Tumors" for more than one reason. First, not only are nontumoral cardiac masses much more frequent than true cardiac tumors, but also nontumoral masses usually require a medical (or no) treatment whereas cardiac surgery is still the preferred therapeutic approach for cardiac tumors. Thus, accurate differentiation between the two conditions is a first requirement for each imaging technique dealing with the diagnosis of cardiac masses. Second, precise knowledge of the normal cardiac anatomy and its variants is required since with the advent of modern cardiac imaging techniques, not only are abnormal masses much more easily and frequently detected, but normal cardiac structures may be interpreted as abnormal by inexperienced people. Therefore the major aims of this chapter are to guide the reader in recognizing the diversity of cardiac tumors, nontumoral masses, and normal variants, to discuss their appearance on MRI, and to highlight the role of MRI in the detection and differentiation of cardiac masses, comparing this technique with the other cardiac imaging techniques.

10.2 Clinical Presentation

The clinical presentation of tumors originating in the heart is often atypical, suggestive more of a systemic illness than a cardiovascular problem (Salcedo et al. 1992). Therefore, a high index of suspicion and a goal-directed diagnostic approach are required. Cardiac tumors can manifest in one of several ways (Table 10.1). They can be an incidental finding on chest radiography, echocardiography, or another cardiovascular diagnostic test. The first symptoms can be constitutional, particularly in patients with myxomas, and a high index of suspicion is needed to make the proper diagnosis. Cardiovascular symptoms, specifically congestive heart failure and thromboembolism, can be the presenting manifestations. Since these are rather nonspecific, a great deal of suspicion is required to direct the clinician toward the proper diagnosis. Finally, patients with noncardiac malignancies can have cardiac involvement with or without cardiovascular symptoms.

In patients with cardiac tumors, the history and clinical findings are determined primarily by the

J. Bogaert, MD, PhD, Department of Radiology, Gasthuisberg University Hospital, University of Leuven, Herestraat 49, B-3000 Leuven, Belgium

anatomic location of the tumor rather than by the histopathology. It can be said that cardiac tumors can be clinically and pathologically benign, but have a "malignant" and fatal outcome, or they can be clinically and pathologically malignant. Generally, tumors manifest symptomatology and clinical signs by virtue of tumor growth that impedes cardiac hemodynamics. Thus, large infiltrative tumors may be clinically silent, while smaller, yet strategically located tumors can produce dramatic symptomatology due to transient obstruction of flow

across the valve. Arrhythmias and interventricular conduction defects may also be encountered as a consequence of tumor infiltrating the conduction system.

10.3
Conventional Imaging Modalities

Whether a cardiac imaging modality is useful in the diagnosis of patients with suspected cardiac masses depends on following requirements: high accuracy (i.e., low rate of false-negative and false-positive results), accurate evaluation of tumor extent and tumor composition (i.e., tissue characterization), and detection of complications (e.g., valvular obstruction). At present, several cardiac imaging techniques are available. Although this chapter is focused on the role of MRI, the advantages and limitations of the other currently available imaging techniques are briefly discussed and summarized in Table 10.2.

Table 10.1. Presentation of cardiac tumors

Systemic illness
Cardiovascular symptoms
  Congestive heart failure
  Thromboembolism
  Arrhythmias/interventricular conduction disturbances
Incidental finding
History of noncardiac malignancy

Table 10.2. Advantages and limitations of current cardiac imaging techniques in the detection of cardiac masses

	Advantages	Limitations

X-ray angiography	Tumor size/shape/mobility/location
	Tumor vascularity
	Nutritive supply
		Radiation/cost
		Invasive
		Dislodgement of tumor fragments
		Only indirect information on
		  – Myocardial masses or invasion
		  – Pericardial effusions/masses
		False-positive/-negative results

TTE	Widely available/portable Accurate/real-time imaging Relatively inexpensive Tumor size/shape/mobility/location	Poor echogenicity in 30% of patients No tissue characterization Poor evaluation of pericardium/extracardiac structures

TEE	Advantages = those of TTE
	Better than TTE in:
	  – Defining tumor attachment and tumor extension
	  – Detecting cardiac thrombi
	  – Evaluation of pericardium and extracardiac structures
		Semi-invasive procedure
		Evaluation of pericardium/extracardiac structures may be insufficient
		No tissue characterization

CT	Noninvasive High spatial resolution High temporal resolution (ultrafast mode) Possibility of multiplanar reconstruction Tumor size/shape/mobility/location Tissue characterization to a limited extent	Radiation Iodinated contrast material required No real multiplanar imaging capability Limited availability of ultrafast CT scanners
MRI	Noninvasive High spatial and temporal resolution Multiplanar imaging capability Large field of view Tumor size/shape/mobility/location Accurate information on tumor extent and tumor vascularity Tissue characterization to a limited extent	Absolute and relative contraindications (such as pacemaker, intracranial vascular clips) Claustrophobia Real-time imaging not yet clinically available

10.3.1
X-ray Angiography

In many cases, the noninvasive imaging modalities (i.e., echocardiography, CT, and MRI) will provide adequate preoperative information on the location and extent of the cardiac tumor, so that no further cardiac catheterization and selective angiocardiography is required. However, in special circumstances information can be needed (a) when inadequate information on the tumor location, attachment, or extent is obtained by the noninvasive imaging methods, (b) when a malignant tumor is considered likely, and (c) when other cardiac lesions (e.g., coronary artery or valvular lesions) may coexist with a cardiac tumor and possibly dictate a different surgical approach (FUEREDI et al. 1989). Cardiac tumors present on X-ray angiography as (a) intracavitary filling defects, (b) compression, displacement, or deformation of the cardiac chambers, (c) increased myocardial wall thickness, or (d) local alteration in wall motion. Furthermore, coronary arteriography may provide information on the vascular pattern of the tumor, its vascular supply, and its relation to the coronary arteries (SINGH et al. 1984). Differentiation with nontumoral conditions such as thrombus, intramuscular hydatid cyst, and aneurysm may not be possible, which yields a high number of false-positive results. Furthermore, x-ray angiocardiography may be false-negative in patients not suspected for cardiac tumor prior to the catheterization. Finally, the invasiveness of this procedure entails the risk of peripheral embolization due to dislodgement of tumor fragments.

10.3.2
Echocardiography

Echocardiography is considered the procedure of choice for the diagnosis of intracardiac tumors. This technique may provide information on the size, mobility, shape, and location of cardiac masses, but it cannot describe histologic features. The transthoracic approach is totally noninvasive and often sufficient for a complete evaluation. However, when TTE provides inadequate images, as in obese patients and patients with obstructive pulmonary disease, TEE or MRI offers a diagnostic alternative. TEE is superior to TTE in the diagnosis of intracardial and peri- or paracardial tumors (HERRERA et al. 1992). Details such as the attachment point of myxomas, compression of cardiac structures, or in-

filtration of the great vessels by a malignant disease in close contact with the heart can be better identified by TEE (ENGBERDING et al. 1993). TEE is also superior to TTE in the detection of left atrial thrombi, especially when located in the left atrial appendage (MUGGE et al. 1991). After surgery, TEE can detect an early recurrence of a tumor, or if a patient receives chemotherapy, the result can be more easily quantified.

While cardiac masses can be very well depicted with echocardiography, additional imaging modalities such as CT or MRI may be required to define the extent of pericardial and extracardiac masses (TESORO TESS et al. 1993; KUPFERWASSER et al. 1994). Absolute contraindications to the performance of TEE include a history of or current pathologic conditions of the esophagus, and recent esophageal operations. In patients with relative contraindications, such as unstable angina, esophageal varices, or active upper gastrointestinal bleeding, an individual assessment must be made before TEE is performed. Complications associated with TEE can be related to the probe, to the procedure, or to drugs used during the examination.

10.3.3
Computed Tomography

Conventional, spiral and ultrafast CT can be applied to detect cardiac and extracardiac masses. They all have a very high spatial resolution, while only ultrafast CT has a sufficiently high temporal resolution (e.g., exposure times of 50 ms) to eliminate cardiac motion artifacts. The latter technique allows rapid multilevel imaging of the heart after injection of iodinated contrast medium for opacification of the heart chambers and vessels. Both intra- and extracardiac masses can be very well depicted, as well as their degree of myocardial or pericardial involvement (STANFORD et al. 1991; BLEIWEIS et al. 1994; KEMP et al. 1996). However, ultrafast CT requires iodinated contrast medium and the availability of ultrafast CT scanners is limited.

10.3.4
Magnetic Resonance Imaging

At present, MRI is one of the preferred imaging modalities in the evaluation of patients with suspected cardiac masses. Major advantages of this technique are the excellent spatial resolution, the large field of

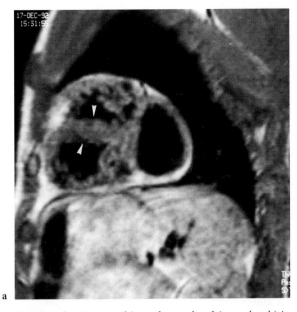

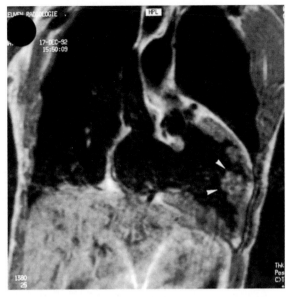

Fig. 10.1 a,b. Hypertrophic moderator band (*arrowheads*) in a patient with transposition of the great arteries. T1-weighted SE images in the cardiac short-axis (**a**) and vertical long-axis (**b**). This MRI study was performed because the patient was suspected on echocardiography to have a thrombus or mass in the right ventricle. The typical location and the signal intensity similar to that of the myocardium allow a correct diagnosis

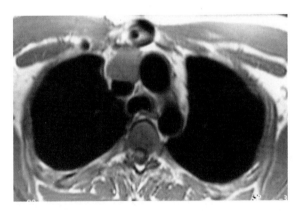

Fig. 10.2. Recurrent synoviosarcoma of the pericardium. Axial turbo SE image. Nodular mass arising anterior to the superior vena cava and lateral to the ascending aorta

view, the inherent natural contrast between flowing blood and the surrounding heart chambers, vessel walls, and tumor masses without the need for contrast administration, the multiplanar imaging capability, and the ability to administer paramagnetic contrast agents in order to obtain a better detection of the tumor borders and the degree of tumor vascularization. These advantages are important in planning the patient's therapy, particularly if surgical intervention is being considered. Using MRI, cardiac tumors can be depicted with a very high accuracy. Not only are abnormal masses easily detected but tumor mimics, e.g., normal anatomic variants, not infrequently misinterpreted as tumor masses by other imaging modalities, are well recognized by means of MRI (Fig. 10.1). A distinct advantage over echocardiography is the large field of view, which allows perfect assessment not only of the intracardiac but also of the extracardiac extent of the tumor. Also, masses originating in the pericardium or in the neighboring lung parenchyma or mediastinum can be much better evaluated. For instance, frequently misinterpreted paracardiac tumors using TEE include diaphragmatic hernias and aneurysmal dilatation of the descending thoracic aorta. MRI may be particularly useful in detecting recurrence in the postoperative period since echocardiography may not be suitable if surgery has decreased the echo window (KAMINAGA et al. 1993) (Fig. 10.2). An advantage over CT is the multiplanar imaging capability by which directly tomographic images in any desired plane can be obtained, which aids in the determination of the location, size, and anatomic relationships of normal and abnormal cardiac structures. Furthermore, MRI can provide contiguous image slices of known thickness and accurately measure cardiac and tissue volumes, and can be used to quantify tumor volume. In comparison with echocardiography, MRI lacks the ability for real-time imaging, though with the advent of faster MRI sequences real-time imaging may become clinically available in the near future.

For the evaluation and tissue characterization of suspected cardiac masses with MRI, basically two types of ECG-triggered sequences are used (for a more extensive description, see Chap. 1). The first is the spin-echo (SE) technique, providing dark blood, while the second is the gradient-echo (GE) technique, providing bright blood. SE MRI allows excellent anatomic evaluation of the heart. By varying the length of the repetition time and the length of the echo time, the SE sequence can be T1- or T2-weighted. A combination of T1- and T2-weighted measurements allows a better description of the composition of cardiac masses, although the initial hope that the pattern of signal intensity would allow differentiation between benign and malignant neoplasms has not been fulfilled. Cystic fluid, e.g., (pleuro)pericardial cyst, has a very low signal on T1-weighted images but a very high signal on T2-weighted images. Masses with a lipomatous composition, e.g., lipomas and lipomatous hypertrophy of the interatrial septum, have a signal intensity that resembles that of epicardial or subcutaneous fat. They have a relatively high signal on T1-weighted sequences and a moderate signal on T2-weighted sequences (AMPARO et al. 1984; SECHTEM et al. 1986; BROWN et al. 1989). Fat suppression techniques, as applied, for instance, in coronary MR angiography, will selectively saturate the signal coming from fat and can be used to prove the fatty composition of cardiac masses. Most soft tissue tumors have relaxation times shorter than fluid, but long enough to produce a relatively low signal on T1-weighted images and a relatively high signal on T2-weighted images (GAMSU et al. 1984). Some cardiac tumors may present a prolongation of T1 and T2 relaxation times as a result of an increased water content (WILLIAMS et al. 1980). Mineral-rich tissues, containing cortical bone and calcifications, and mature fibrotic tissue have few mobile protons, resulting in low signal regardless of the repetition time and echo time used. Subacute and chronic hemorrhage will show a high signal intensity on both T1-weighted and T2-weighted MRI (MITCHELL et al. 1987).

The distinction of intramural tumors from normal myocardium may be equivocal because of the similarity of signal intensity between tumor and normal myocardium on SE images (FUNARI et al. 1991). Paramagnetic contrast agents, such as gadolinium-diethylene triamine penta-acetic acid (Gd-DTPA), may be administered for improved visualization of cardiac tumors. Differences in perfusion and wash-out of these contrast agents between normal and tumoral tissue may facilitate demonstration of the extent of pathology. Gd-DTPA usually accumulates in higher concentrations in tissues which contain augmented vascularization or a substantial proportion of interstitial space (BRASCH et al. 1984). Paramagnetic contrast agents can also provide information about the internal architecture, i.e., nonvascularized, necrotic or cystic areas, of a tumor, because they do not accumulate contrast medium (NEUERBURG et al. 1989). This may be of clinical importance, since the presence of such regions inside a mass may help to formulate the differential diagnosis or to assess the efficacy of radiotherapeutic or chemotherapeutic treatment on follow-up MRI studies (FUNARI et al. 1991). Gd-DTPA may also be helpful to differentiate tumor from acute and subacute thrombus, since the latter does not have vascularization and therefore cannot be enhanced by contrast media. However, on rare occasions chronic thrombi do acquire vascularization, so potentially they can enhance after administration of contrast medium (JOHNSON et al. 1988).

Gradient-echo MRI is usually applied as a single-slice multiphase approach and provides bright blood. In a single tomographic section throughout the heart, images are obtained at different time points during the cardiac cycle. These images are loaded in a cine loop display providing dynamic information on the heart contraction, i.e., cine MRI. Although cine MRI still does not provide real-time imaging as obtained with echocardiography for instance, it is a very useful technique to evaluate the mobility of cardiac masses, to detect the site of implantation, to detect atrioventricular obstruction, to differentiate slow flow from thrombus, and to evaluate the effects of cardiac masses on myocardial contractility. Calcifications which are "invisible" on SE MRI because they cannot be differentiated from the surrounding black blood can be very well detected on cine MRI as areas devoid of signal surrounded by bright blood (GLAZER et al. 1985; DE ROOS et al. 1989b) (Fig. 10.3).

Magnetic resonance techniques such as MR myocardial tagging and MR phase imaging can be applied to improve the differentiation between tumor and, respectively, myocardium and intracavitary blood (Fig. 10.4). MR myocardial tagging allows a selective saturation of myocardial tissue, in this fashion creating tag lines or a grid pattern on the myocardium (ZERHOUNI et al. 1988). This technique has been applied to differentiate normal contractile myocardium from noncontractile tumor in a neonate with a cardiac rhabdomyoma (BOUTON et al. 1991). Phase imaging techniques can be used to dis-

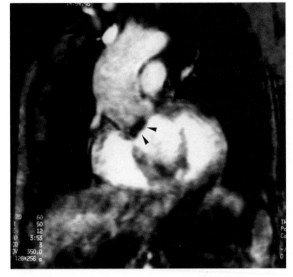

Fig. 10.3. Calcified aortic valve. Coronal GE image. The aortic valve calcifications are visible as an area devoid of signal (*arrowheads*) clearly in contrast with the surrounding bright blood

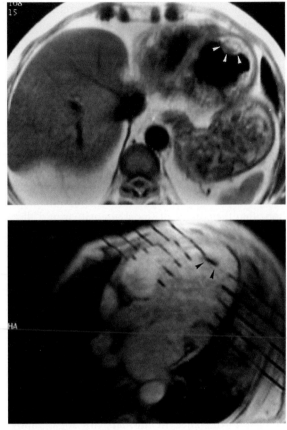

Fig. 10.4 a,b. Mural thrombus in the LV apex in a patient with a dilated cardiomyopathy. **a** Axial HASTE image. **b** Four-chamber view with MR myocardial tagging. Persistence of the tag (*arrowheads*) throughout the cardiac cycle in the thrombus allows differentiation from stagnant or slow-flowing blood in a hypokinetic dilated left ventricle

tinguish cardiac masses, e.g., tumor tissue or thrombus, from moving blood adjacent to the cardiac mass (RUMANCIK et al. 1988; KAMINAGA et al. 1993). SE magnitude images alone are not an accurate indicator in differentiating intracavitary tumor or thrombus from flow-related enhancement. Phase images, however, are sensitive for identifying flow, and this technique is complementary to conventional SE magnitude images in helping to distinguish flow-related signal from intraluminal pathologic conditions (RUMANCIK et al. 1988; HATABU et al. 1994).

10.4
Classification

Cardiac masses are divided into neoplasms and nonneoplastic conditions. Cardiac tumors can be primary or secondary. Primary cardiac tumors may be benign or malignant while secondary tumors may involve the heart by direct extension, venous extension, lymphatic extension, or metastatic spread. The heterogeneous group of nonneoplastic conditions includes all nontumoral cardiac masses and other abnormalities which may present as cardiac masses on cardiac imaging. This group also includes normal anatomic variants which may mimic cardiac masses. The MRI characteristics of the most common cardiac masses are shown in Table 10.3.

10.4.1
Primary Cardiac Tumors

Primary tumors of the heart and pericardium are extremely rare, with an incidence of between 0.0017% and 0.28% in unselected patients at autopsy, while metastatic tumors to the heart are 20–40 times more common than primary tumors (HEATH 1968; MCALLISTER and FENOGLIO 1978). Three-quarters of the primary tumors are benign. Nearly half the benign tumors are myxomas, and the majority of the rest are lipomas, papillary fibroelastomas, and rhabdomyomas. Whereas myxomas are the most common primary tumors in adults, rhabdomyomas clearly predominante in children.

Table 10.3. MRI characteristics of the most common cardiac masses

	Preferential location	SE (T1)	SE (T2)	GE	Contrast enhancement	Appearance
Benign cardiac tumors						
Myxoma	Left atrium (IAS)	Variable	Variable	Low	Yes	Heterogeneous sharp border
Lipoma	No	High	High	Medium	No	Homogeneous, sharp border
Papillary fibroelastoma	Cardiac valves	Medium	Medium	Low	?	Small (less than 1 cm)
Rhabdomyoma	Atrium Intramural/ intracavitary	Medium/ high	Medium	Low	Similar to myocardium	Multiple
Fibroma	Ventricles Intramural	Medium	Medium	Low	Variable	Usually single
Pheochromocytoma	Intrapercardial (roof of left atrium)		High		Yes	
Hemangioma	Ventricles Intramural/ intracavitary	Medium	Very high	Variable	Yes Variable	Heterogeneous Sharp border
Malignant cardiac tumors						
Angiosarcoma	Right atrium Pericardial and myocardial invasion	Variable (mixed)	Variable (mixed)	Low	Yes	Heterogeneous "Cauliflower" appearance
Rhabdomyosarcoma	No	Medium	High	?	Yes	
Malignant fibrous histiocytoma	Left atrium (posterior wall)	Medium	High	?	?	Slightly heterogeneous
Lymphoma	Pericardial effusion Intracardiac masses	Medium	Medium	Low	Yes	Variable
Malignant pericardial mesothelioma	Pericardium	Medium	High	Low	Yes	Heterogeneous (no myocardial invasion)
Nontumoral cardiac masses and mimics						
Thrombus	Atrium (valve disease) Ventricles (if diseased)	Medium to high	Medium to high	Low	No (possible if chronic)	Appearance related to age of thrombus
Valvular vegetations	Cardiac valves	Not visible	Not visible	Low	No	
Lipomatous hypertrophy of the interatrial septum	Interatrial septum	High	High	Medium	Low	"Camel hump" or "dumbbell" shaped, sparing the fossa ovalis
Hydatid cyst	Left ventricle (IVS)	Low	Very high		No	Low signal intensity peripheral border (pericyst)
Pleuropericardial cyst	Right cardiophrenic angle	Low	Very high		No	Sharply defined

The signal intensity of the cardiac masses on SE sequences is compared with the signal intensity of myocardium. The signal intensity of the cardiac masses on GE sequences is compared with the signal intensity of flowing blood

IAS, Interatrial septum; IVS, interventricular septum; GE, gradient-echo; SE, spin-echo.

10.4.1.1
Benign Cardiac Tumors

10.4.1.1.1
MYXOMA

Cardiac myxoma, the most frequent primary cardiac tumor, is an intracavitary neoplasm that can occur anywhere in the heart. Seventy-five percent of myxomas occur in the left atrium, and 75% of these have a pedunculated attachment to the atrial septum near the fossa ovalis (HANSON 1992) (Fig. 10.5). Twenty percent of myxomas occur in the right atrium, without the predilection for the fossa ovalis (MCALLISTER 1979). Five percent of myxomas are found in either the right or the left ventricle.

The typical patient diagnosed with this condition is a middle-aged female presenting to her physician or referred to a cardiologist with vague complaints such as atypical chest pains, palpitations, or intermittent shortness of breath with few if any clinical findings. Before the widespread use of modern diagnostic imaging, the majority of patients were di-agnosed late and were moderately or severely symptomatic. Today, myxomas are frequently discovered in the asymptomatic or nearly asymptomatic patient who is essentially free of clinical findings.

Depending on their size and mobility, myxomas commonly give rise to signs of obstructed filling of the left and right ventricle with subsequent dyspnea, recurrent pulmonary edema, and right heart failure. These signs mimic the clinical picture of mitral or tricuspid valve stenosis. Embolism occurs in 30%–40% of patients with myxomas. It is suggested that myxomas with high mobility or gelatinous consistency might present a higher incidence of embolization (ENGBERDING et al. 1993). Since most myxomas are located in the left atrium, systemic embolism is particularly frequent. In the majority of cases, the cerebral arteries, including the retinal arteries, are affected. The differential diagnosis of peripheral embolism should therefore include myxoma. The rate of growth of myxomas is unknown but they generally appear to grow rather quickly. Myxomas have a malignant counterpart,

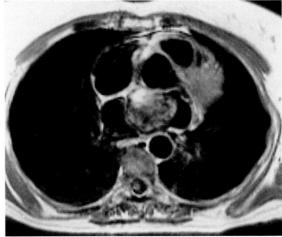

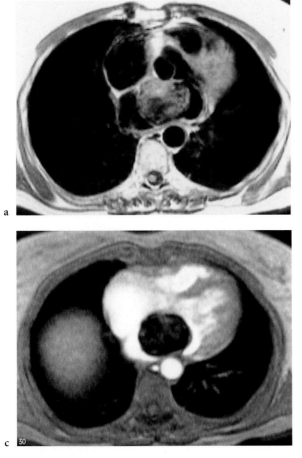

Fig. 10.5 a–c. Left atrial myxoma. T1-weighted axial SE images before (a) and after (b) administration of Gd-DTPA. There is a well-defined large inhomogeneous mass in the left atrium attached to the interatrial septum. The tumor demonstrates an inhomogeneous enhancement pattern after contrast administration. c Axial GE image: the myxoma appears strongly hypointense, surrounded by the bright intracavitary blood. There is no evidence of atrioventricular entrapment during ventricular filling during cine MRI

"myxosarcomas", which also arise in the left atrium (KLIMA et al. 1986; BURKE et al. 1992).

The signal characteristics of cardiac myxomas on MRI depend on the tumor composition. Areas of high signal in the myxoma correspond with subacute intratumoral hemorrhage, while areas with low signal intensity correspond with calcification or deposition of hemosiderin (i.e., chronic hemorrhage) (DE ROOS et al. 1989b; WATANABE et al. 1994) (Fig. 10.5). Additionally, the surface of the tumor is often covered by thrombus (SEMELKA et al. 1992). Massive hemosiderin deposition in a cardiac myxoma was reported by Lie and Watanabe (LIE 1989; WATANABE et al. 1994). Its presence may lead to an apparent enlargement of the tumor volume on cine MRI compared with the tumor volume on SE MRI. Though calcification of myxomas is reported to be rare, occurring more commonly in myxomas of the right atrium, in a recent paper by FUERIDI et al. (1989), up to one-third of all myxomas in the left atrium were calcified. After administration of paramagnetic contrast agents, myxomas may exhibit a homogeneous or heterogeneous enhancement pattern depending on the histologic characteristics of the tumor (MATSUOKA et al. 1996). Areas of enhancement correspond with histologic myxoma or inflammation, while unenhanced regions reflect necrosis of cystic changes. In addition, myxomas are highly vascular, showing tortuosity of the vessels within the tumor; this may explain the significant enhancement after Gd-DTPA administration (FUEREDI et al. 1989). On cine MRI, myxomas have a low signal intensity and this technique may be used to depict atrioventricular tumor entrapment and to detect tumor attachment.

Differential diagnosis of myxoma primarily encompasses other benign and malignant primary tumors, metastatic tumors, and organized atrial thrombi. Valvular vegetations are also an important part of the differential diagnosis. In cases of right atrial masses, a prominent eustachian valve and an aneurysm of the interatrial septum must be considered, in addition to tumors, sessile or mobile, and vegetations on the tricuspid valve. As mentioned later in this chapter, normal variants which may mimic cardiac masses can be easily recognized with MRI.

10.4.1.1.2
LIPOMA
Cardiac lipomas account for approximately 10% of all cardiac neoplasms and about 14% of benign cardiac tumors (HANANOUCHI and GOFF 1990). True lipomas are less frequent than lipomatous hypertrophy of the interatrial septum (see Sect. 10.4.4.4).

Lipomas are benign tumors of encapsulated mature adipose cells. Lipomas can be intracavitary, intramyocardial, or intrapericardial (WOLF et al. 1987). The left ventricle and right atrium are the most frequent locations. Lipomas are usually asymptomatic and in most cases require no treatment or surgical intervention. Symptoms may be produced depending on the size and the location of the tumor. Characteristic is the very low density (average −100 Hounsfield units) on CT. MRI is the most informative imaging technique in that it reveals the nature, size, location, and blood flow pattern of the tumor. T1- and T2-weighted MRI can be compared to clearly differentiate fat from other surrounding tissue. Differential diagnosis includes subacute hemorrhage. Both entities have a high signal intensity on T1-weighted MRI. On T2-weighted MRI, lipomas have an intermediate signal intensity whereas subacute hemorrhage has a high signal intensity. The use of fat suppression techniques may be useful to further differentiate fatty tissue from subacute hemorrhage.

10.4.1.1.3
PAPILLARY FIBROELASTOMA
Papillary fibroelastoma are rare cardiac benign tumors, but they are the most common primary tumor of the cardiac valves (EDWARDS et al. 1991) (Fig. 10.6). The lesions occur on any of the cardiac valves or endothelial surfaces of the heart, such as the apex of the left ventricle, the chordae tendineae, or the outflow tract (UCHIDA et al. 1992; SHAHIAN et al. 1995; COLUCCI et al. 1995). They are discovered accidentally or when neurologic or cardiologic complications occur due to emboli with stroke or coronary artery occlusion and myocardial infarction (McFADDEN and LACY 1987; KASARSKIS et al. 1988; PINELLI et al. 1995). They do not cause valvular dysfunction (KLARICH et al. 1997). Papillary fibroelastomas are small tumors, with a mean diameter of 12 × 9 mm, that are usually pedunculated and mobile (KLARICH et al. 1997). TTE and TEE are the preferred imaging modalities for detection. In addition, MRI can also be used (GROTE et al. 1995; PINELLI et al. 1995). The embolic risks justify the surgical treatment of these lesions while anticoagulation therapy can be suggested as a substitute for surgery in high-risk patients (KLARICH et al. 1997).

10.4.1.1.4
RHABDOMYOMA
Rhabdomyoma is the commonest cardiac tumor in early childhood, representing 75% of all primary

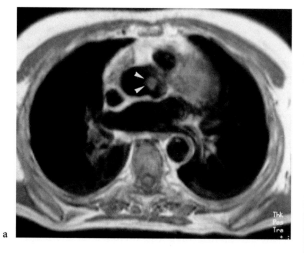

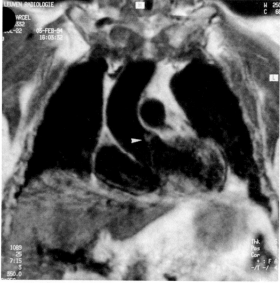

Fig. 10.6 a,b. Papillary fibroelastoma attached on the left coronary cusp of the aortic valve. Axial (**a**) and coronal (**b**) T1-weighted SE images. A small pedunculated mass (*arrowheads*) is present in the proximal part of the ascending thoracic aorta, causing repetitive systemic emboli

cardiac tumors arising in the neonatal period (YANAGISAWA 1991; AGGOUN et al. 1992). Rhabdomyoma is not infrequently considered as a hamartoma rather than a true tumor, since it may regress spontaneously by the age of 2 years (MATTEUCCI et al. 1997). This tumor may have similar clinical features as a fibroma (see Sect. 10.4.1.1.5). However, rhabdomyomas are frequently multiple, involve both atria and ventricles, and, while usually located intramurally, can have an intracavitary location. Fibromas, in contrast, are infrequently multiple or located in the atria. Rhabdomyomas rarely calcify. A most important differential feature is the association of rhabdomyomas with tuberous sclerosis (Bourneville's tuberous sclerosis). MRI is very helpful in locating and determining the extent of the tumor. Cardiac rhabdomyomas have an intermediate to high signal intensity on T1-weighted MRI and an intermediate signal intensity on T2-weighted images. The postcontrast enhancement of the tumor is similar to the surrounding myocardium (SEMELKA et al. 1992). BOUTON et al. (1991) used MRI tagging to differentiate viable myocardium from tumor in a pediatric patient with intramyocardially located rhabdomyoma.

10.4.1.1.5
FIBROMA

In the large series of 533 cases of primary cardiac tumors reported by the Armed Forces Institute of Pathology, fibromas constituted only 3.2% of the total (MCALLISTER and FENOGLIO 1978; PARMLEY et al. 1988). Fibromas are predominantly found in the pediatric age group, though they may be detected in adolescents and adults (BURKE et al. 1994). Very likely cardiac fibroma is a congenital tumor, since it is usually manifest at birth or in early infancy or childhood. Fibromas primarily arise in the ventricles and are commonly located intramurally, i.e., in the anterior wall and intraventricular septum. These tumors not infrequently calcify. The high frequency of sudden death and the potential for preventing this occurrence emphasize the need for early diagnosis and appropriate surgical and medical therapy (PARMLEY et al. 1988). The major tumors requiring differentiation are myxoma, lipoma, and rhabdomyoma. Echocardiography and MRI are very sensitive in the diagnosis and preoperative assessment (PARMLEY et al. 1988; BURKE et al. 1994). The signal characteristics on SE sequences are similar to the surrounding myocardium while after contrast administration fibromas demonstrate a heterogeneous enhancement with a lower intensity central area surrounded by a peripheral hyperintense rim (FUNARI et al. 1991). The central area likely corresponds to a poorly vascularized fibrous region.

10.4.1.1.6
INTRAPERICARDIAL PARAGANGLIOMA
(PHEOCHROMOCYTOMA)

Intrapericardial paraganglioma (pheochromocytoma) is a catecholamine-secreting tumor causing persistent or paroxysmal hypertension. The incidence of pheochromocytoma is less than 1% of the hypertensive population. Ninety percent of pheochromocytomas arise from the chromaffin cells of the adrenal medulla and about 10% of the tumors originate from other parts of the adrenal glands, retroperitioneally in the para-aortic region, the urinary bladder, or rarely the chest (less than 2% of tumors) or neck (less than 0.1% of tumors) (MANGER and GIFFORD 1990). The majority of tumors in the chest occur in the posterior mediastinum and originate from the paravertebral sympathetic ganglia. Cardiac pheochromocytomas are exceedingly rare, and are usually found intrapericardially, most often in relation to the roof of the left atrium, and less frequently arise in the interatrial septum (HAOUZI et al. 1989; KAWASUJI et al. 1989; GOMI et al. 1994). For initial detection, regional location of these extra-adrenal tumors and detection of distant metastases by means of metaiodobenzylguanidine (MIBG) scintigraphy is recommended. MRI can then provide detailed anatomic delineation before surgical resection (FISHER et al. 1985; HAMILTON et al. 1997). Pheochromocytomas usually have a high signal intensity on T2-weighted pulse sequences (VARGHESE et al. 1997). They usually reveal a marked enhancement after administration of paramagnetic contrast agents (ICHIKAWA et al. 1995).

10.4.1.1.7
(HEM)ANGIOMA

Hemangiomas are vascular tumors composed of blood vessels that can be either capillaries, i.e., capillary hemangioma, or large cavernous vascular channels, i.e., cavernous hemangioma. Hemangiomas are most frequently localized in the skin and subcutaneous muscles, and their localization in the heart is extremely rare (MOSTHAF et al. 1991; BRIZARD et al. 1993). The most common localizations are the lateral walls of the left ventricle, the anterior wall of the right ventricle, and the septum, while in 30% of cases multiple locations were found. Half of these tumors grow intramurally while the other 50% have an intracavitary localization. On coronary angiography, these tumors have a typical vascular blush. MRI may be helpful in demonstrating the vascular nature of the tumor and in evaluating the surgical resectability (BRIZARD et al. 1993). Hemangiomas generally present on MRI as heterogeneous masses. They have an intermediate signal intensity on T1-weighted images and a very high signal intensity on T2-weighted images. After contrast administration, the increase in signal intensity depends on the blood flow through the tumor. High-flow angiomas will demonstrate a much lower increase in signal intensity than low-flow angiomas (KAPLAN and WILLIAMS 1987; KONERMANN et al. 1989).

10.4.1.1.8
TERATOMA

Teratomas are generally benign tumors typically occurring in infancy. These tumors are not infrequently detected during intrauterine life by means of fetal ultrasonography. Teratomas are intrapericardially located pedunculated tumors, arising from the root of the ascending aorta, and may cause large pericardial effusion with cardiac tamponade (ARCINIEGAS et al. 1980; BENETAR et al. 1992). They consist of the three germ layers and may be cystic as well as solid. Early surgical removal is usually curative. The experience with MRI in the detection and diagnosis of cardiac teratomas is very limited. BARAKOS et al. (1989a) noted a high signal intensity on T1-weighted images in a patient with an intrathoracic teratoma.

10.4.1.2
Malignant Cardiac Tumors

Primary malignant cardiac tumors can be divided into three major groups, i.e., sarcomas, lymphomas, and mesotheliomas.

10.4.1.2.1
SARCOMAS

Soft tissue sarcoma is the most common malignant neoplasm of the heart, pericardium, and great vessels. Its presentation is infrequent, nonspecific, and subtle, and may mimic other diseases. New noninvasive techniques such as echocardiography and MRI aid in the diagnosis and preoperative assessment (RAAF and RAAF 1994). Overall survival is poor. At this time, aggressive and complete surgical resection seems to offer the best hope for palliation and survival in an otherwise fatal disease.

Angiosarcoma. In adults approximately 25% of all primary cardiac tumors are malignant. One-third of these tumors are angiosarcomas (HERRMANN et al. 1992; BURKE et al. 1992). This highly aggressive malignant tumor can develop from the endothelium of lymphatics, i.e., lymphangiosarcoma, or blood vessels, i.e., hemangiosarcoma. In a review study by NAKA et al. (1995), 12 out of 99 angiosarcomas arose in the heart. Most cardiac angiosarcomas arise in the right atrium (75%), although the reasons for this remain unclear (JANIGAN et al. 1986) (Fig. 10.7). They present as single or multiple nodules, filling the right atrium and/or infiltrating the myocardium and pericardium (MCALLISTER and FENOGLIO 1978; URBA and LONGO 1986). The pericardial sac is filled by hemorrhage and blood. Since the presentation is often nonspecific, diagnosis is delayed and at the time of the diagnosis cardiac angiosarcomas have usually metastasized, most frequently to the lung (URBA and LONGO 1986; AOUATE et al. 1988). The pulmonary metastases most frequently have irregular margins due to peripheral hemorrhages. Calcified and cavitary metastases have been reported but are seldom and have to be differentiated from calcified pulmonary metastases arising from the colon, breast, ovary, and thyroid gland. Cardiac angiosarcomas

have a dismal prognosis, with a mean survival of 6 months after presentation.

Angiosarcomas usually present on MRI as heterogeneous masses (Fig. 10.7). A characteristic presentation of angiosarcomas is the mosaic pattern, consisting of nodular areas of increased signal intensity interspersed with areas of intermediate signal intensity on T1-weighted images. The high signal areas result from intratumoral hemorrhage. T2-weighted images usually show a clear demarcation of the tumor from the normal myocardium (SATO et al. 1995). Angiosarcomas may have a "cauliflower" appearance on MRI, with focal areas of increased signal intensity probably related to thrombosis or hemorrhage (KIM et al. 1989). Hemangiopericytomas, a much rarer primary cardiac sarcoma, may have a similar appearance on MRI and their distinction relies on pathologic examination (SATO et al. 1995).

Rhabdomyosarcoma. Rhabdomyosarcoma is the second most frequent primary malignant tumor of the heart. These tumors are composed of malignant

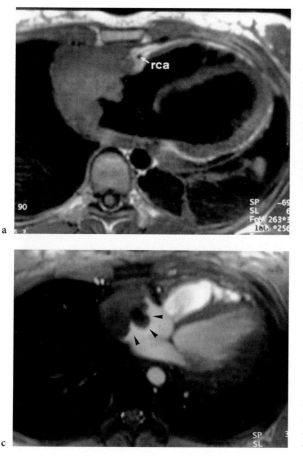

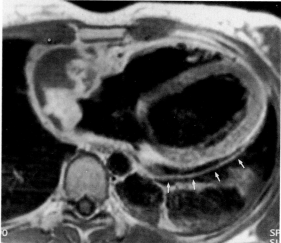

Fig. 10.7 a–c. Angiosarcoma of the right atrium with massive pericardial invasion. Axial T1-weighted SE images before (**a**) and after (**b**) administration of Gd-DTPA. **c** Axial GE image. A large mass originating in the lateral right atrial wall is invading the pericardium. Pericardial effusion and malignant pericardial thickening (*small arrows*) are present. After contrast administration the tumor borders can be better delineated and the tumor better differentiated from the adjacent pericardial effusion. The nodular appearance of the tumor can be well appreciated on the GE image (*black arrowheads*). *rca,* Right coronary artery

cells from striated muscle and occur singly or in multiples anywhere in the heart (Szucs et al. 1991). The right and left side of the heart are involved with equal frequency, and in a third to a half of the cases the pericardium is involved by direct extension from the myocardium. The prognosis is generally poor. MRI is not only helpful in quantifying the initial extent of the tumor, but also in evaluating its response to chemotherapy (Szucs et al. 1991). The most common appearance of rhabdomyosarcomas is that of a homogeneous mass, isointense or minimally hyperintense to muscle on T1-weighted images and hyperintense to muscle on T2-weighted images. After Gd-DTPA administration, these tumors enhance markedly (Yousem et al. 1990).

Malignant Fibrous Histiocytoma. Malignant fibrous histiocytoma is the most common soft tissue sarcoma in adults, but is distinctly rare as a primary tumor of the heart (Murphey et al. 1994; Fang et al. 1996). Malignant fibrous histiocytomas are not infrequently anchored onto the posterior wall in the left atrium while right-sided tumors are extremely rare (Norita et al. 1992; Teramoto et al. 1995). This tumor may demonstrate clinical similarities with myxoma, and careful anatomopathologic examination of multiple sections of the tumor is necessary to distinguish it from benign tumors, especially myxomas (Ouzan et al. 1990; Kasugai et al. 1990). However, this tumor is far more aggressive than a myxoma and exhibits a greater tendency for local recurrence and infiltration. The tumors exhibit an intermediate, slightly heterogeneous signal intensity on T1-weighted im-

ages and a high signal intensity on T2-weighted images (Mahajan et al. 1989; Kim et al. 1989).

Other Cardiac Sarcomas. The heart is occasionally the primary site of other rare sarcomas, including undifferentiated sarcomas, liposarcomas, osteosarcomas, fibrosarcomas, synovial sarcomas, neuro-fibrosarcomas, leiomyosarcomas, chrondrosarcomas, and Kaposi's sarcomas. In a study by Burke et al., in a total of 75 primary cardiac sarcomas, 18 were undifferentiated sarcomas and nine were osteosarcomas; all of the latter tumors arose in the left atrium (Burke et al. 1991, 1992). Liposarcomas of the heart and pericardium are very rare, while cardiac metastasis of liposarcoma seems to occur more frequently. Most liposarcomas of the heart are tumors with diffuse cardiac involvement. The right ventricle is most frequently involved (Papa et al. 1994). In contrast to lipomas, liposarcomas display a signal intensity less than that of fat on T1-weighted images, or evidence of inhomogeneity if of high intensity (Conces et al. 1985; Dooms et al. 1985) (Fig. 10.8). Metastases are common by the time of diagnosis. Leiomyosarcomas predominate in the muscular arteries and great veins, while primary cardiac involvement is extremely rare (Lupetin et al. 1986; Raaf and Raaf 1994). Leiomyosarcomas of the inferior and superior vena cava may directly involve the right atrium. Primary cardiac leiomyosarcomas are usually located in the atria and may invade the pericardium (Borner et al. 1990; Takamizawa et al. 1992; Kuo et al. 1997). Cardiac Kaposi's sarcoma has been found in patients with AIDS and in immuno-

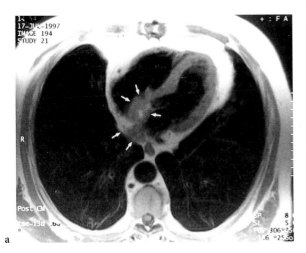
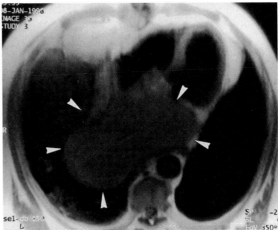

Fig. 10.8 a,b. Recurrence of myxoid liposarcoma in the left atrium. **a** Follow-up MRI study 1 year after surgery for left atrial myxoid liposarcoma; axial T1-weighted SE image. **b** Similar image 5 months later. On **a** there is inhomogeneously thickened interatrial septum and posterior left atrial wall, highly suggestive for tumor recurrence (*arrows*). Five months later (**b**) huge growth of the tumor recurrence has occurred (*arrowheads*)

suppressed organ transplant recipients (Lanza et al. 1983; Raaf and Raaf 1994). Kaposi's sarcoma of the heart may present as cardiac masses or as widely disseminated with infiltration of the heart and great vessels (Corallo et al. 1988; Langer et al. 1988).

10.4.1.2.2
LYMPHOMA

Primary cardiac lymphomas are extremely rare while metastatic involvement of the heart in patients with malignant lymphoma is far more common and results from retrograde lymphatic spread, hematogenous spread, and direction extension from other primary tumor masses. However, since primary cardiac lymphoma is associated with AIDS, an increase in primary cardiac lymphomas may be expected (Balasubramanyam et al. 1986; Gill et al. 1987). Primary lymphoma of the heart is defined as lymphoma involving only the heart and pericardium (Curtinsinger et al. 1989; Castelli et al. 1989). The clinical course in most patients with primary lymphoma of the heart is remarkably acute in onset and short in duration, and the diagnosis is often not made antemortem. Primary cardiac lymphoma presents with pericardial effusion, intracardiac masses, arrhythmias, and other nonspecific cardiac manifestations (Fig. 10.9) (Gill et al. 1987; Chao et al. 1995; Bogaert et al. 1995a). The intracardiac masses not infrequently arise in the ventricles (Gill et al. 1987). Imaging techniques are helpful for diagnosis but lack specificity (Chou et al. 1983; Coghlan et al. 1989; Rob-

erts et al. 1990; Bogaert et al. 1995a). Cytologic examination of the pericardial fluid or pericardial biopsy seems to be most suitable for diagnosis because of the frequent involvement of the pericardium. MRI provides accurate information on the cardiac masses and the extent of pericardial fluid, and can be repeated at follow-up.

10.4.1.2.3
MALIGNANT PERICARDIAL MESOTHELIOMA

The incidence of malignant pericardial mesothelioma is approximately 15% of all malignant cardiac tumors (Salcedo et al. 1992) (see Sect. 4.9 and Fig. 4.7) Mesotheliomas usually cover the visceral and parietal pericardium diffusely, encasing the heart, but generally do not invade the heart. Unlike malignant pleural mesotheliomas, the cardiac variety has no association with prior exposure to asbestos. Although they may be very extensive, they can sometimes be resected. MRI is helpful in depicting tumor localization and expansion, and in delineating the anatomic extent of malignant pericardial mesothelioma. On T1-weighted images the signal intensity is equal to or a little higher than that of the myocardium, and on T2-weighted images it is the same as or higher than that of fat tissue (Gossinger et al. 1988; Lund et al. 1989; Vogel et al. 1989; Kaminaga et al. 1993). A heterogeneous signal on T2-weighted images is related to the presence of intratumoral necrosis. Gd-DTPA administration is useful in clarifying the border between the tumor and myocar-

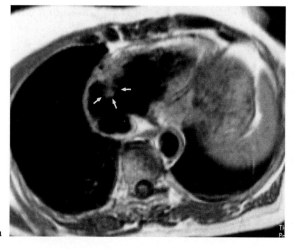

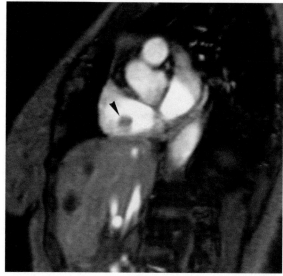

a

b

Fig. 10.9 a,b. Primary cardiac lymphoma. **a** Axial T1-weighted SE image. **b** Short-axis GE image. Primary cardiac lymphoma, presenting as a small mass in the right atrium (*arrowheads*). This patient died 4 months later from massive tumor emboli in the pulmonary arteries. [From J. Bogaert et al. (1995) Röfo 162:186–188; reprinted with permission from Fortschritte Röentgenstr, Georg Thieme Verlag]

dium (KAMINAGA et al. 1993). The location and MRI signal intensity of pericardial mesothelioma resembles those of fibrosarcoma and some metastatic tumors in the pericardial space. However, the latter are more invasive than malignant mesothelioma and tend to invade the intracardiac structures (SALCEDO et al. 1992; KAMINAGA et al. 1993).

10.4.2
Secondary Cardiac Tumors

Secondary tumors of the heart are 20–40 times more frequent than primary tumors of the heart. They may result from direct extension, hematogenous or venous extension, or retrograde flow by lymphatic vessels.

10.4.2.1
Direct Extension

Direct extension of a malignant tumor in the pericardium or in the heart occurs from tumors originating in the lung, mediastinum, or breast. Bronchial carcinoma may directly invade the mediastinum, the pericardium, or the heart (Fig. 10.10). Pericardial

involvement alone is characterized by a pericardial disruption associated with focal pericardial thickening and pericardial effusion. Irregular thickening of the atrial or ventricular myocardium is the hallmark of myocardial involvement (BARAKOS et al. 1989b). As many as 20% of all patients who die of lymphoma are found to have cardiac involvement at autopsy. The vast majority of these patients, however, do not have symptoms referable to cardiac involvement. The most frequent site of involvement is the pericardium, including the subepicardial fat (TESORO TESS et al. 1993). The atrioventricular groove is the most common site of epicardial invasion and often very large deposits occur in it. The cardiac chambers are less frequently involved. Not infrequently tumor may extend through the entire wall of a cardiac chamber or through the atrial septum (ROBERTS et al. 1968). Determination of lymphomatous involvement of the paracardiac spaces, the pericardium, and the heart is important for patients who are treated with radiation therapy. Generally, lung and cardiac blocks are placed to protect normal heart and lung, but these blocks are modified in the presence of pericardial involvement (JOCHELSON et al. 1983). Also, if the paracardiac disease encompasses a too great area, chemotherapy may be used in addition to radiation therapy.

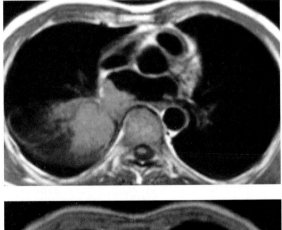

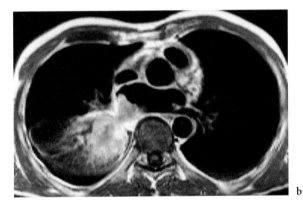

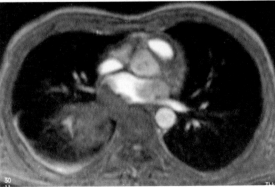

Fig. 10.10 a–c. Squamous cell carcinoma of the right lower lobe invading the left atrium. T1-weighted axial SE images before (**a**) and after (**b**) administration of Gd-DTPA. The lung tumor can be staged as T4, i.e., inoperable. Differentiation from an adjacent thrombus in the left atrium is feasible after contrast administration since the intracardiac part of the mass exhibits a similar enhancement pattern to the intrapulmonary part of the tumor. **c** Axial GE image: on cine MRI, the intracardiac mass is fixed to the rest of the tumor, and does not move with the rest of the heart

10.4.2.2
Hematogenous Extension

The incidence of cardiac metastases ranges from 1.5% to 20.6% (average 6%) in autopsies on patients with malignant diseases (ROSENTHAL and BRAUNWALD 1992). There has been a gradual increase in the frequency of cardiac metastases, perhaps as a consequence of the rising frequency of cancer plus the existence of reliable noninvasive diagnostic tests. Cardiac metastases are usually found in patients with disseminated tumors. Despite their frequent occurrence in patients with malignant disease, cardiac metastases are usually clinically silent (HEATH 1968). Isolated metastases occurring only in the heart are very unusual. Surgical resection of isolated cardiac metastases can be attempted to improve survival in patients whose primary tumor is well controlled (LEE and FISHER 1989). The most common tumors that metastasize to the heart are of bronchial and breast origin, followed by melanomas, lymphoma, and leukemia (LAGRANGE et al. 1986; HALLALI and HAIAT 1987). Malignant melanoma has a peculiar predilection for metastatic cardiac involvement (accounting for 60% of cases of cardiac metastasis). The pericardium is most frequently affected, while isolated involvement of the myocardium is seldom seen. Intracardiac metastases from neuroendocrine tumors of the carcinoid type may mimic benign cardiac tumors (e.g., myxoma) and this entity has to be differentiated from valvular abnormalities seen in some patients with carcinoid syndrome.

Magnetic resonance imaging may be of benefit in defining the size, shape, and extent of metastatic cardiac neoplasms (LEE and FISHER 1989; PAPA et al. 1994). Metastatic deposits present as focal nodular lesions of the pericardium or myocardium. Adjacent pleural effusion or flowing blood provides marked signal contrast, so that myocardial and pericardial lesions are visualized easily, as is the extension of the tumor in the cardiac chamber (BARAKOS et al. 1989b).

10.4.2.3
Venous Extension

Intracaval extension is a well-known but rare complication of benign tumors such as leiomyomatosis arising from a uterine myoma or from the wall of the vessel itself (BASSISH 1974; ROSENBERG et al. 1988; DUNLAP and UDJUS 1990; STEINMETZ et al. 1996) and malignant tumors, e.g., adrenocortical carcinoma (RITCHEY et al. 1987; GODINE et al. 1990), hepatocellu-

lar carcinoma (KANEMATSU et al. 1994), Wilms' tumor (GIBSON et al. 1990), renal cell carcinoma (PAUL et al. 1975), recurrent pheochromocytoma (ROTE et al. 1977), endometrial stromal carcinoma (PHILLIPS et al. 1995), and thyroid carcinoma (THOMPSON et al. 1978). Its presence is potentially hazardous because it can cause caval obstruction, extension of the tumor thrombus into the right-atrium causing atrial occlusion, and tumor embolization (Fig. 10.11). Intracardiac leiomyomatosis is a rare complication of right-sided obstruction and should be considered in the differential diagnosis if the patient is of reproductive age and is found to have a mass lesion in the right side of the heart.

Complete excision of tumors showing intracaval extension is necessary to avoid recurrence. Preoperative diagnosis of caval involvement is essential for planning the extent of surgery. For instance, intravascular extension of adrenocortical carcinoma is not a contraindication to radical surgery. Accurate identification is essential to plan treatment and to avoid complications. MRI is perfectly suited to detect the presence and extension of an intracaval tumor thrombus. Although differentiation between the tumor component and the accompanying bland thrombus is still difficult with MRI, NGUYEN et al. (1996) recently reported the presence of a patchy flow signal within the cavoatrial thrombus as a pattern of tumoral neovascularity in a patient with a renal granular cell carcinoma.

10.4.2.4
Retrograde Flow by Lymphatic Vessels

This fourth pathway of cardiac involvement occurs from spread from noncontiguous mediastinal lymph nodes via the lymphatic vessels to the heart with predominant epicardial involvement and variable myocardial invasion. Retrograde spread has been shown to be the most common mechanism in lymphomas and may also be seen in cases of lung and breast carcinoma (DELOACH and HAYNES 1953) (Fig. 10.12). Disease spreads from the anterior mediastinum to the paracardiac area and pericardium; the hilus may be bypassed and may remain uninvolved, since it is not necessarily part of the drainage (JOCHELSON et al. 1983).

The lymphatics of the visceral pericardium and the heart drain into larger lymphatic vessels which run within the subepicardial fat and drain either to the nodes situated at the base of the heart, between the transverse part of the aorta and the left pulmo-

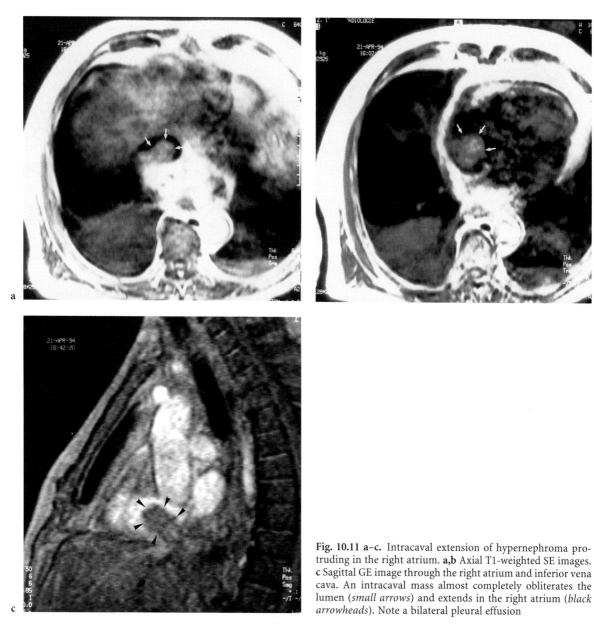

Fig. 10.11 a–c. Intracaval extension of hypernephroma protruding in the right atrium. **a,b** Axial T1-weighted SE images. **c** Sagittal GE image through the right atrium and inferior vena cava. An intracaval mass almost completely obliterates the lumen (*small arrows*) and extends in the right atrium (*black arrowheads*). Note a bilateral pleural effusion

nary artery, or directly into the anterosuperior mediastinal nodes. The lymphatics of the parietal pericaridium are scanty and run upward along the phrenic nerve over the lateral aspect of the cardiac silhouette and into the anterior mediastinal nodes. A chain of nodes may also be seen posteriorly, running along the pulmonary ligament to the hilus. Lymph nodes that are sometimes present on the parietal pericardial surface, usually in the right hemithorax, are associated with the lymph drainage from the central part of the diaphragm. Therefore, the nodal areas referred to as pericardiac and paracardiac include the inferior internal mammary, diaphragmatic,

paraphrenic, posterior pulmonary ligament, and paraesophageal nodes.

10.4.3
Para- and Extracardiac Tumors

Though an extensive description of the para- and extracardiac tumors is beyond the scope of this chapter, a brief summary will be given. Not only are these tumors more frequent than primary cardiac tumors but due to their close relation with the pericardium and heart, knowledge of their presenta-

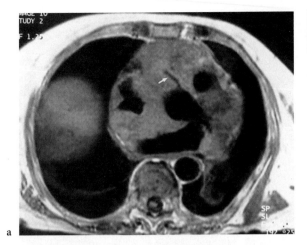
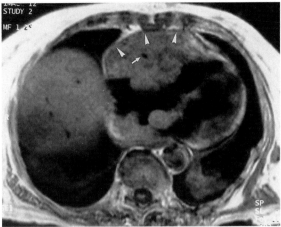

a

b

Fig. 10.12 a,b. High-grade mediastinal non-Hodgkin lymphoma diffusely infiltrating the heart. T1-weighted axial SE images. The anterior subepicardial fat and the anterior atrioventricular groove are entirely invaded by lympho- matous tissue, surrounding the right coronary artery (*arrow*). There is narrowing of the right atrium due to a tumoral thick- ening of the lateroposterior wall and the interatrial septum. The pericardial sac is displaced anteriorly (*arrowheads*)

tion is required. Paracardial tumors typically arise within the mediastinum, coming into close contact with the heart by direct growth. Pericardial and myo- cardial involvement occurs by external compression or tumor invasion. Mediastinal masses often abut the pericardium without penetration of the pericar- dium. The presence of a normal pericardium and pericardial sinuses provides a natural cleavage plane between the heart and the mediastinal mass. In these cases, usually no pericardial effusion is seen (BARAKOS et al. 1989b). Tumors located in the anterior mediastinum include thymomas, thymo- lipomas, lymphomas, germ cell tumors, and tumor or masses originating from the thyroid gland (Fig. 10.13). Tumors located in the middle and poste- rior mediastinum are mostly neurogenic, arise from the esophagus (e.g., esophageal cancer, enteric cyst/duplication), or are related to the trachea or bronchi (e.g., bronchogenic cyst or bronchial cancer).

Magnetic resonance imaging is perfectly suited to describe the relation of the tumor to the heart, and to evaluate cardiac or vascular compression or invasion by the tumor (Fig. 10.13). Furthermore, the signal characteristics on MRI can be used for tissue charac- terization. For instance, a bronchogenic cyst has a relatively high signal intensity on T1-weighted imag- ing and a very high signal intensity on T2-weighted imaging (NAKATA et al. 1993). A fluid-fluid level in the cyst may be caused by an intracystic hemorrhage or precipitation of calcium in the dependent part of the cyst (BARGALLO et al. 1993; AYDINGOZ et al. 1997). Thymolipomas are anterior mediastinal masses that

may conform to the shape of the adjacent structures, and thus may simulate cardiomegaly or diaphrag- matic elevation on chest radiographs. MRI typically demonstrates a mixture of fat and soft tissue signal intensity characteristics (ROSADO DE CHRISTENSON et al. 1994). MRI can be helpful in determining the malig- nancy of thymomas (SAKAI et al. 1992; ENDO et al. 1993; KUSHIHASHI et al. 1996). Benign thymomas are well-defined round or oval masses in the anterior mediastinum with a homogeneous or slightly inhomogeneous signal on T2-weighted images. On the other hand, invasive thymomas usually have an inhomogeneous signal intensity, a multinodular appearance, and a lobulated internal architecture or fibrous septa, and often display irregular borders. Thymic carcinomas demonstrate low signal intensi- ties on both T1- and T2-weighted images and irregu- lar margins, but lack fibrous septa or lobutated internal architecture. Although MRI appears prom- ising, histology is still essential to distinguish benign from malignant mediastinal lesions (MASSIE et al. 1997).

10.4.4
Nontumoral Cardiac Masses and Mimics

10.4.4.1
Thrombus

Cardiac thrombi are much more frequent than car- diac tumors. The formation of thrombi usually oc- curs in patients with regional or global wall motion

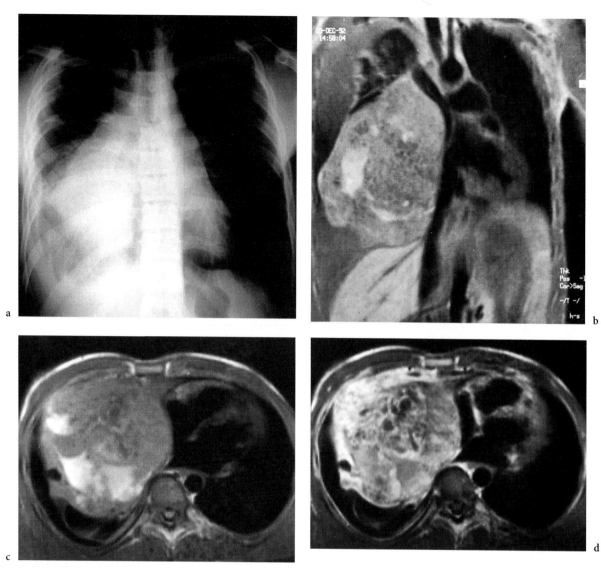

Fig. 10.13 a–d. Mediastinal germ cell tumor. **a** Frontal chest radiograph; **b,c** nonenhanced coronal (**b**) and axial (**c**) T1-weighted SE images; **d** contrast-enhanced axial T1-weighted SE image. A large inhomogeneous mass is present in the right paracardiac space with compression of the right atrium and inferior and superior vena cava. There is no evidence of cardiac or diaphragmatic invasion. Associated right-sided pleural effusion is observed

abnormalities, such as those that develop after myocardial infarction and in association with dilated cardiomyopathy or atrial fibrillation, especially if mitral valve disease and enlarged atrium are present (DePace et al. 1981). Left atrial thrombi are generally attached to the posterior left atrial wall by a broad base, so that they are immobile. If they are pedunculated and mobile, distinguishing them from a myxoma may be difficult. Right atrial thrombi are often found in patients with generalized poor condition (Fig. 10.14). Ventricular thrombi are exceedingly rare in patients with normal ventricular function (DeGroat et al. 1985; Chin et al. 1988). Left ventricular thrombi are often attached to the apex or within a discrete aneurysm or dyskinetic ventricular wall (Keeley and Hillis 1996) (Fig. 10.15). The majority of thrombi are immobile but occasionally slight motion of the thrombus can simulate a tumor such as a myxoma.

The primary screening modality for patients with suspected cardiac thrombus is two-dimensional echocardiography. However, false-negative, false-

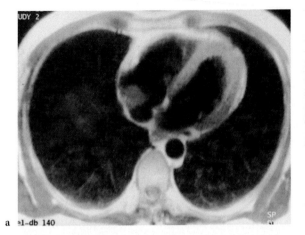 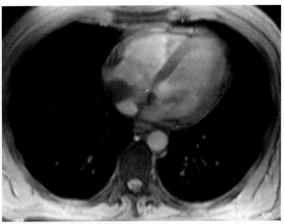

Fig. 10.14 a,b. Right atrial thrombus in a patient receiving chemotherapy for testis carcinoma. **a** Axial HASTE image; **b** axial GE image. Thrombi arising in the right atrium are rare but are not infrequently found in patients with intravenous catheters. In this patient a massive thrombus was shown at the tip of the catheter

positive, or equivocal findings are not uncommon, and are related to inadequate echocardiograms caused by anatomic abnormalities of the patients or to certain characteristics of the thrombus (STRATTON et al. 1982; JUNGEHULSING et al. 1992). For instance, large, echogenic, irregular, mobile mural thrombi are easy to detect on echocardiography, while laminated mural thrombi may be difficult to distinguish from myocardium, and slowflowing blood in aneurysm may be confused with thrombus.

Magnetic resonance imaging has a great potential in the diagnosis of suspected cardiac thrombi (JOHNSON et al. 1988). Cardiac thrombi usually have higher signal intensity than the normal myocardium on SE MRI, especially on the second echo (DOOMS and HIGGINS 1986). Differentiation between thrombus and slow-flowing blood on SE MRI, however, may be difficult because of the increased MR signal produced by slow-flowing blood (GOMES et al. 1987; SECHTEM et al. 1989).

Gradient-echo MRI permits improved differentiation of thrombi from the surrounding blood pool and myocardium (JUNGEHULSING et al. 1992). On GE MRI, thrombus always shows a lower signal intensity than does blood. The differentiation between thrombus and myocardium on GE MRI is more difficult because the thrombus is iso- to hyperintense compared with the adjacent surrounding myocardium. Since the thrombotic material differs according to its age and degree of organization, the signal intensity of the thrombus will change due to loss of water, condensation of paramagnetic iron complexes, and sometimes calcification (BAUMGARTNER 1973). Another advantage of GE images is the capability for cine display of cardiac motion and blood flow, i.e., cine MRI. Signal intensity from blood changes slightly during the cardiac cycle, whereas normal anatomic structures or thrombus maintain a nearly constant signal intensity. Alternative methods to distinguish slowly moving blood from thrombus are MRI phase imaging and MRI tagging (see Sect. 10.3.4) (RUMANCIK et al. 1988; AXEL and DOUGHERTY 1989).

10.4.4.2
Valvular Vegetations

Valvular vegetations can also be confused as mass lesions by echocardiography. However, in these instances, the echoes generally appear small and movement is limited. Furthermore, the vegetations follow the motion of the valvular cusp to which they are attached. MRI may be useful in clarifying echocardiographic findings and establishing the diagnosis in previously undiagnosed patients. Vegetations are usually not visible on SE MRI but are clearly visible on cine MRI, appearing as areas of low signal at valve leaflets in contrast to the bright flowing blood (CADUFF et al. 1996) (Fig. 10.16).

Libman-Sacks endocarditis, or the endocardial involvement in patients with systemic lupus erythematosus, is found in up to 50% of hearts at autopsy (see also Sect. 5.5.4). It presents as small verrucous vegetations (3–4 mm in size) appearing on the valvular or mural endocardial surface. The posterior leaflet of the mitral valve is most frequently involved. Infrequently, such vegetations may become massive thrombotic lesions, up to 10 mm, or even larger (DOHERTY and SIEGEL 1985). Libman–Sacks endocar-

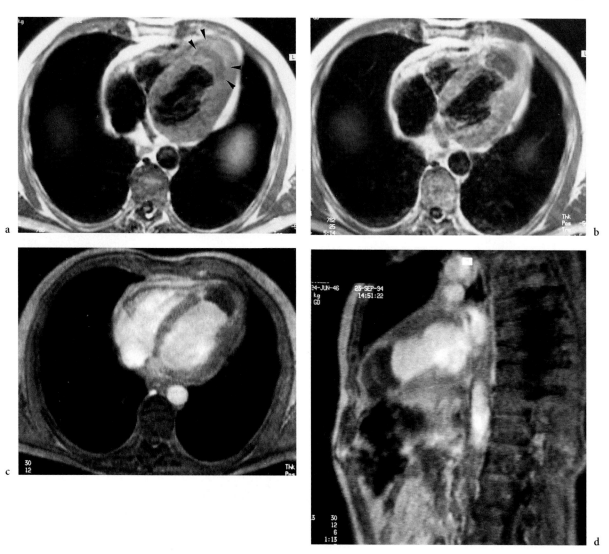

Fig. 10.15 a–d. Mural thrombus in the left ventricular (LV) apex in a patient with a history of acute apical myocardial infarction. **a,b** T1-weighted axial SE images before (**a**) and after (**b**) Gd-DTPA administration. **c,d** Axial (**c**) and vertical long-axis (**d**) GE images. On the precontrast SE images the thrombus in the LV apex is slightly hypointense compared with the adjacent myocardium (*arrowheads*). On the postcontrast images the thrombus can be clearly differentiated from the myocardium. On GE MRI, the thrombus is hypointense compared with the myocardium and surrounding blood

ditis may predispose to infective endocarditis. As in other causes of valvular vegetations, MRI can be helpful in visualization of the valve or mural lesions (Fig. 10.17).

10.4.4.3
Perivalvular Extension of Infection

Perivalvular extension of infection (i.e., cardiac abscess and pseudoaneurysm) is a not infrequent and potentially fatal complication of bacterial endocarditis (CARPENTER 1991). Cardiac abscesses are observed in 20%–30% of cases of infective endocarditis and in at least 60% of cases of prosthetic valve endocarditis (THOMAS et al. 1993). The aortic valve ring is more frequently affected than the mitral valve ring. The perivalvular extension of infection (usually involving the mitral-aortic intervalvular fibrosa) may present as a closed purulent collection (i.e., cardiac abscess) or as a cavity contiguous with a cardiac chamber (i.e., pseudoaneurysm). Subsequent rup-

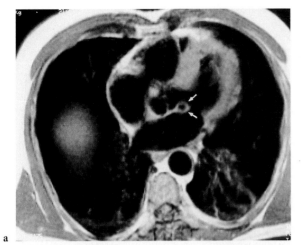

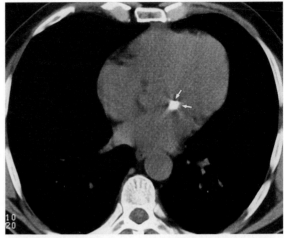

a

b

Fig. 10.16 a,b. Chronic vegetation of the mitral valve. **a** Axial T1-weighted SE image; **b** non-contrast-enhanced CT. Small, nodular, centrally hypointense mass at the anterior mitral valve leaflet (*arrows*). The calcified nature as suggested by the absence of signal on SE images is proven on CT

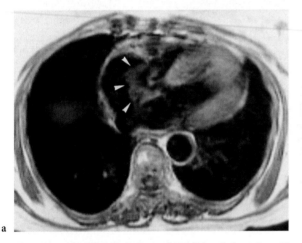

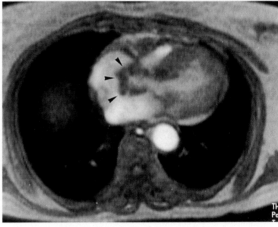

a

b

Fig. 10.17 a,b. Libman-Sacks endocarditis of the tricuspid valve. **a** Axial T1-weighted SE MRI; **b** axial GE image. A large vegetation in the right atrium arising on the tricuspid valve (*arrowheads*) was erroneously mistaken for an atrial tumor on echocardiography and MRI (diagnosis confirmed during cardiac surgery). The mass demonstrated strong enhancement after Gd-DTPA administration (not shown)

ture of the infected zone of mitral-aortic intervalvular fibrosa or subaortic aneurysm into the left atrium may occur, a condition which should be differentiated from ruptured aneurysm of the sinus of Valsalva (BANSAL et al. 1990) (see Sect. 10.4.4.6).

Although transesophageal echocardiography is the imaging method of choice for the diagnosis of valvular vegetations in infectious endocarditis, the diagnosis of an associated ring abscess is sometimes difficult, especially in patients with valvular prostheses or calcifications, which are an important source of artifacts. MRI may be useful to detect the paravalvular abscess and infectious pseudoaneurysms (JEANG et al. 1986; WINKLER and HIGGINS 1986; FURBER et al. 1997). A cardiac abscess is visible as a

heterogeneous low signal intensity zone on T1-weighted MRI and as high intensity signal on T2-weighted MRI. The inflammatory origin is responsible for the increase in signal after injection of paramagnetic contrast agents. Cine MRI is helpful to detect the presence or absence of communication between the abscess cavity and the cardiac chambers.

10.4.4.4
Lipomatous Hypertrophy of the Interatrial Septum

Lipomatous hypertrophy of the interatrial septum is, pathogenetically, a hypertrophy of preexisting fat,

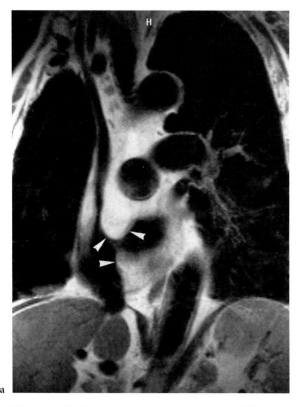

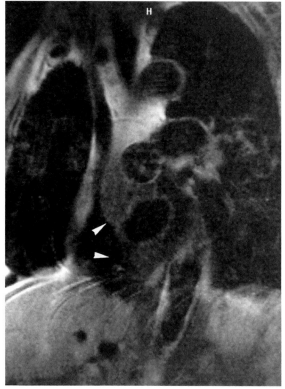

a   b

Fig. 10.18 a,b. Lipomatous hypertrophy of the atrial septum (LHAS). **a** Short-axis T1-weighted turbo SE; **b** similar image with fat suppression. LHAS is visible on T1-weighted images as a hyperintense bilobated appearance of the atrial septum sparing the fossa ovalis (*arrowheads*). The fatty nature can be depicted by means of fat suppression techniques which will selectively reduce the signal of fat

and not a true neoplasm (see Sect. 10.4.1.1.2), and it is not infrequently associated with increased epicardial fat (MEANY et al. 1997). This poorly recognized, but not rare, benign condition represents a fat accumulation within the interatrial septum in continuity with the epicardial fat. It is usually anterior to the fossa ovalis. There may be a component posterior to the fossa. Since there is no fat accumulation in the fossa ovalis, lipomatous hypertrophy of the interatial septum often has a typical bilobed "camel-humped" or "dumbbell-shaped" appearance (Fig. 10.18). The typical appearance and the lipomatous nature, presenting as fat attenuation on CT and high signal intensity on T1-weighted MRI, should suggest lipomatous hypertrophy of the atrial septum and obviate biopsy or excision (LEVINE et al. 1986; APPLEGATE et al. 1987; FISHER and EDMONDS 1988). The differential diagnosis includes nonacute hematoma, lipoma, liposarcoma, hemangioma, and hemorrhage into a preexisting mass. Liposarcoma has a lower signal intensity than that of fat, or evidence of inhomogeneity if of high intensity (DOOMS et al. 1985). In addition, selective fat suppression techniques can be used to demonstrate the fatty nature and to differentiate lipomatous hypertrophy of the atrial septum from other nonlipomatous conditions (Fig. 10.18).

10.4.4.5
Atrial Septal Aneurysm

An aneurysm of the atrial septum is defined as a diffuse or a localized protrusion of the interatrial septum into the right or left atrium, or both, caused by a bulging of the whole interatrial septum or a bulging of the primary component of the septum through the fossa ovalis. It is an uncommon anomaly and may be associated with other congenital cardiac malformations or with acquired diseases that result in elevated pressures in one atrial chamber with bulging of the septum to the opposite side (HANLEY et al. 1985). Atrial septal aneurysms have been associated with septal defects, atrial arrhythmias, systolic clicks, atrioventricular valve prolapse, systemic and pulmonary embolism, and atrial tumors, and they usually occur at the fossa ovalis (HANLEY et al. 1985; GALLET et al. 1985, BOGAERT et al. 1995b). HANLEY et al. (1985) observed three types of fossa ovalis aneurysm and one type of aneurysm involving the entire atrial

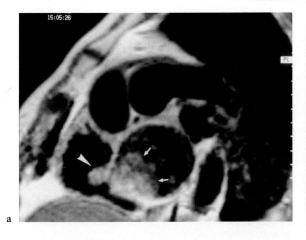

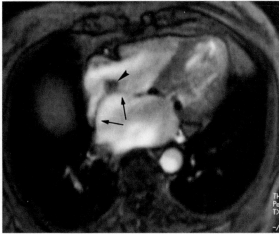

Fig. 10.19 a,b. Aneurysm of the atrial septum with concomitant right atrial tumor. **a** Short-axis T1-weighted SE image; **b** four-chamber view GE image. There is localized bulging of the atrial septum to the right (type Ib according to Hanley) (*black arrows*). A small tumorous mass is attached to the right side of the atrial septum (*arrowhead*). On SE images, stagnant blood or turbulent flow in the concavity of the aneurysm should not be mistaken for thrombus or tumor (*white arrows*)

septum. Systemic and pulmonary thromboembolic events in the presence of an atrial septal aneurysm are probably due to thrombus formation within the concave aspect of the aneurysm. The frequently associated atrial septal defect may result in paradoxical emboli (SCHNEIDER et al. 1990).

Diagnosis is usually made by echocardiography, though stagnant blood flow within the cavity of the aneurysm may mimic a cystic mass (SMITH et al. 1990). MRI is helpful in detecting atrial septal aneurysms, though it should be mentioned that low flow or stagnant flow may appear on SE MRI as signal rich rather than signal void, thus mimicking a cardiac mass (SMITH et al. 1990) (Fig. 10.19). Cine MRI may overcome this shortcoming, and may allow a better description of the type and movement of aneurysm (BOGAERT et al. 1995b).

10.4.4.6
Aneurysm of the Sinus of Valsalva

Aneurysms of the sinus of Valsalva are uncommon entities and although they are not truly cardiac masses, it is worth mentioning this condition in the differential diagnostic list of cardiac masses (Fig. 10.20). They usually originate from the right coronary sinus, and much less frequently from the noncoronary and the left coronary sinus (DEV et al. 1993). The aneurysms are usually congenital but infrequently they can be acquired (usually endocarditis associated). This condition is usually detected

in adults as an incidental finding or by virtue of a complication due to the aneurysm. The most frequent complication is rupture of the aneurysm, usually into the right ventricular outflow tract, right ventricular cavity, or right atrium, and less frequently into the other cardiac chambers or dissecting into the interventricular septum (DEV et al. 1993; ABAD 1995). Other less frequent complications are embolization, compression of the coronary arteries by the aneurysm with subsequent myocardial infarction, and thrombosis of the aneurysm (REID et al. 1990; WIEMER et al. 1996).

The diagnosis is usually made by transthoracic and transesophageal echocardiography, though MRI may be very helpful to demonstrate the aneurysm and to depict the communication between the aorta and the cardiac chambers (OGAWA et al. 1991; RAFFA et al. 1991; HO et al. 1995; KULAN et al. 1996). The latter will be visible on cine MRI as a hypo-intense jet directed from the aorta into one of the cardiac chambers.

10.4.4.7
Hydatid Cyst

Echinococcosis is endemic in several countries around the Mediterranean Sea. Cardiac involvement in hydatid disease is rare, representing 0.5%–2% of all clinical forms of this condition (CACOUB et al. 1991). Because of the risk of potentially lethal complications (due to cyst rupture and massive embo-

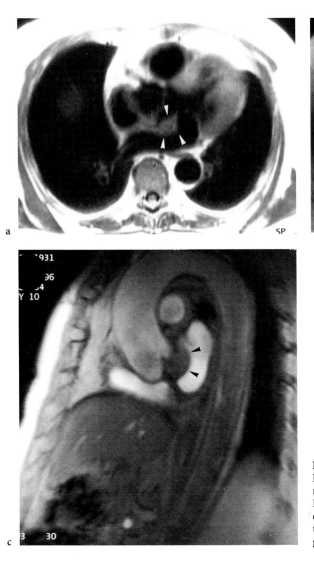

a

b

c

Fig. 10.20 a–c. Aneurysm of the sinus of Valsalva. a Axial HASTE image; b axial GE image; c short-axis GE image. Abnormal "mass" on the ventral side of the left atrium on the HASTE image. Cine MRI shows a bulging of the posterior wall of the aortic root with slow flow. The diagnosis of aneurysm of the sinus of Valsalva was confirmed during coronary bypass graft surgery

lism), early diagnosis and adequate treatment are very important (PASAOGLU et al. 1994). The diagnosis of cardiac echinococcosis is difficult and is based on a series of findings amongst which hydatid serology and cardiac imaging are particularly important. Hydatid cysts most frequently involve the left ventricular myocardial wall and interventricular septum (KARDARAS et al. 1996). MRI, together with echocardiography and CT, is of considerable importance in the detection of intramyocardial hydatid cysts (ELKOUBY et al. 1990; KULAN et al. 1995; KARDARAS et al. 1996; MACEDO et al. 1997). MRI also allows diagnosis of noncardiac lesions, e.g., pulmonary, hepatic, splenic, and renal involvement, and is helpful in planning surgical intervention.

The detection of intramyocardial cystic lesions is virtually pathognomomic for hydatid disease. These hydatid cysts have a fluid content with a homoge-

neously hypointense signal intensity on T1-weighted and a homogeneously hyperintense signal on T2-weighted images (KOTOULAS et al. 1996) (Fig. 10.21). The pericyst, a thick fibrotic membrane surrounding the hydatid cyst, has a low-signal intensity on T1- and T2-weighted images and this allows differentiation from nonparasitic epithelial cysts (VANJAK et al. 1990; CACOUB et al. 1991; CANTONI et al. 1993; ÜNAL et al. 1995).

10.4.4.8
(Pleuro)pericardial Cyst

Very likely pericardial cysts can be considered as nontumoral masses (see also Sect. 4.5.2 and Fig. 4.2). They are usually asymptomatic and most frequently arise in the right cardiophrenic angle, followed by the

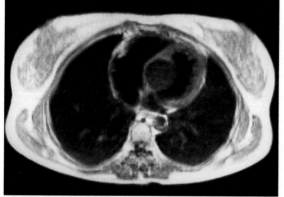

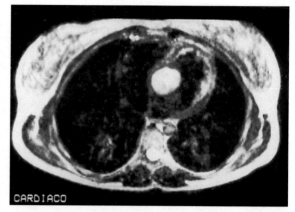

Fig. 10.21 a,b. Hydatid cyst of the interventricular septum of the heart. T1-weighted SE image (**a**) shows a hypointense mass bulging into the left ventricle. T2-weighted SE image (**b**) shows the characteristic high signal intensity of cystic lesions. [From CANTONI et al. (1993) Am J Roentgenol 161:753–754. Reprinted with permission of the American Roentgen Ray Society]

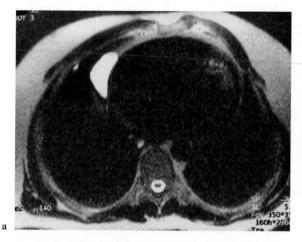

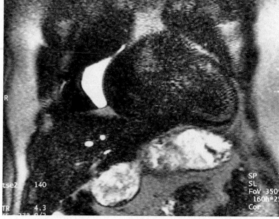

Fig. 10.22 a,b. Pericardial cyst. T2-weighted HASTE images: **a** axial, **b** coronal. Well-defined hyperintense structure in the right cardiophrenic angle. On these strongly T2-weighted images, the intracystic fluid is strongly hyperintense, similar to the cerebrospinal fluid

left cardiophrenic angle and, rarely, the anterior or posterior mediastinum. They are usually unilocular and present with a variable diameter. Pericardial cysts are usually discovered during routine radiography. MRI may be very helpful in detecting the water content (VINEE et al. 1992). Pericardial cysts have a low signal intensity on T1-weighted images and a very high signal intensity on T2-weighted images (Fig. 10.22). No enhancement effect of Gd-DTPA is observed. MRI is also helpful in differentiattion from other cystic mediastinal structures such as bronchogenic cyst, cystic teratoma, cystic neurogenic tumor, and thymus cyst. Differences in signal intensities on T1-weighted imaging can help in the differentiation since pericardial cysts have a pure water content with low signal intensities, while the others may have a higher signal intensity due to intracystic

hemorrhage or the presence of sebaceous fluid (MURAYAMA et al. 1995) Furthermore, cystic teratomas typically contain fat and calcifications.

10.4.4.9
Gossypiboma or Textiloma

Gossypibomas or textilomas are an iatrogenic cause of cardiac, pericardial, or extracardiac masses. They represent a foreign body reaction surrounding a retained surgical sponge composed of a cotton matrix. Gossypibomas are rare occurrences which are infrequently reported in the literature because of legal implications (BHAT et al. 1997). Their manifestations and complications are so variable that diagnosis is difficult and patient morbidity is significant. A

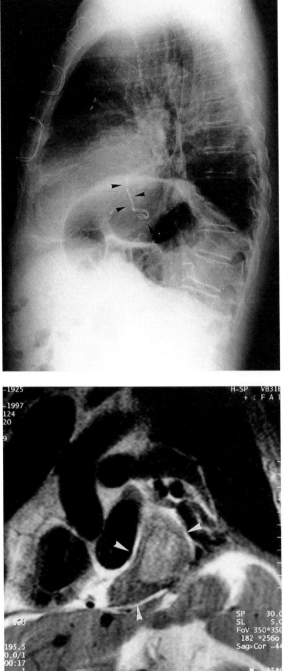

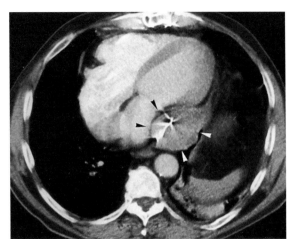

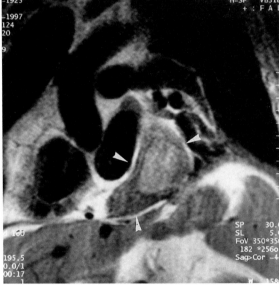

Fig. 10.23 a–c. Gossypiboma. **a** Lateral chest x-ray; **b** contrast-enhanced CT image; **c** short-axis turbo SE image. Intrapericardial gossypiboma or textiloma following coronary bypass graft surgery 25 years previously. The surgical sponge can be easily detected by its radiopaque marker on standard radiographs (*arrowheads*). Both CT and MRI demonstrate very nicely the foreign tissue granuloma and the compression of the left heart. Note the elevation of the left hemidiaphragm

high index of suspicion in a patient who has previously been operated upon will greatly aid in the diagnosis of this unfortunate complication. Most surgical sponges have radiopaque markers that have a characteristic appearance on plain radiographs (Fig. 10.23). However, the marker may disintegrate over long periods, or sponges used in some countries may not have markers (LERNER and DANG 1997).

Computed tomography, echocardiography, and MRI are particularly important in localizing gossypibomas. Gossypibomas have a typical spongiform pattern on CT; gas bubbles are the most specific sign for the detection of textilomas but do not indicate abscess formation (KOPKA et al. 1996). The MRI appearances of gossypibomas include masses with low signal intensity on T1- and T2-weighted images, high signal intensity on T1- and T2-weighted images, and heterogeneous signal intensity on T2-weighted images on which the internal architecture suggests retained surgical sponge (MOCHIZUKI et al. 1992; KUWASHIMA et al. 1993; LERNER and DANG 1997). As a result of a pericardial gossypiboma one or several heart chambers may be compressed (Fig. 10.23). Gossypibomas should be differentiated from postoperative scar formation and tumors (VAN GOETHEM et al. 1991).

10.4.5
Normal Cardiac Anatomy and Variants

Several normal intracardiac structures can mimic pathologic masses. Knowledge of these normal variants will reduce the number of false-positively diagnosed cardiac masses. This is particularly important since with the currently available cardiac imaging modalities, even the smallest cardiac structures are almost perfectly visible. Therefore, the most common normal variants will be described for each cardiac chamber separately and for the pericardium (see also Chap. 2).

10.4.5.1
Right Atrium

Nodular thickening of the posterior right atrial wall is a common finding on cardiac MRI and may resemble a mass lesion (MIROWITZ and GUTIERREZ 1992). Anatomically this nodular thickening corresponds to the *crista terminalis*, which marks the embryologic division between the portion of the right atrium that is derived from the sinus venosus, i.e., smooth-walled sinus venarum, and that which is derived from the embryonic atrium, i.e., trabeculated atrium proper and auriculum. The crista terminalis is a prominent muscular ridge that extends along the posterolateral aspect of the right atrium between the orifices of the superior and inferior venae cavae (Fig. 10.24). Inferiorly, it merges with the valve of the inferior vena cava (*eustachian valve*) and the valve of the coronary sinus (*thebesian valve*). In addition, strand-like fibrous structures, known as the *Chiari network*, may arise from the region of the inferior crista terminalis and/or eustachian valve and extend into the right atrial chamber. These structures, which are of variable prominence and have a similar signal intensity to myocardial tissue, are routinely observed on cardiac MRI and should not be mistaken

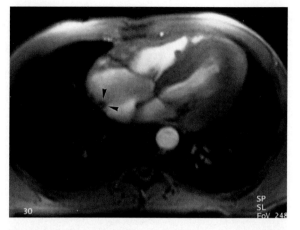

Fig. 10.24. Crista terminalis. Axial GE image. Nodular thickening of the posterolateral right atrial wall (*arrowheads*)

for neoplasms, thrombosis, or inflammation (MEIER and HARTNELL 1994).

10.4.5.2
Right Ventricle

The *moderator band,* a thin muscular band, is unique for the right ventricle, which can be very helpful in differentiating the right from the left ventricle in congenital heart malformations. This muscular structure extends from the midinterventricular septum through the cavity of the right ventricle and attaches near the base of the anterior papillary muscle on the free wall of the right ventricle. It may become very prominent in patients with right ventricular enlargement or hypertrophy or both, and may be mistaken for a right ventricular thrombus or tumor (Fig. 10.1). MRI allows detection of the muscular nature of the moderator band, with signal intensities similar to the surrounding myocardium.

10.4.5.3
Left Atrium

While the left atrium has a smooth wall delineation, the left atrial appendage is lined with small, equally spaced muscular pectinate ridges. These pectinate ridges must be distinguished from thrombi. Furthermore, a variety of extracardiac abnormalities such as hiatal hernia, esophageal carcinoma,

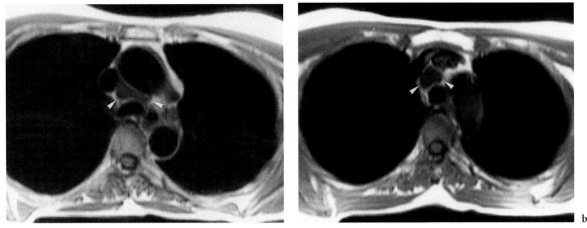

a   b

Fig. 10.25 a,b. Highly extending superior pericardial sinus presenting as a nodular mass (*arrowheads*). Axial T1-weighted SE images

bronchogenic cyst, or tortuous descending aorta can simulate masses in the left atrium on echocardiography (MENEGUS et al. 1992). The exact location of these "masses" can be determined by means of MRI.

10.4.5.4
Left Ventricle

Besides the normal papillary muscles and chordae tendinae, in a minority of the population false tendons or false chordae occur as normal variants in the left ventricle. Rather than connecting the papillary muscles with the valve leaflets, the false chordae are linear structures attached at both ends to the endomyocardium (KEREN et al. 1984). They are asymptomatic and usually accidental findings on echocardiography.

10.4.5.5
Pericardium

Knowledge of the normal appearance of the pericardium on MRI is necessary to adequately interpret cardiovascular MRI studies (see also Chap. 4). The superior pericardial sinus may not be mistaken for an aortic dissection, anomalous vascular structure, or a nodular mass on MRI (BLACK et al. 1993) (Fig. 10.25).

10.4.6
Prosthetic Valves and Other Foreign Devices

Metallic objects, such as metallic heart valves, stents, cardiac occluders, vascular clips, and catheters, may induce artifacts on the MR images (see also Sect. 11.3.6). The artifacts are variable and depend on the type and the amount of metal used in the implant and on the type of MRI sequence (SHELLOCK and MORISOLI 1994a,b). Metallic implants induce an alteration of the local magnetic field which leads to loss of signal from the surrounding tissue. For metallic heart valves studied with SE MRI, artifacts are minimal since the prosthetic valves cannot be differentiated from the surrounding dark blood (Fig. 10.26). SE MRI is advantageous in the depiction of anatomic structures like paravalvular abscesses (BACHMANN et al. 1991). Artifacts, however, are accentuated on GE MRI (cine MRI). Metallic heart valves are therefore visible as dark areas surrounded by bright blood (Fig. 10.26). Nevertheless, in a majority of cases qualitative analysis of the valve function and accurate measurement of the blood velocity downstream of the prosthetic heart valve can be performed (DI CESARE et al. 1995; WALKER et al. 1995). Physiologic valvular regurgitation can be differentiated from pathologic or valvular regurgitation. Artifacts caused by other foreign cardiac devices, such as intravascular or coronary stents, are similar to those caused by prosthetic valves (MOHIADDIN et al. 1995) (Fig. 10.27).

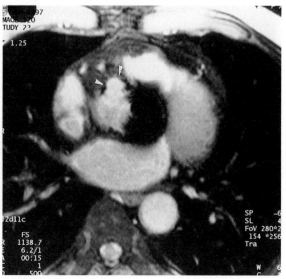

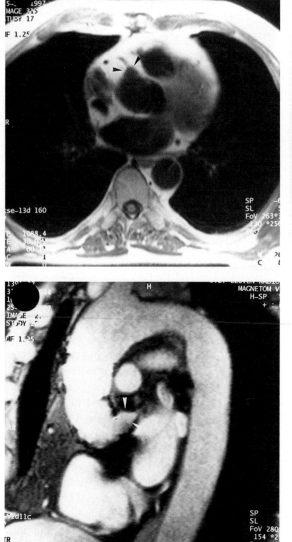

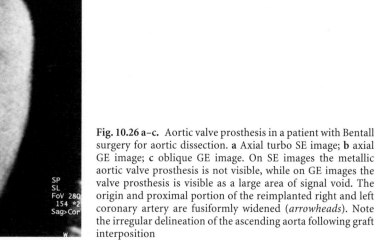

Fig. 10.26 a–c. Aortic valve prosthesis in a patient with Bentall surgery for aortic dissection. **a** Axial turbo SE image; **b** axial GE image; **c** oblique GE image. On SE images the metallic aortic valve prosthesis is not visible, while on GE images the valve prosthesis is visible as a large area of signal void. The origin and proximal portion of the reimplanted right and left coronary artery are fusiformly widened (*arrowheads*). Note the irregular delineation of the ascending aorta following graft interposition

10.5
Conclusions

With the advent of several noninvasive or minimally invasive cardiac imaging modalities such as echocardiography, CT, and MRI, detailed morphologic description of the heart, pericardium, great vessels, and mediastinum has become a reality. Even small normal anatomic structures can be very well recognized and differentiated from pathologic structures. The location and extent of cardiac tumors can be precisely evaluated, and the response to treatment can be accurately followed. Though differentiation between benign and malignant tumors, or between

tumoral and nontumoral conditions, is often not feasible without histologic proof, cardiac masses can be very accurately depicted or ruled out. Rather than being a primary imaging modality in patients suspected of having a cardiac tumor, MRI can be considered as an excellent "second-line" imaging modality which can be applied to confirm the findings on echocardiography, to determine precisely the tumor location and extent, for tissue characterization, for follow-up of patients under treatment, and to detect early tumor recurrence.

Acknowledgements. The author would like to thank S. Dymarkowski, MD, and B. Claikens, MD, for their help in the preparation of this chapter; Mr. W. Desmedt for producing

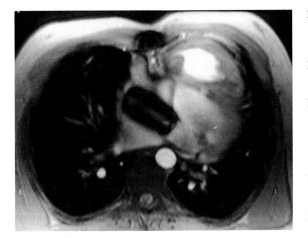

Fig. 10.27. Stent in a venous baffle in a patient with transposition of the great arteries. Axial GE image. A venous baffle conducts the systemic venous blood to the left heart and pulmonary arteries. The metallic stent in the "leg" coming from the superior vena cava is visible as a tubular hypointense structure. The lumen of the stent is patent though the intraluminal diameter cannot be exactly assessed as a consequence of metallic susceptibility artifacts

illustrations; F. Van de Werf, MD, PhD, from the department of Cardiology, M. Gewillig from the Department of Pediatric Cardiology, and other colleagues for their cooperation in the patient MRI studies.

References

Abad C (1995) Congenital aneurysm of the sinus of Valsalva dissecting into the interventricular septum. Cardiovasc Surg 3:563–564

Aggoun Y, Hunkeler N, Destephen M, et al. (1992) Cardiac rhabdomyomatosis and Bourneville's tuberous sclerosis in the fetus. A propos of 2 cases (in French). Arch Mal Coeur Vaiss 85:609–613

Amparo EG, Higgins CB, Farmer D, Gamsu G, McNamara M (1984) Gated MRI of cardiac and paracardiac masses: initial experience. Am J Roentgenol 143:1151–1156

Aouate P, Artigou JY, Rovany X, et al. (1988) Contribution of nuclear magnetic resonance in right atrial angiosarcoma. Apropos of a case (in French). Arch Mal Coeur Vaiss 81:1543–1546

Applegate PM, Tajik AJ, Ehman RL, Julsrud PR, Miller FAJ (1987) Two-dimensional echocardiographic and magnetic resonance imaging observations in massive lipomatous hypertrophy of the atrial septum. Am J Cardiol 59:489–491

Arciniegas E, Hakimi M, Farooki ZQ, Green EW (1980) Intrapericardial teratoma in infancy. J Thorac Cardiovasc Surg 79:306–311

Axel L, Dougherty L (1989) Heart wall motion: improved method for spatial modulation of magnetization for me imaging. Radiology 172:349–350

Aydingoz U, Ariyurek M, Selcuk ZT, Demirkazik FB, Baris YI (1997) Calcium within a bronchogenic cyst with a fluid level. Br J Radiol 70:761–763

Bachmann R, Deutsch HJ, Jungehulsing M, Sechtem U, Hilger HH, Schicha H (1991) Magnetic resonance imaging in patients with heart valve prostheses. Rofo Fortschr Rontgenstr 155:499–505

Balasubramanyam A, Waxman M, Kazal HL, Lee MH (1986) Malignant lymphoma of the heart in acquired immune deficiency syndrome. Chest 90:243–246

Bansal RC, Graham BM, Jutzy KR, Shakudo M, Shah PM (1990) Left ventricular outflow tract to left atrial communication secondary to rupture of mitral-aortic inter valvular fibrosa in infective endocarditis: diagnosis by transesophageal echocardiography and color flow imaging. J Am Coll Cardiol 15:499–504

Barakos JA, Brown JJ, Brescia RJ, Higgins CB (1989a) High signal intensity lesions of the chest in MR imaging. J Comput Assist Tomogr 13:797–802

Barakos JA, Brown JJ, Higgins CB (1989b) MR imaging of secondary cardiac and paracardiac lesions. Am J Roentgenol 153:47–50

Bargallo J, Luburich P, Garcia Barrionuevo J, Sanchez Gonzalez M (1993) Fluid-fluid level in bronchogenic cysts. Radiology 186:427–428

Bassish MS (1974) Mesenchymal tumors of the uterus. Clin Obstet Gynecol 17:51–88

Baumgartner HR (1973) The role of blood flow in platelet adhesion, fibrin deposition, and formation of mural thrombi. Microvasc Rev 5:167–179

Benetar A, Vaughan J, Nicolini U, Trotter S, Corrin B, Lincoln C (1992) Prenatal pericardiocentesis: its role in the management of intrapericardial teratoma. Obstet Gynecol 79:856–859

Bhat HS, Mahesh G, Ramgopal KS (1997) "Gossypiboma": an unusual cause of perinephric abscess. J R Coll Surg Edinb 42:277–278

Black CM, Hedges LK, Javitt MC (1993) The superior pericardial sinus: normal appearance on gradient-echo MR images. Am J Roentgenol 160:749–751

Bleiweis MS, Georgiou D, Brundage BH (1994) Detection and characterization of intracardiac masses by ultrafast computed tomography. Am J Card Imag 8:63–68

Bogaert J, Rademakers F, Cappelle L, Moerman P, Van de Werf F, Baert AL (1995a) High-grade immunoblastic sarcoma: an unusual type of a primary cardiac non-Hodgkin lymphoma. Rofo Fortschr Rontgenstr 162:186–188

Bogaert J, De Man F, Rademakers F, et al. (1995b) Right atrial tumor arising on an atrial septal aneurysm. Assessment by MR imaging. Clin Imaging 19:172–175

Borner C, Haberbosch W, Hagl S, Mechtersheimer G, Kretzschmar U, Hild R (1990) Primary leiomyosarcoma of the right atrium in an adult patient. Z Kardiol 79:865–869

Bouton S, Yang A, McCrindle BW, Kidd L, McVeigh ER, Zerhouni EA (1991) Differentiation of tumor from viable myocardium using cardiac tagging with MR imaging. J Comput Assist Tomogr 15:676–678

Brasch RC, Weinmann HJ, Wesbey GE (1984) Contrast-enhanced NMR imaging: animal studies using gadolinium-DTPA complex. Am J Roentgenol 142:625–630

Brizard C, Latremouille C, Jebara VA, et al. (1993) Cardiac hemangiomas (see comments). Ann Thorac Surg 56:390–394

Brown JJ, Barakos JA, Higgins CB (1989) Magnetic resonance imaging of cardiac and paracardiac masses. J Thorac Imaging 4:58–64

Burke AP, Virmani R (1991) Osteosarcomas of the heart. Am J Surg Pathol 51:289–295

Burke AP, Cowan D, Virmani R (1992) Primary sarcomas of the heart. Cancer 69:387–395

Burke AP, Rosado de Christenson M, Templeton PA, Virmani R (1994) Cardiac fibroma: clinicopathologic correlates and surgical treatment. J Thorac Cardiovasc Surg 108:862–870

Cacoub P, Chapoutot L, Du Boutin LT, et al. (1991) Hydatid cyst of the interventricular septum. Contribution of magnetic resonance imaging (in French). Arch Mal Coeur Vaiss 84:1857–1860

Caduff JH, Hernandez RJ, Ludomirsky A (1996) MR visualization of aortic valve vegetations. J Comput Assist Tomogr 20:613–615

Cantoni S, Frola C, Gatto R, Loria F, Terzi MI, Vallebona A (1993) Hydatid cyst of the interventricular septum of the heart: MR findings. Am J Roentgenol 161:753–754

Carpenter JL (1991) Perivalvular extension of infection in patients with infectious endocarditis. Rev Infect Dis 13:127–138

Castelli MJ, Mihalov ML, Posniak HV, Gattuso P (1989) Primary cardiac lymphoma initially diagnosed by routine cytology: case report and literature review. Acta Cytol 30:662–664

Chao TY, Han SC, Nieh S, Lan GY, Lee SH (1995) Diagnosis of primary cardiac lymphoma. Report of a case with cytologic examination of pericardial fluid and imprints of transvenously biopsied intracardiac tissue. Acta Cytol 39:955–959

Chin WW, Van Tosh A, Hecht SR, Berger M (1988) Left ventricular thrombus with normal left ventricular function in ulcerative colitis. Am Heart J 116:562–563

Chou ST, Arkles LB, Gill GD, Pinkus N, Parkin A, Hicks JD (1983) Primary lymphoma of the heart: a case report. Cancer 52:744–747

Coghlan JG, Paul VE, Mitchell AG (1989) Cardiac involvement by lymphoma: diagnostic difficulties. Eur Heart J 10:765–768

Colucci V, Alberti A, Bonacina E, Gordini V (1995) Papillary fibroelastoma of the mitral valve. A rare cause of embolic events. Tex Heart Inst J 22:327–331

Conces DJ, Vix VA, Klatte EC (1985) Gated MR imaging of left atrial myxomas. Radiology 156:445–447

Corallo S, Mutinelli MR, Moroni M, et al. (1988) Echocardiographic detects myocardial damage in AIDS: prospective study in 102 patients. Eur Heart J 9:887–892

Curtinsinger CR, Wilson MJ, Yoneda K (1989) Primary cardiac lymphoma. Cancer 64:521–525

DeGroat TS, Parameswaran R, Popper PM, Kotler MN (1985) Left ventricular thrombi in association with normal left ventricular wall motion in patients with malignancy. Am J Cardiol 56:827–828

DeLoach JF, Haynes JW (1953) Secondary tumors of the heart and pericardium. Review of subject and report of 137 cases. Arch Intern Med 91:224–249

DePace NL, Soulen RL, Kotler MN, Mintz GS (1981) Two dimensional echocardiographic detection of intraatrial masses. Am J Cardiol 48:954–960

de Roos A, Reichek N, Axel L, Kressel HY (1989a) Cine MR imaging in aortic stenosis. J Comput Assist Tomogr 13:421–425

de Roos A, Weijers E, van Duinen S, Van der Wall EE (1989b) Calcified right atrial myxoma demonstrated by magnetic resonance imaging. Chest 95:478–479

Dev V, Goswami KC, Shrivastava S, Bahl VK, Saxena A (1993) Echocardiographic diagnosis of aneurysm of the sinus of Valsalva. Am Heart J 126:930–936

Di Cesare E, Enrici RM, Paparoni S, et al. (1995) Low-field magnetic resonance imaging in the evaluation of mechanical and biological heart valve function. Eur J Radiol 20:224–228

Doherty NE, Siegel RJ (1985) Cardiovascular manifestations of systemic lupus erythematosus. Am Heart J 110:1257–1265

Dooms GC, Higgins CB (1986) MR imaging of cardiac thrombi. J Comput Assist Tomogr 10:415–420

Dooms GC, Hricak H, Sollitto RA, Higgins CB (1985) Lipomatous tumors and tumors with fatty components: MR imaging potential and comparison of MR and CT results. Radiology 157:479–483

Drake WM, Jenkins PJ, Phillips RR, et al. (1997) Intracardiac metastases from neuroendocrine tumours. Clin Endocrinol (Oxf) 46:517–522

Dunlap HJ, Udjus K (1990) Atypical leiomyoma arising in an hepatic vein with extension into the inferior vena cava and right atrium. Report of a case in a child. Pediatr Radiol 20:202–203

Edwards FH, Hale D, Cohen A, Thompson L, Pezzella AT, Virmani R (1991) Primary cardiac valve tumors. Ann Thorac Surg 52:1127–1131

Elkouby A, Vaillant A, Comet B, Malmejac C, Houel J (1990) Cardiac hydatidosis. Review of recent literature and report of 15 cases (in French). Ann Chir 44:603–610

Endo M, Adachi S, Kusumoto M, et al. (1993) A study of the utility of the MR image for the diagnosis of thymic tumors – imaging and pathologic correlation. Nippon Igaku Hoshasen Gakkai Zasshi 53:1–10

Engberding R, Daniel WG, Erbel R, et al. (1993) Diagnosis of heart tumours by transoesophageal echocardiography: a multicentre study in 154 patients. European Cooperative Study Group. Eur Heart J 14:1223–1228

Fang CY, Fu M, Chang JP, Eng HL, Hung JS (1996) Malignant fibrous histiocytoma of the left ventricle: a case report. Chang Keng I Hsueh 19:187–190

Fisher MS, Edmonds PR (1988) Lipomatous hypertrophy of the interatrial septum. Diagnosis by magnetic resonance imaging. J Comput Tomogr 12:267–269

Fisher MR, Higgins CB, Andereck W (1985) MR imaging of an intrapericardial pheochromocytoma. J Comput Assist Tomogr 9:1103–1105

Fueredi GA, Knechtges TE, Czarnecki DJ (1989) Coronary angiography in atrial myxoma: findings in nine cases. Am J Roentgenol 152:737–738

Funari M, Fujita N, Peck WW, Higgins CB (1991) Cardiac tumors: assessment with Gd-DTPA enhanced MR imaging. J Comput Assist Tomogr 15:953–958

Furber A, Geslin P, Le Jeune JJ, et al. (1997) Value of MRI with injection of gadolinium in the diagnosis of mitral ring abscess. Apropos of a case (in French). Arch Mal Coeur Vaiss 90:399–404

Gallet B, Malergue MC, Adams C, et al. (1985) Atrial septal aneurysm – a potential cause of systemic embolism. Br Heart J 53:292–297

Gamsu G, Starck D, Webb WR, Moore EH, Sheldon PE (1984) Magnetic resonance of benign mediastinal masses. Radiology 151:709–713

Gibson JM, Hall CM, Dicks MC, Finn JP (1990) Intracardiac extension of Wilms' tumour: demonstration by magnetic resonance. Br J Radiol 63:568–569

Gill PS, Chandraratna AN, Meyer PR, Levine AM (1987) Malignant lymphoma: cardiac involvement at initial presentation. J Clin Oncol 5:216–224

Glazer HS, Gutierrez FR, Levitt RG, Lee JK, Murphy WA (1985) The thoracic aorta studied by MR imaging. Radiology 157:149–155

Godine LB, Berdon WE, Brasch RC, Leonidas JC (1990) Adrenocortical carcinoma with extension into inferior vena cava and right atrium: report of 3 cases in children. Pediatr Radiol 20:166–168

Gomes AS, Lois JF, Child JS, Brown K, Batra P (1987) Cardiac tumors and thrombus: evaluation with MR imaging. AJR Am J Roentgenol 49:895–899

Gomi T, Ikeda T, Sakurai J, Toya Y, Tani M (1994) Cardiac pheochromocytoma. A case report and review of the literature. Jpn Heart J 35:117–124

Gossinger HD, Siostrzonek P, Zangeneh M, et al. (1988) Magnetic resonance imaging findings in a patient with pericardial mesothelioma. Am Heart J 115:1321–1322

Grote J, Mugge A, Schfers HJ, Daniel WG, Lichtlen PR (1995) Multiplane transoesophageal echocardiography detection of a papillary fibroelastoma of the aortic valve causing myocardial infarction. Eur Heart J 16:426–429

Grotz J, Steiner G, Josephs W, Sorge B, Wiechmann HW, Beyer HK (1986) Demonstration of intra- and paracardiac space-occupying lesions by magnetic resonance tomography. Dtsch Med Wochenschr 111:1594–1598

Hallali P, Haiat R (1987) Tumeurs malignes du coeur et du péricarde. In: Actualités en Cardiologie. Sandoz, Paris, pp 1–12

Hamilton BH, Francis IR, Gross BH, et al. (1997) Intrapericardial paragangliomas (pheochromocytomas): imaging features. Am J Roentgenol 168:109–113

Hananouchi GI, Goff WB (1990) Cardiac lipoma: six-year follow-up with MRI characteristics, and a review of the literature. Magn Reson Imaging 8:825–828

Hanley PC, Tajik AJ, Hynes JK, et al. (1985) Diagnosis and classification of atrial septal aneurysm by two-dimensional echocardiography: report of 80 consecutive cases. J Am Coll Cardiol 6:1370–1382

Hanson EC (1992) Cardiac tumors: a current perspective. N Y State J Med 92:41–42

Haouzi A, Danchin N, Renoult E, et al. (1989) Cardiac pheochromocytoma. Failure of classic non-invasive diagnostic methods (in French). Arch Mal Coeur Vaiss 82: 97–100

Hatabu H, Gefter WB, Axel L, et al. (1994) MR imaging with spatial modulation of magnetization in the evaluation of chronic central pulmonary thromboemboli. Radiology 190:791–796

Heath D (1968) Pathology of cardiac tumors. Am J Cardiol 21:315–327

Herrera CJ, Mehlman DJ, Hartz RS, Talano JV, McPherson DD (1992) Comparison of transesophageal and transthoracic echocardiography for diagnosis of right sided cardiac lesions. Am J Cardiol 70:964–966

Herrmann MA, Shankerman RA, Edwards WD, Shub C, Schaff HV (1992) Primary cardiac angiosarcoma: a clinicopathologic study of six cases. J Thorac Cardiovasc Surg 103:655–664

Ho VB, Kinney JB, Sahn DJ (1995) Ruptured sinus of Valsalva aneurysm: cine phase-contrast MR characterization. J Comput Assist Tomogr 19:652–656

Ichikawa T, Ohtomo K, Uchiyama G, Fujimoto H, Nasu K (1995) Contrast-enhanced dynamic MRI of adrenal masses: classification of characteristic enhancement patterns. Clin Radiol 50:295–300

Janigan DT, Husain A, Robinson NA (1986) Cardiac angiosarcomas. A review and a case report. Cancer 57: 852–859

Jeang MK, Fuentes F, Gately A, Byrnes J, Lewis M (1986) Aortic root abscess. Initial experience using magnetic resonance imaging. Chest 89:613–615

Jochelson MS, Balikian JP, Mauch P, Liebman H (1983) Peri- and paracardial involvement in lymphoma: a radiographic study of 11 cases. Am J Roentgenol 140: 483–488

Johnson DE, Vacek J, Gollub SB, Wilson DB, Dunn M (1988) Comparison of gated cardiac magnetic resonance imaging and two-dimensional echocardiography for the evaluation of right ventricular thrombi: a case report with autopsy correlation. Cathet Cardiovasc Diagn 14:266–268

Jungehulsing M, Sechtem U, Theissen P, Hilger HH, Schicha H (1992) Left ventricular thrombi: evaluation with spin-echo and gradient-echo MR imaging. Radiology 182:225–229

Kaminaga T, Yamada N, Imakita S, Takamiya M, Nishimura T (1993) Magnetic resonance imaging of pericardial malignant mesothelioma. Magn Reson Imaging 11: 1057–1061

Kanematsu M, Imaeda T, Minowa H, et al. (1994) Hepatocellular carcinoma with tumor thrombus in the inferior vena cava and right atrium. Abdom Imaging 19:313–316

Kaplan PA, Williams SM (1987) Mucocutaneous and peripheral soft tissue hemangiomas. MR findings. Radiology 163:163–168

Kardaras F, Kardara D, Tselikos D, et al. (1996) Fifteen year surveillance of echinococcal heart disease from a referral hospital in Greece. Eur Heart J 17:1265–1270

Kasarskis EJ, O'Connor W, Earle G (1988) Embolic stroke from cardiac papillary fibroelastomas. Stroke 19: 1171–1173

Kasugai T, Sakurai M, Yutani C, et al. (1990) Sequential malignant transformation of cardiac myxoma. Acta Pathol Jpn 40:687–692

Kawasuji M, Matsunaga Y, Iwa T (1989) Cardiac phaeochromocytoma of the interatrial septum. Eur J Cardiothorac Surg 3:175–177

Keeley EC, Hillis LD (1996) Left ventricular mural thrombus after acute myocardial infarction. Clin Cardiol 19:83–86

Kemp JL, Kessler RM, Raizada V, Williamson MR (1996) Case report. MR and CT appearance of cardiac hemangioma. J Comput Assist Tomogr 20:482–483

Keren A, Billingham ME, Popp RL (1984) Echocardiographic recognition and implications of ventricular hypertrophic trabeculations and aberrant bands. Circulation 70:836–842

Kim EE, Wallace S, Abello R, et al. (1989) Malignant cardiac fibrous histiocytomas and angiosarcomas: MR features. J Comput Assist Tomogr 13:627–632

Klarich KW, Enriquez-Sarano M, Gura GM, Edwards WD, Tajik AJ, Seward JB (1997) Papillary fibroelastoma: echocardiographic characteristics for diagnosis and pathologic correlation. J Am Coll Cardiol 30:784–790

Klima T, Milam JD, Bossart MI, Cooley DA (1986) Rare primary sarcomas of the heart. Arch Pathol Lab Med 110:1155–1159

Konermann M, Sorge HB, Grotz J, Josephs W, Hotzinger H (1989) Hemangioma of the left coronary artery with a fistula into the pulmonary artery (in German). Dtsch Med Wochenschr 114:1363–1366

Kopka L, Fischer U, Gross AJ, Funke M, Oestmann JW, Grabbe E (1996) CT of retained surgical sponges (textilomas): pitfalls in detection and evaluation. J Comput Assist Tomogr 20:919–923

Kotoulas GK, Magoufis GL, Gouliamos AD, et al. (1996) Evaluation of hydatid disease of the heart with magnetic resonance imaging. Cardiovasc Intervent Radiol 19: 187–189

Kulan K, Tuncer C, Kulan C, et al. (1995) Hydatid cyst of the interventricular septum and contribution of magnetic resonance imaging. Acta Cardiol 50:477–481

Kulan K, Kulan C, Tuncer C, Komsuoglu B, Zengin M (1996) Echocardiography and magnetic resonance imaging of sinus of Valsalva aneurysm with rupture into the ventricle. J Cardiovasc Surg Torino 37:639–641

Kuo CS, Hsu HC, Huang CH, Liu SM, Ho CH (1997) Leiomyosarcoma of the left atrium: a case report. Chung Hua I Hsueh Tsa Chih 59:136–140

Kupferwasser I, Mohr-Kahaly S, Erbel R, et al. (1994) Three-dimensional imaging of cardiac mass lesions by transesophageal echocardiographic computed tomography. J Am Soc Echocardiogr 7:561–570

Kushihashi T, Fujisawa H, Munechika H (1996) Magnetic resonance imaging of thymic epithelial tumors. Crit Rev Diagn Imaging 37:191–259

Kuwashima S, Yamato M, Fujioka M, Ishibashi M, Kogure H, Tajima Y (1993) MR findings of surgically retained sponges and towels: report of two cases. Radiat Med 11:98–101

Lagrange JL, Despins P, Spielman M, et al. (1986) Cardiac metastases. Case report on an isolated cardiac metastasis of a myxoid liposarcoma. Cancer 58:2333–2337

Langer E, Mischke U, Stommer P, Harrer T, Stoll R (1988) Kaposi's sarcoma with pericardial tamponade in AIDS. Dtsch Med Wochenschr 29:1187–1190

Lanza RP, Cooper DK, Cassidy MJ, Barnard CN (1983) Malignant neoplasms occurring after cardiac transplantation. JAMA 249:1746–1748

Lee R, Fisher MR (1989) MR imaging of cardiac metastases from malignant fibrous histiocytoma. J Comput Assist Tomogr 13:126–168

Lerner CA, Dang HP (1997) MR imaging of a pericardial gossypiboma (letter). Am J Roentgenol 169:314

Levine RA, Weyman AE, Dinsmore RE, et al. (1986) Noninvasive tissue characterization: diagnosis of lipo-matous hypertrophy of the atrial septum by nuclear magnetic resonance imaging. J Am Coll Cardiol 7:688–692

Lie JT (1989) Petrified cardiac myxoma masquerading as organized atrial mural thrombus. Arch Pathol Lab Med 113:742–745

Lund JT, Ehman RL, Julsrud PR, Sinak LJ, Tajik AJ (1989) Cardiac masses: assessment by MR imaging. Am J Roentgenol 152:469–473

Lupetin AR, Dash N, Beckman I (1986) Leiomyosarcoma of the superior vena cava: diagnosis by cardiac gated MR. Cardiovasc Intervent Radiol 9:103–105

Macedo AJ, Magalhaes MP, Tavares NJ, Bento L, Sampayo F, Lima M (1997) Cardiac hydatid cyst in a child. Pediatr Cardiol 18:226–228

Mahajan H, Kim EE, Wallace S, Abello R, Benjamin R, Evans HL (1989) Magnetic resonance imaging of malignant fibrous histiocytoma. Magn Reson Imaging 7:283–288

Manger WM, Gifford RWJ (1990) Pheochromocytoma. In: Laragh JH, Brenner BM (eds) Hypertension. Raven Press, New York, pp 1639–1650

Massie RJ, Van Asperen PP, Mellis CM (1997) A review of open biopsy for mediastinal masses. J Paediatr Child Health 33:230–233

Matsuoka H, Hamada M, Honda T, et al. (1996) Morphologic and histologic characterization of cardiac myxomas by magnetic resonance imaging. Angiology 47:693–698

Matteucci C, Busi G, Biferali F, Paventi S (1997) Tardive pseudo-ischemic presentation of cardiac rhabdomyoma (in Italian). G Ital Cardiol 27:583–587

McAllister HGJ (1979) Primary tumors and cysts of the heart and pericardium. Curr Probl Cardiol 4:1–11

McAllister HA, Fenoglio JJ (1978) Tumors of the cardiovascular system. Armed Forces Institute of Pathology, Washington DC, pp 1–39

McFadden PM, Lacy JR (1987) Intracardiac papillary fibroelastoma: an occult cause of embolic neurologic deficit. Ann Thorac Surg 43:667–669

Meany JFM, Kazerooni EA, Jamadar DA, Korobkin M (1997) CT appearance of lipomatous hypertrophy of the interatrial septum. Am J Roentgenol 168:1081–1084

Meier RA, Hartnell GG (1994) MRI of right atrial pseudomass: is it really a diagnostic problem? J Comput Assist Tomogr 18:398–401

Menegus MA, Greenberg MA, Spindola-Franco H, Fayemi A (1992) Magnetic resonance imaging of suspected atrial tumors. Am Heart J 123:1260–1268

Mirowitz SA, Gutierrez FR (1992) Fibromuscular elements of the right atrium: pseudomass at MR imaging. Radiology 182:231–233

Mitchell DG, Burk DL, Vinitski S, Rifkin MD (1987) The biophysical basis of tissue contrast in extracranial MR imaging. Am J Roentgenol 149:831–837

Mochizuki T, Takehara Y, Ichijo K, Nishimura T, Takahashi M, Kaneko M (1992) Case report: MR appearance of a retained surgical sponge. Clin Radiol 46:66–67

Mohiaddin RH, Roberts RH, Underwood R, Rothman M (1995) Localization of a misplaced coronary artery stent by magnetic resonance imaging. Clin Cardiol 18:175–177

Mosthaf FA, Gieseler U, Mehmel HC, Fischer JT, Gams E (1991) Left bundle-branch block and primary benign heart tumor (in German). Dtsch Med Wochenschr 116:134–136

Mugge A, Daniel WG, Haverich A, Lichtlen PR (1991) Diagnosis of noninfective cardiac mass lesions by two-dimensional echocardiography. Comparison of the transthoracic and transesophageal approaches. Circulation 83:70–78

Murayama S, Murakami J, Watanabe H, et al. (1995) Signal intensity characteristics of mediastinal cystic masses on T1-weighted MRI. J Comput Assist Tomogr 19:188–191

Murphey MD, Gross TM, Rosenthal HG (1994) From the archives of the AFIP. Musculoskeletal malignant fibrous histiocytoma: radiologic-pathologic correlation. Radiographics 14:807–826

Naka N, Ohsawa M, Tomita Y, Kanno H, Uchida A, Aozasa K (1995) Angiosarcoma in Japan. Cancer 75:989–996

Nakata H, Egashira K, Watanabe H, et al. (1993) MRI of bronchogenic cysts. J Comput Assist Tomogr 17:267–270

Neuerburg JM, Bohndorf K, Sohn M, Teufl F, Guenther RW, Davis HJ (1989) Urinary bladder neoplasms: evaluation with contrast-enhancement MR imaging. Radiology 172:739–743

Nguyen BD, Westra WH, Zerhouni EA (1996) Renal cell carcinoma and tumor thrombus neovascularity: MR demonstration with pathologic correlation. Abdom Imaging 21:269–271

Norita H, Ohteki H, Todaka K, Hisanou R, Yoshitake K, Yamada M (1992) Malignant fibrous histiocytoma of the heart. Nippon Kyobu Geka Gakkai Zasshi 40:1933–1937

Ogawa T, Iwama Y, Hashimoto H, Ito T, Satake T (1991) Noninvasive methods in the diagnosis of ruptured aneurysm of Valsalva. Usefulness of magnetic resonance imaging and Doppler echocardiography. Chest 100:579–581

Ouzan J, Joundi A, Chapoutot L, et al. (1990) Malignant histiocytofibroma of the heart simulating myxoma of the left atrium (in French). Arch Mal Coeur Vaiss 83:1011–1013

Papa MZ, Shinfeld A, Klein E, Greif F, Ben AG (1994) Cardiac metastasis of liposarcoma. J Surg Oncol 55:132–134

Parmley LF, Salley RK, Williams JP, Head G3 (1988) The clinical spectrum of cardiac fibroma with diagnostic and surgical considerations: noninvasive imaging enhances management. Ann Thorac Surg 45:455–465

Pasaoglu I, Dogan R, Pasaoglu E, Tokgozoglu L (1994) Surgical treatment of giant hydatid cyst of the left ventricle and diagnostic value of magnetic resonance imaging. Cardiovasc Surg 2:114–116

Paul JG, Rhodes DB, Skow JR (1975) Renal cell carcinoma presenting as right atrial tumor with successful removal using cardiopulmonary bypass. Ann Surg 181:471–473

Phillips MR, Bower TC, Orszulak TA, Hartmann LC (1995) Intracardiac extension of an intracaval sarcoma of endometrial origin. Ann Thorac Surg 59:742–744

Pinelli G, Carteaux JP, Mertes PM, Civit T, Trinh A, Villemot JP (1995) Mitral valve tumor revealed by stroke. J Heart Valve Dis 4:199–201

Putnam JBJ, Sweeney MS, Colon R, Lanza LA, Frazier OH, Cooley DA (1991) Primary cardiac sarcomas. Ann Thorac Surg 51:906–910

Raaf HN, Raaf JH (1994) Sarcomas related to the heart and vasculature. Semin Surg Oncol 10:374–382

Raffa H, Mosieri J, Sorefan AA, Kayali MT (1991) Sinus of Valsalva aneurysm eroding into the interventricular septum. Ann Thorac Surg 51:996–998

Reid PG, Goudevenos JA, Hilton CJ (1990) Thrombosed saccular aneurysm of a sinus of Valsalva: unusual cause of a mediastinal mass. Br Heart J 63:183–185

Ritchey ML, Kinard R, Novicki DE (1987) Adrenal tumors: involvement of the inferior vena cava. J Urol 38:1134–1136

Roberts CS, Gottdiener JS, Roberts WC (1990) Clinically undetected cardiac lymphoma causing fatal congestive heart failure. Am Heart J 120:1239–1242

Roberts WC, Glancy DL, De Vita VT (1968) Heart in malignant lymphoma (Hodgkin's disease, lymphosarcoma, reticulum cell sarcoma and mycosis fungoides). A study of 196 autopsy cases. Am Heart J 22:85–108

Rosado de Christenson ML, Pugatch RD, Moran CA, Galobardes J (1994) Thymolipoma: analysis of 27 cases. Radiology 193:121–126

Rosenberg JM, Marvasti MA, Obeid A, Johnson LW, Bonaventura M (1988) Intravenous leiomyomatosis: a rare cause of right sided cardiac obstruction. Eur J Cardiothorac Surg 2:58–60

Rosenthal DS, Braunwald E (1992) Cardiac manifestations of neoplastic disease. Saunders, Philadelphia, pp 1752–1760

Rote AR, Flint LD, Ellis FH (1977) Intracaval extension of pheochromocytoma extending into the right atrium: surgical management using intracorporeal circulation. N Engl J Med 296:1269–1271

Rumancik WM, Naidich DP, Chandra R, et al. (1988) Cardiovascular disease: evaluation with MR phase imaging. Radiology 166:63–68

Sakai F, Sone S, Kiyono K, et al. (1992) MR imaging of thymoma: radiologic-pathologic correlation. Am J Roentgenol 158:751–756

Salcedo EE, Cohen GI, White RD, Davison MB (1992) Cardiac tumors: diagnosis and management. Curr Probl Cardiol 17:73–137

Sato Y, Togawa K, Ogawa K, Hashimoto M, Sakamaki T, Kanmatsuse K (1995) Magnetic resonance imaging of cardiac hemangiopericytoma. Heart Vessels 10:328–330

Schneider B, Hanrath P, Vogel P, Meinertz T (1990) Improved morphologic characterization of atrial septal aneurysm by transesophageal echocardiography: relation to cerebrovascular events. J Am Coll Cardiol 16:1000–1009

Schrem SS, Colvin SB, Weinreb JC, Glassman E, Kronzon I (1990) Metastatic cardiac liposarcoma: diagnosis by

transesophageal echocardiography and magnetic resonance imaging. J Am Soc Echocardiogr 3:149–153

Sechtem U, Tscholakoff D, Higgins CB (1986) MRI of the abnormal pericardium. Am J Roentgenol 147:245–252

Sechtem U, Theissen P, Heindel W, et al. (1989) Diagnosis of left ventricular thrombi by magnetic resonance imaging and comparison with angiocardiography, computed tomography and echocardiography. Am J Cardiol 64:1195–1199

Semelka RC, Shoenut JP, Wilson ME, Pellech AE, Patton JN (1992) Cardiac masses: signal intensity features on spin-echo, gradient-echo, gadolinium-enhanced spin-echo, and TurboFLASH images. J Magn Reson Imaging 2:415–420

Shahian DM, Labib SB, Chang G (1995) Cardiac papillary fibroelastoma (see comments). Ann Thorac Surg 59:538–541

Shellock FG, Morisoli SM (1994a) Ex vivo evaluation of ferromagnetism, heating, and artifacts produced by heart valve prostheses exposed to a 1.5-T MR system. J Magn Reson Imaging 4:756–758

Shellock FG, Morisoli SM (1994b) Ex vivo evaluation of ferromagnetism and artifacts of cardiac occluders exposed to a 1.5-T MR system. J Magn Reson Imaging 4:213–215

Singh RN, Burkholder JA, Magovern GJ (1984) Coronary arteriography as an aid in the diagnosis of angiosarcoma of the heart. Cardiovasc Intervent Radiol 7:40–43

Smith AJ, Panidis IP, Berger S, Gonzales R (1990) Large atrial septal aneurysm mimicking a cystic right atrial mass. Am Heart J 120:714–716

Stanford W, Galvin JR, Weiss RM, Hajduczok ZD, Skorton DJ (1991) Ultrafast computed tomography in cardiac imaging: a review. Semin Ultrasound CT MR 12:45–60

Steinmetz OK, Bedard P, Prefontaine ME, Bourke M, Barber GG (1996) Uterine tumor in the heart: intravenous leiomyomatosis. Surgery 119:226–229

Stratton JR, Ligthy GW, Pearlman AS (1982) Detection of left ventricular thrombus by two-dimensional echocardiography: sensitivity, specificity, and causes of uncertainty. Circulation 66:156–164

Szucs RA, Rehr RB, Yanovich S, Tatum JL (1991) Magnetic resonance imaging of cardiac rhabdomyosarcoma. Quantifying the response to chemotherapy. Cancer 67:2066–2070

Takamizawa S, Sugimoto K, Tanaka H, Sakai O, Arai T, Saitoh A (1992) A case of primary leiomyosarcoma of the heart. Intern Med 31:265–268

Teramoto N, Hayashi K, Miyatani K, et al. (1995) Malignant fibrous histiocytoma of the right ventricle of the heart. Pathol Int 45:315–319

Tesoro Tess JD, Biasi S, Balzarini L, et al. (1993) Heart involvement in lymphomas. The value of magnetic resonance imaging and two-dimensional echocardiography at disease presentation. Cancer 72:2484–2490

Thomas D, Desruennes M, Jault F, Isnard R, Gandjbakhch I (1993) Cardiac and extracardiac abscesses in bacterial endocarditis (in French). Arch Mal Coeur Vaiss 86:1825–1835

Thompson NW, Brown J, Orringer M, Sisson J, Nishiyama R (1978) Follicular carcinoma of the thyroid with massive angioinvasion: extension of tumor thrombus to the heart. Surgery 83:451–457

Uchida S, Obayashi N, Yamanari H, Matsubara K, Saito D, Haraoka S (1992) Papillary fibroelastoma in the left ventricular outflow tract. Heart Vessels 7:164–167

Ünal M, Tuncer C, Serce K, Bostan M, Erem C, Gökce M (1995) A cardiac giant hydatid cyst of the interventricular septum masquerading as ischemic heart disease: role of MR imaging. Acta Cardiol 50:323–326

Urba WJ, Longo DL (1986) Primary solid tumors of the heart. In: Kapoor AS (ed) Cancer and the heart. Springer, New York Berlin Heidelberg, pp 62–75

Van Goethem JW, Parizel PM, Perdieus D, Hermans P, de Moor J (1991) MR and CT imaging of paraspinal textiloma (gossypiboma). J Comput Assist Tomogr 15:1000–1003

Vanjak D, Moutaoufik M, Leroy O, et al. (1990) Cardiac hydatidosis: contribution of magnetic resonance imaging. Report of a case (in French). Arch Mal Coeur Vaiss 83:1739–1742

Varghese JC, Hahn PF, Papanicolaou N, Mayo-Smith WW, Gaa JA, Lee MJ (1997) MR differentiation of phaechromocytoma from other adrenal lesions based on qualitative analysis of T2 relaxation times. Clin Radiol 52:603–606

Vinee P, Stover B, Sigmund G, et al. (1992) MR imaging of the pericardial cyst. J Magn Reson Imaging 2:593–596

Vogel HJ, Wondergem JH, Falke TH (1989) Mesothelioma of the pericardium: CT and MR findings. J Comput Assist Tomogr 13:543–544

Walker PG, Pedersen EM, Oyre S, et al. (1995) Magnetic resonance velocity imaging: a new method for prosthetic heart valve study. J Heart Valve Dis 4:296–307

Watanabe M, Takazawa K, Wada A, et al. (1994) Cardiac myxoma with Gamna-Gandy bodies: case report with MR imaging. J Thorac Imaging 9:185–187

Wiemer J, Winkelmann BR, Beyersdorf F, et al. (1996) Multiplicity of clinical symptoms and manifestations of unruptured aneurysms of the sinus of Valsalva. Three case reports. Z Kardiol 85:221–225

Williams ES, Kaplan JI, Thatcher F, Zimmerman G, Knoebel SB (1980) Prolongation of proton spin lattice relaxation times in regionally ischemic tissue from dog hearts. J Nucl Med 21:449–453

Winkler ML, Higgins CB (1986) MRI of perivalvular infectious pseudoaneurysms. Am J Roentgenol 147:253–256

Wolf JE, Lambert B, Pilichowski P, et al. (1987) Value of magnetic resonance imaging in a lipoma of the left ventricle (in French). Arch Mal Coeur Vaiss 80:1801–1805

Yanagisawa H (1991) Left ventricular intramyocardial rhabdomyoma suggested by coronary angiography. Cardiology 79:146–150

Yousem DM, Lexa FJ, Bilaniuk LT, Zimmerman RI (1990) Rhabdomyosarcomas in the head and neck: MR imaging evaluation. Radiology 177:683–686

Zerhouni EA, Parish DM, Rogers WJ, Yang A, Shapiro EP (1988) Human heart: tagging with MR imaging – a new method for noninvasive assessment of myocardial motion. Radiology 169:59–63

11 Valvular Heart Disease

A.M. Taylor and D.J. Pennell

CONTENTS

11.1
Introduction

In general when clinicians ask for investigations of the cardiac valves they require information that can be divided into four categories. First, clarification of the affected valve after auscultation of the heart. Second, definition of the valvular anatomy (leaflet thickness, the number of valve leaflets, the presence of infective endocarditis). Third, assessment of valvular function (degree of valvular stenosis or regurgitation). And finally, definition of the effect of the valvular dysfunction on other cardiac structures and function (ventricular size, function and mass, pulmonary artery pressure). These points can be addressed by combining echocardiography with x-ray angiography. However, magnetic resonance imaging (MRI) can now provide much of the required information in a single investigation that is safe, non-invasive and without x-rays.

In this chapter we will discuss the advantages and limitations of MRI and the conventional imaging modalities for investigating valvular heart disease. We will also present an overview of the MRI techniques that are currently used in the assessment of valvular heart disease, and identify new areas of development in this field.

11.2
Conventional Imaging Modalities

11.2.1
Transthoracic Echocardiography

Transthoracic echocardiography remains the most important and easily accessible investigation in the assessment of valvular heart disease. The technique is non-invasive, safe, portable and accurate at localising the diseased valve. Quantification of valvular stenosis and valve area can be easily performed; however, echocardiography is poor at quantifying valvular regurgitation (Hatle and Angelson 1992). A semiquantitative assessment can be achieved by measuring the regurgitant jet length and width, but there is poor correlation to x-ray angiographic measurements (Abbasi et al. 1980; Quinones et al. 1980; Bolger et al. 1988). Several echocardiography methods have been developed in an attempt to quantify valvular regurgitation, but all have their limitations. The regurgitant fraction can be calculated, but this is time consuming, only patients with isolated valvular regurgitation can be readily assessed (Rockey et al. 1987), and echocardiography only provides an estimate of ventricular function (Boehrer et al. 1992). Imaging of the proximal isovelocity surface area has been proposed. However, this technique relies on the assumption that the regurgitant jet orifice is both flat and circular, which is not the case for most patients

A.M. Taylor, MA, MRCP, Research Fellow, Magnetic Resonance Unit, Royal Brompton Hospital, Sydney Street, London, SW3 6NP, UK
D.J. Pennell, MD, FRCP, FACC, FESC, Clinical Director, Magnetic Resonance Unit, Royal Brompton Hospital, Sydney Street, London, SW3 6NP, UK

(UTSUNOMIYA et al. 1991). More recently, laser Doppler anemometry has been used to characterise the central laminar core (DIEBOLD et al. 1996). Though this technique is based on sound physical principles, current Doppler colour flow imagers are not capable of displaying the laminar core because of aliasing at velocities of 0.5–1.0 cm/s (RODRIGUEZ et al. 1992). A final limitation of transthoracic echocardiography is that the imaging plane may be restricted by the lack of good acoustic windows.

11.2.2
Transoesophageal Echocardiography

Transoesophageal echocardiography is valuable in the assessment of left atrial thrombus (MANNING et al. 1993), atrial septal wall defects (HAUSMANN et al. 1992) and aortic dissection (TICE and KISSLO 1993; LAISSY et al. 1995). In the assessment of valvular heart disease the technique may clarify valvular anatomy in patients with infective endocarditis (PEDERSEN et al. 1991) or in patients with poor acoustic windows. With regard to functional assessment it is less accurate than transthoracic echocardiography because of difficulties with Doppler alignment and has all the limitations of transthoracic echocardiography in the assessment of valvular regurgitation, in addition to being an invasive procedure. A unique use for transesophageal echocardiography is in the intraoperative assessment of valvular function for monitoring and evaluating surgical and percutaneous interventions (FIX et al. 1993; BRYAN et al. 1995).

11.2.3
X-ray Angiography

X-ray angiography has been regarded as the "gold standard" investigation of valvular heart disease, against which other imaging modalities should be compared (SANDLER et al. 1963; SELLERS et al. 1964; CARROLL 1993). Valvular stenosis can be quantified by calculating the transvalvular gradients and valve areas using the Gorlin formula (GORLIN and GORLIN 1951). However, the grading system used for the assessment of valvular regurgitation is both imprecise and inaccurate. Although generally regarded as safe, the technique is associated with a mortality of approximately 0.1%, and other complications occur such as myocardial infarction, arterial embolisation, thrombosis and dissection (DAVIS et al. 1979). Also

the use of ionising radiation during the procedure is not ideal (COHEN 1991). In general, x-ray angiography should only be regarded as necessary if the pulmonary artery pressure needs accurate measurement, if the coronary artery anatomy needs defining, or if there is a discrepancy between the clinical symptoms and the non-invasive investigations.

11.2.4
Radionuclide Angiography

The main use of radionuclide angiography is in the monitoring of ventricular function in order to assess when interventions should take place (RIGO et al. 1979; SORENSON et al. 1980). The technique can also be used to calculate the regurgitant fraction, but again only when regurgitation in a single valve is present. As with x-ray angiography, the use of ionising radiation is not ideal, especially as serial measurements of ventricular function are necessary.

11.3
Magnetic Resonance Imaging of Cardiac Valves

Magnetic resonance imaging can provide good functional information about both valvular stenosis and regurgitation, and allows accurate assessment of the ventricular function and relevant cardiac anatomy.

11.3.1
Morphology

11.3.1.1
Normal Valves

Normal valves are only occasionally seen on spin-echo (SE) images because of averaging, which hinders the visualisation of fast-moving, low proton density, fine structures. When thickened and immobile their identification is more common (Fig. 11.1). In gradient-echo (GE) cine imaging, the moving leaflets are easily seen as blood flowing over the valve tips leads to signal loss, secondary to eddies and mild turbulence (Fig. 11.2). Thus, despite the superior spatial resolution of MRI, echocardiography remains the investigation of choice for imaging valvular anatomy.

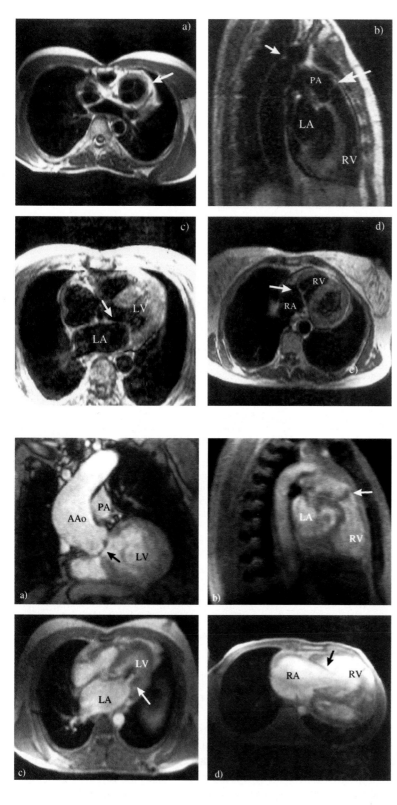

Fig. 11.1 a–d. SE images of the valves. **a** Transaxial image in a patient with transposition of the great arteries. The right-sided aorta (*arrow*) and its three valve cusps can be seen clearly, with a small central perforation. **b** Sagittal image of the pulmonary valve (*large arrow*) in a patient with coarctation of the aorta (*small arrow*). *LA*, Left atrium; *RV*, right ventricle; *PA*, pulmonary artery. **c** Transaxial image (systole) of the closed mitral valve. **d** Transaxial image (systole) of the tricuspid valve (*arrow*). *RA*, Right atrium

Fig. 11.2 a–d. GE images of the valves. **a** Oblique coronal image of the aorta (*arrow*). *AAo*, Ascending aorta; *LV*, left ventricle; *PA*, pulmonary artery. **b** Sagittal image of the pulmonary valve (*arrow*). *LA*, left atrium; *RV*, right ventricle. **c** Transaxial image of the mitral valve (*arrow*) in a patient with mitral stenosis. **d** Transaxial image in a patient with Uhl's anomaly. The right ventricle and atrium (*RA*) are hugely dilated. The leaflets of the tricuspid valve are clearly seen (*arrow*)

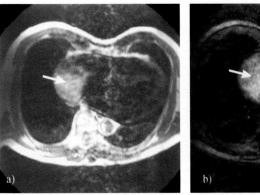
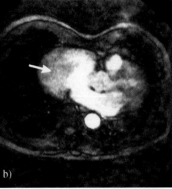

Fig. 11.3. **a** Transaxial SE images reveal a mass in the right atrium (bright pixels in the right atrium, *arrow*). **b** Transaxial GE images show blood flow (brighter pixels) adjacent to the mass (*arrow*), and not stagnant blood flow. The overall appearance is consistent with atrial thrombus

11.3.1.2
Thrombus

It is important to identify the presence of thrombus in the atria, particularly in the presence of mitral stenosis or valvular disease with atrial fibrillation. Conventional SE imaging can identify atrial thrombus, but care must be taken to distinguish between slow-moving blood which may appear as increased signal on these images (DOOMS and HIGGINS 1986). GE imaging and velocity mapping should thus be used to confirm the presence and size of any apparent mass (Fig. 11.3). Thrombus can also be distinguished from other atrial masses using gadolinium-based contrast agents (WEINMANN et al. 1984).

11.3.1.3
Endocarditis

Only very large vegetations can be demonstrated by SE MRI. Fast GE imaging has been shown to be helpful in clarifying echocardiographic findings in aortic valve vegetations (CADUFF et al. 1996). MRI can be invaluable in the identification of abscesses (Fig. 11.4) (JEANG et al. 1986) or if infection has spread outside the heart.

11.3.2
Valvular Regurgitation

Currently none of the conventional imaging techniques can accurately define valvular regurgitation and it is here that MRI has particular value. MRI can image the regurgitant jet in any plane and thus a 3D appreciation of the jet can be acquired. Furthermore, MRI can quantify the regurgitant volume, either as an absolute value or as the regurgitant fraction. Such

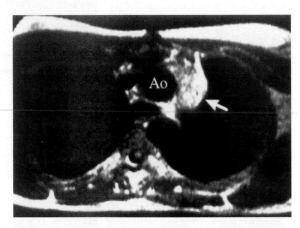

Fig. 11.4. Aortic root abscess on the left of the aorta (*arrow*). This 23-year-old man had had an aortic valve replacement and become pyrexial 3 weeks postoperatively. Conventional non-invasive imaging had revealed no abscess. Infective abscess was confirmed at surgery *Ao*, Aorta

a non-invasive quantification of the degree of valvular regurgitation, in combination with information about ventricular function, is of particular clinical relevance for the timing of valve replacement.

11.3.2.1
Qualitative Assessment
with Cine Gradient-Echo Imaging

In GE cine imaging, dephasing of the proton spins, secondary to turbulent flow, leads to signal loss (EVANS et al. 1988). Imaging over 16 frames enables accurate assessment of the turbulent flow, throughout the cardiac cycle. For regurgitant lesions the signal loss can be graded in a similar way to x-ray angiography; grade 1 = signal loss close to the valve; grade 2 = signal loss extending into the proximal chamber; grade 3 = signal loss filling the whole of the

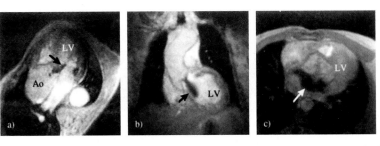

Fig. 11.5 a–c. GE images. **a** Horizontal long-axis. Grade 1 aortic regurgitation adjacent to the anterior leaflet of the mitral valve (*arrow*). There is some signal loss at the level of the valve secondary to calcification of the aortic valve cusps. *Ao,* Aorta; *LV,* left ventricle **b** Oblique coronal plane. Grade 2 aortic regurgitation (*arrow*). **c** Transaxial plane. Grade 3 mitral regurgitation (*arrow*)

proximal chamber; grade 4 = signal loss in the receiving chamber throughout the relevant half of the cardiac cycle (Fig. 11.5) (UNDERWOOD et al. 1987a; SECHTEM et al. 1987). This qualitative method has been validated but is unable to separate turbulent volumes when dual valve disease exists (e.g. aortic regurgitation and mitral stenosis), and there remains poor reproducibility of the technique between centres (SECHTEM et al. 1988; WAGNER et al. 1989; GLOBITS et al. 1991). In addition, signal loss is very dependent on MR parameters such as echo time (TE), and jet size is easily underestimated when it impinges on the myocardial wall, as has been known for echocardiography for some years.

11.3.2.2
Quantitative Evaluation of Ventricular Volume Measurement

Magnetic resonance imaging can now be regarded as the "gold standard" for the measurement of ventricular volumes (DULCE et al. 1993; SAKUMA et al. 1993). Using a set of short-axis cuts covering the length of the ventricles, the stroke volumes of both the right and the left ventricle can be measured (Fig. 11.6). In normal individuals there is a 1:1 relationship between these stroke volumes. Any discrepancy between the ventricular volumes in a patient with regurgitation will identify the regurgitant volume. The main limitation of this technique, when used alone, is that only patients with a single regurgitant valve can be assessed. A further limitation is the long overall acquisition time required for a short-axis stack of GE images (30 min). However, with the continued improvement of MR hardware, faster imaging techniques such as segmented k-space fast low-angle shot (FLASH) can be used to acquire 16 frame cines in a single breath-hold, reducing the

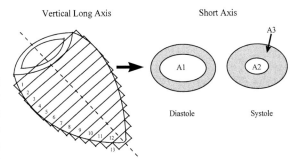

Fig. 11.6. Schematic diagram for the calculation of LV volumes and mass. The left ventricle is divided into multiple short-axis slices of 1 cm thickness, from the mitral valve to the apex. The LV end-diastolic volume (LVEDV) for each slice is thus given by the area A1 (cm^2) × 1 cm, i.e. A1 (ml). The LV end-systolic volume for each slice is A2 (ml). The ventricular volumes for the entire left ventricle are the sum of all the slice volumes, e.g. LVEDV = A1$_1$ + A1$_2$ + ... A1$_{13}$. The LV mass can be calculated for each slice by subtracting the endocardial area from the epicardial area to give the area A3. The sum of these areas is then multiplied by the specific gravity of myocardium (1.05 kg/l) to give a measurement in grams

overall image time to less than 10 min (BOGAERT et al. 1995; WIESMANN et al. 1998).

11.3.2.3
Quantitative Evaluation with Velocity Mapping

For velocity mapping, phase information and not magnitude information is displayed. The application of short-lived magnetic gradients allows each point in the imaging plane to be encoded with a phase shift that is directly proportional to the velocity at that point. Because phase shifts can arise from other factors, a second velocity-compensated phase image is acquired, and subtraction yields the actual phase relationship of the protons (NAYLER et al. 1986; UNDERWOOD et al. 1987b). Velocity encoding can be

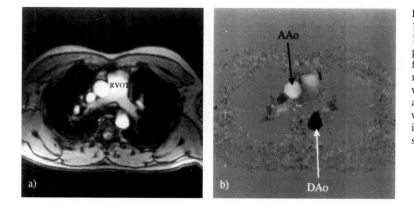

Fig. 11.7 a,b. GE velocity map, TE 14 ms, velocity encoding window ± 1.5 m/s. **a** Magnitude image at level of pulmonary bifurcation. *RVOT*, RV outflow tract. **b** Velocity image. Stationary material is represented as mid-grey whilst flow towards the head in the ascending aorta (*AAo*) is represented by white pixels, and flow towards the feet in the descending aorta (*DAo*) is represented by black pixels

applied in any direction (through plane, left to right, up and down) and the size of the velocity window defined for increased sensitivity. Stationary material is represented as mid-grey whilst increasing velocities in either direction are shown in increasing grades of black or white (Fig. 11.7).

Measurement of the spatial mean velocity for all pixels in a region of interest of known area makes possible the calculation of the instantaneous flow volume at any point in the cardiac cycle. Calculation of the flow volume per heart beat can be made by integrating the instantaneous flow volumes for all frames throughout the cardiac cycle. This technique has been validated in vitro and in vivo, and is extremely accurate and reproducible (FIRMIN et al. 1987; MEIER et al. 1988; BOGREN et al. 1989a). It now represents the gold standard for flow measurements in vivo. Quantification of the right ventricular (RV) and left ventricular (LV) outputs can be compared using through-plane flow measurements from the proximal ascending aorta and pulmonary trunk (1:1 ratio in normal individuals) (KONDO et al. 1991).

11.3.2.4
Aortic Regurgitation

A protocol for imaging patients with aortic regurgitation is shown in Fig. 11.8. Regurgitant aortic jets are best visualised in the coronal or oblique coronal plane. Estimation of the signal void volume is possible (AURIGEMMA et al. 1991; NISHIMURA 1992; OHNISHI et al. 1992), but care must be taken to ensure that all the jet has been visualised. The most accurate method for quantifying the regurgitant fraction is with velocity encoding in the slice direction, in an oblique transaxial plane above the aortic valve. A through-plane velocity window of ±1.5 m/s should be set if there is isolated aortic

regurgitation. If significant aortic stenosis is present a dual velocity window, with a high systolic setting of ±5 m/s, changing to ±1.5 m/s for the diastolic frames, may be necessary. Aortic regurgitation is represented by the amount of retrograde diastolic flow, and is measured in ml/beat or l/min (Fig. 11.9).

A good correlation has been demonstrated between ventricular volume measurements and velocity mapping in the ascending aorta, for the calculation of aortic regurgitant fractions (SONDERGAARD et al. 1993). Interstudy reproducibility has been demonstrated to be high and thus the technique is ideal for long-term patient follow-up (DULCE et al. 1992).

Some debate still remains as to the positioning of the plane across the aorta. Current in vivo experience suggests that a position between the coronary ostia and the aortic valve may be most accurate (CHATZIMAVROUDIS et al. 1997). Positions above the coronary ostia lead to inaccuracies secondary to coronary flow and aortic compliance. Further in vivo studies need to be performed to confirm these findings.

Velocity mapping in the ascending aorta has now been performed to analyse the therapeutic effects of ACE inhibition in patients with aortic regurgitation (GLOBITS et al. 1996). MRI demonstrated the beneficial effects of the therapy and was able to identify those patients with aortic regurgitation who responded favourably to ACE inhibition.

11.3.2.5
Mitral Regurgitation

There is good correlation between the signal loss caused by mitral regurgitation on GE cine images and Doppler and x-ray angiographic grading (AURIGEMMA et al. 1990). The regurgitant jet is best

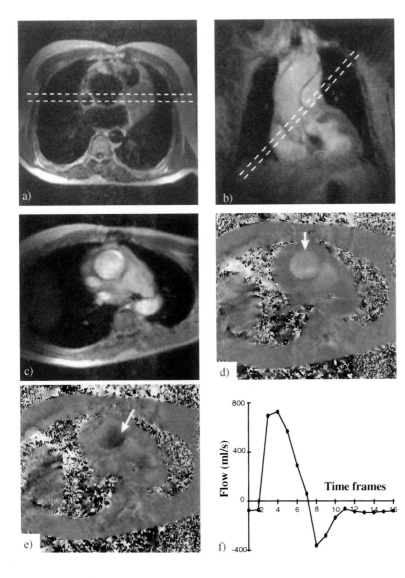

Fig. 11.8 a–f. Aortic regurgitation imaging protocol. A set of anatomical SE (or turbo SE images) in the transaxial plane is acquired. **a** A coronal plane through the aortic valve and LV outflow tract is defined from the SE images. **b** A GE cine image (TE = 14 ms) in the coronal plane is performed to identify the presence of a signal void in the left ventricle during diastole. An oblique transaxial plane is then defined in the ascending aorta, above the aortic valve, perpendicular to the ascending aorta. Velocity mapping is then performed in the oblique transaxial plane (velocity encode window = ±1.5 m/s). **c** Magnitude image. **d** Velocity map in early systole; antegrade aortic flow is represented by bright pixels (*arrow*). **e** Velocity map in diastole; retrograde flow is represented by dark pixels (arrow). **f** Flow versus time plot for the ascending aorta. Antegrade flow calculated at 140 ml/beat, retrograde flow 80 ml/beat, and aortic regurgitant fraction 57%

visualised in either the horizontal or the vertical long-axis plane. MRI has the advantage of being able to define lesions in subjects with poor acoustic windows.

For isolated mitral regurgitation, however, ventricular volume measurements provide an accurate method for quantifying mitral regurgitation (HUNDLEY et al. 1995):

Regurgitant volume (ml/beat)

$$= \text{LVSV (ml/beat)} - \text{RVSV (ml/beat)}, \qquad (1)$$

Regurgitant fraction (%)

$$= \frac{\text{Regurgitant volume (ml/beat)} \times 100}{\text{LVSV (ml/beat)}}, \qquad (2)$$

[where LVSV = left ventricular stroke volume and RVSV = right ventricular stroke volume.]

Secondly, when other valvular disease is present, the mitral regurgitant volume can be calculated from the LV stroke volume and velocity mapping flow measurements in the aorta:

Regurgitant volume (ml/beat)

$$= \text{LVSV} - (\text{total Ao flow}$$

$$+ \text{Ao diastolic flow}), \qquad (3)$$

where Ao = aorta.

Equation 3 can be simplified to:

Regurgitant volume (ml/beat)

$$= \text{LVSV} - \text{Ao systolic flow}. \qquad (4)$$

A third proposed method for quantifying mitral regurgitation involves calculation of the difference between ventricular outflow and ventricular inflow. Velocity mapping in the ascending aorta can be used

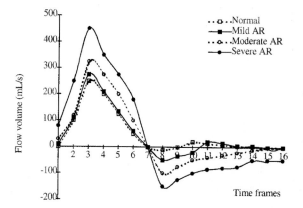

Fig. 11.9. Plots of flow volume versus time frames per cardiac cycle. Measurements were made in the ascending aorta for a normal subject and patients with increasing severity of aortic regurgitation (*AR*). Each point on the graphs represents the blood flow in the aorta for each image in the cardiac cycle. Negative values represent retrograde flow during diastole. Integration of the area under the curve for antegrade and retrograde flow enables calculation of the regurgitant volume per cardiac cycle (mL/beat)

to assess ventricular outflow, whilst velocity mapping at the mitral valve annulus during diastole can be used to assess inflow (Fig. 11.10). Results in 19 patients with mitral regurgitation demonstrated significantly different regurgitant volumes for groups with mild, moderate and severe mitral regurgitation, defined at echocardiography. There was also good correlation between the calculated regurgitant fraction and the grading of mitral regurgitation severity at Doppler echocardiography (FUJITA et al. 1994).

11.3.2.6
Mixed Valvular Regurgitation

The measurement of both RV and LV stroke volumes with GE cine imaging, in combination with velocity mapping measurement of pulmonary and aortic flow, permits the quantification of valvular regurgitation in all four valves, even if aortic, mitral, pulmo-

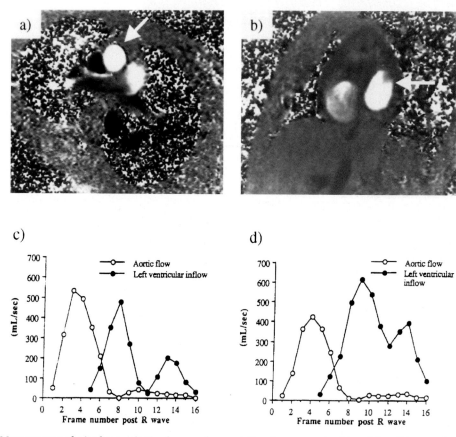

Fig. 11.10. Measurement of mitral regurgitation by use of velocity-encoded MRI to measure the difference between outflow across the proximal ascending aorta and in flow across the mitral annulus (**a** and **b**). Phase images acquired at the level of the proximal part of ascending aorta (*arrow* in **a**) and the mitral annulus (*arrow* in **b**). The graphs show the flow volume versus time frame for mitral inflow and aortic

inflow in a normal subject (**c**) and in a patient with mitral regurgitation (**d**). The difference in the areas under the two curves is the volume of mitral regurgitation. [Reprinted with permission from the American College of Cardiologists: Journal of the American College of Cardiology (1994) 23:951–958, FUJITA et al. 1994]

nary, and tricuspid regurgitation are all present. Aortic and pulmonary regurgitation are calculated from the velocity maps and diastolic reverse flow, and subtraction of the total systolic forward flow from the LVSV and RVSV yields the amount of mitral and tricuspid regurgitation respectively.

11.3.3
Valvular Stenosis

The presence of valvular stenosis can be identified by signal loss seen in GE cine images. Velocity mapping may then be used to establish an accurate peak velocity across the valve to quantify the severity of the stenosis. The use of the mean velocity across the caval veins and mitral valve can be used to describe the inflow curves for the atrioventricular valves (MOHIADDIN et al. 1990).

11.3.3.1
Qualitative Assessment with Cine Gradient-Echo Imaging

For stenotic lesions, the degree of signal loss is dependent on the degree of stenosis and the echo time used. Thus, for shorter echo times less proton spin dephasing can take place and more signal is recovered (DEROOS et al. 1989; KILNER et al. 1991). Figure 11.11 demonstrates the relationship between the echo time and the peak velocity across a stenosis. Thus in more severe stenosis, a lower echo time must be used to prevent signal loss in the images.

11.3.3.2
Quantitative Evaluation with Velocity Mapping

Direct measurement from the velocity map enables the measurement of the peak velocity across the valve, and application of the modified Bernoulli equation,

$$\Delta P = 4\,V^2, \tag{5}$$

[where P = the pressure drop across the stenosis (mmHg) and V = velocity (m/s)] enables an estimate of the gradient across the valve. The technique is comparable to Doppler echocardiography valvular stenosis measurements and has an in vitro accuracy of 4% (SIMPSON et al. 1993). The main advantage of the technique over echocardiography is that the velocity jet can be easily aligned in any direction without the limitation of acoustic windows.

11.3.3.3
Aortic Stenosis

A protocol for investigating aortic stenosis is outlined in Fig. 11.12. The alignment of the jet, the choice of TE, and definition of the velocity encode window are all important variables. The jet core appears as high signal sandwiched between two jets of low signal. In general, selection of the TE and velocity window should aim for greatest signal to noise and velocity sensitivity; however, if the shortest TE and largest velocity window are defined, most clinically significant jets will be accounted for. Good in vivo agreement has been demonstrated for a wide

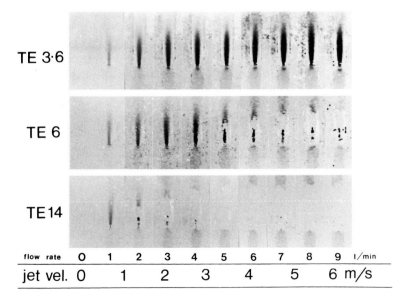

Fig. 11.11. In vitro jet velocity mapping. Velocity maps obtained with MRI of flow – increased from left to right – through the test stenosis, showing the significance of shortening the TE from 14 ms (*bottom*) to 6 ms (*centre*) and 3.6 ms (*top*). Only the 3.6 ms TE sequence allows mapping of high-velocity jets, up to a maximum tested velocity of 6.0 m/s [Reprinted with permission from KILNER et al. (1991) Valve and great vessel stenosis: assessment with MR jet velocity mapping. Radiology 178:229–235]

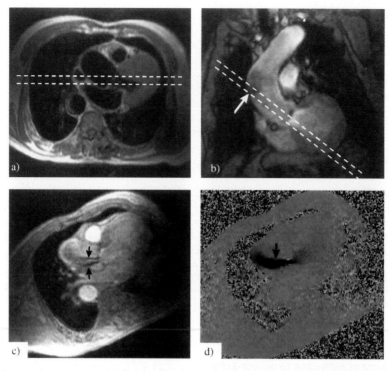

Fig. 11.12 a–d. Aortic stenosis imaging protocol. A set of anatomical SE (or turbo SE images) in the transaxial plane is acquired. **a** A coronal plane through the aortic valve and LV outflow tract is defined from the SE images. **b** A GE cine image (TE = 14 ms) in the oblique coronal plane is performed to identify the presence of a signal void in the ascending aorta. In this case the stenotic jet was only partially in plane in the oblique coronal plane (signal loss at the tip of the *white arrow*). A velocity map in an oblique plane was therefore per-formed through the aortic valve and the signal void. **c** The magnitude images (TE = 3.6 ms) demonstrate a posterior aortic flow jet. The central core of the jet is clearly seen as bright signal sandwiched between two turbulent areas of lower signal (*black arrows*). **d** The velocity map (TE = 3.6 ms, velocity encode window = ±8 m/s) shows black pixels in the region of the jet (peak velocity = 4 m/s, calculated gradient across aortic valve = 64 mmHg)

range of pressure gradients across the aortic valve (3–148 mmHg) between MR velocity mapping and Doppler echocardiography and x-ray angiography (EICHENBERGER et al. 1993). In our own institution we have found it easiest to interpret velocity maps parallel to the jet, as this reveals the jet length in relationship to pre- and post-stenotic flows (KILNER et al. 1993a).

In patients with aortic stenosis, MRI can also be used to calculate the LV volume and mass.

11.3.3.4
Mitral Stenosis

Peak velocity measurements at MRI across the mitral valve (short-axis view below the mitral valve) correlate well with Doppler measurements at echocardiography (HEIDENREICH et al. 1995). Because of the complicated shape of the stenotic jet in most patients, through plane measurements of velocity are more accurate than in-plane measurements. Valve area can also be measured (Fig. 11.13).

Velocity mapping flow curves show loss of the normal dual peaks, with high velocities throughout diastole (Fig. 11.14). The flow curves can be used to determine the mitral pressure half-time (the time taken for the pressure gradient to fall to half its peak value), a useful echocardiographic indicator of mitral stenosis severity:

$$\text{Valve area} \left(\text{cm}^2 \right) = \frac{220}{\text{Pressure half time (ms)}}. \quad (6)$$

The severity of mitral stenosis can also be estimated by measuring pulmonary vein flow. In severe mitral stenosis this flow is reversed (MOHIADDIN et al. 1991a).

As previously mentioned, left atrial size and the presence of atrial thrombus can also be noted.

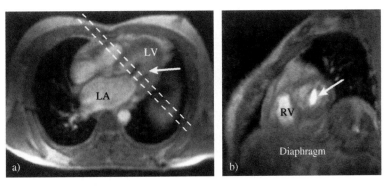

Fig. 11.13 a,b. Mitral stenosis. **a** Transaxial GE image in mid diastole. Turbulent flow is seen through the mitral valve (*arrow*). *Dotted white lines* represent the image plane for the short-axis image. **b** Short-axis GE image in mid diastole. Flow through the mitral valve is shown as bright pixels (*arrow*). The valve orifice area can be easily measured. *LA*, Left atrium; *LV*, left ventricle; *RV*, right ventricle

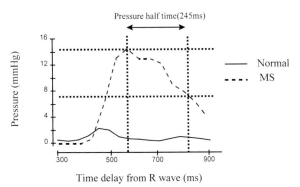

Fig. 11.14. Plot of pressure against time for mitral valve in a normal subject and a patient with mitral stenosis (*MS*). Velocity mapping was performed across the mitral valve annulus. For the normal subject two peaks are seen in early ventricular diastole and atrial contraction. In the patient with mitral stenosis there is persistent high peak velocity throughout diastole, with a pressure half time of 245 ms and a calculated valve area of 0.9 cm^2

11.3.4
Pulmonary Valve

Difficulties with the alignment of the acoustic window for Doppler echocardiographic investigation has made MR velocity mapping a useful tool in the investigation of the pulmonary valve and pulmonary arteries (BOGREN et al. 1989b; MOHIADDIN et al. 1991b; REBERGEN et al. 1993). The imaging protocols for aortic stenosis and regurgitation apply for investigation of the pulmonary valve. For pulmonary stenosis measurement (Fig. 11.15) and the visualisation of pulmonary regurgitation imaging is best performed in a sagittal or oblique sagittal plane. For the quantification of pulmonary regurgitation and right ventricular outflow curves, imaging the main pulmonary trunk in cross-section in a coronal or oblique transaxial plane is most accurate (Fig. 11.16).

11.3.5
Tricuspid Valve

Examination of the tricuspid valve is as for the mitral valve. The regurgitant jet of tricuspid regurgitation is best visualised in the transverse plane. Velocity mapping in the superior vena cava can demonstrate tricuspid regurgitation (Fig. 11.17). It must be noted that trivial tricuspid regurgitation is a common finding in normal subjects (WAGGONER et al. 1981). As with echocardiography, the peak velocity can be measured from right ventricle to right atrium, across the tricuspid valve, in secondary tricuspid regurgitation. If there is no pulmonary artery stenosis the addition of an estimate of the right atrial pressure to the calculated pressure difference between the right atrium and right ventricle can give an estimate of the pulmonary artery pressure.

The tricuspid valve orifice is larger than the mitral orifice. Tricuspid stenosis is uncommon, but can be easily diagnosed on GE cine images. Tricuspid atresia is easily identified on SE images.

11.3.6
Prosthetic Valves

For non-biological prosthetic valves and stented biological valves the applied magnetic field is distorted

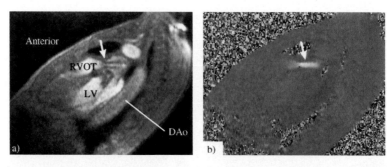

Fig. 11.15 a,b. Velocity mapping in an oblique sagittal plane (TE = 6 ms, velocity encode window = ±8 m/s). This patient had recently undergone a "Ross" procedure (pulmonary homograft, aortic autograft). **a** In the magnitude image the pulmonary trunk is clearly narrowed with significant flow jet distal to the narrowing (again, the central core easily seen). *RVOT*, Right ventricular outflow tract; *LV*, left ventricle; *DAo*, descending aorta. **b** The velocity map confirms significant stenosis (peak velocity = 3.9 m/s, gradient 61 mmHg)

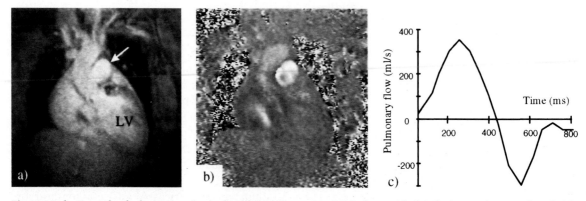

Fig. 11.16 a,b. Example of velocity mapping in the pulmonary trunk in a patient with pulmonary regurgitation. **a** Magnitude image in the coronal plane. *Arrow* points to the pulmonary artery. *LV*, Left ventricle. **b** Velocity map in same plane, bright pixels in the pulmonary artery indicate forward flow. **c** Flow curve for pulmonary regurgitation; regurgitant fraction is 41%

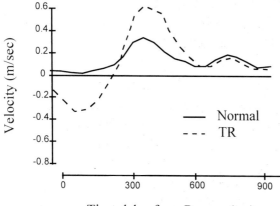

Fig. 11.17. Plot of velocity against time for tricuspid valve in a normal subject and a patient with tricuspid regurgitation (*TR*). Velocity mapping was performed in the superior vena cava. For the normal subject two velocity peaks are seen in early ventricular diastole and atrial contraction. In the patient with tricuspid regurgitation there is reverse flow during systole

by differences in the local magnetic fields between the prosthesis and the biological tissue, and by eddy currents induced in the valve. These phenomena lead to signal loss around the prosthesis. These artefacts can be very severe on GE images, and may degrade the image significantly. This makes imaging turbulent jets in the vicinity of the prosthesis difficult; however, velocity mapping distal to the image artefact can still be accurately performed. Homografts, autografts and stentless porcine valve replacements do not cause signal artefact and can be imaged normally. All valvular prostheses can be safely imaged, at current field strengths, except for Starr-Edwards mitral pre-6000 series valves used from 1960 to 1964, at field strengths of greater than 0.35 T (RANDALL et al. 1988; SHELLOCK 1988; SHELLOCK et al. 1993). Very few of the aforementioned prosthetic valves still remain in situ.

Magnetic resonance imaging offers an ideal method for the non-invasive follow-up of patients

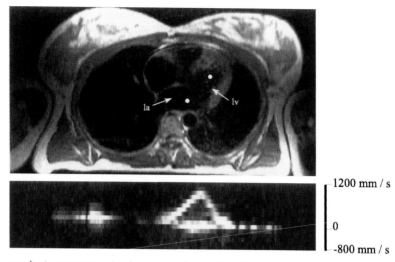

1200 mm / s

0

-800 mm / s

Fig. 11.18. *Upper panel*: A transverse SE image at the midventricular level. The two markers on the left atrium (*la*) and the left ventricle (*lv*) define the position and direction of the Fourier velocity (FV) image for the mitral valve. *Lower panel*: A selected frame from the complete cine acquisition of FV across the mitral valve acquired at peak ventricular filling with velocity through the valve plotted vertically and position along the cylinder plotted horizontally. [Reprinted with permission from MOHIADDIN et al. (1997) Cine MR Fourier velocimetry of blood flow through cardiac valves: comparison with Doppler echocardiography. J Magn Reson Imaging 7:657–663]

after valvular surgery (DEUTSCH et al. 1992). In vitro, the accuracy of MR velocity measurements distal to a wide variety of valvular prostheses has been confirmed by laser Doppler anemometry (FONTAINE et al. 1996). The assessment of prosthetic valve function at low field strength (0.2 T) has also been demonstrated (DICESARE et al. 1995). Useful clinical follow-up has been reported in patients following aortic root reconstruction, where not only was prosthetic valve function assessed, but the aortic graft, LV outflow tract and proximal coronary arteries were all evaluated (LEPORE et al. 1996).

11.3.7
Magnetic Resonance Spectroscopy

There is limited experience with MR spectroscopy and valvular heart disease in the clinical setting (see Sect. 9.4.4). It is known that a reduction in the phosphocreatinine to ATP (PCr/ATP) ratio occurs in patients with heart failure. A preliminary study has been performed to establish whether a decrease in the PCr/ATP ratio could be used to guide the timing of valve replacement in aortic valve disease (CONWAY et al. 1991). A large prospective study, with measurement of both pre- and post-valve replacement PCr/ATP ratios, needs to be performed.

11.4
Future Directions

11.4.1
Ultrafast Imaging

Ultrafast imaging techniques [segmented k-space fast low-angle shot (FLASH), rectilinear echoplanar (EPI) and spiral echoplanar (Spiral)] will enable the acquisition of multi-slice short-axis ventricular volume studies in a matter of 10 min or less (WIESMANN et al. 1998).

Interleaved GE EPI has been used to improve the identification of valvular morphology. In a recent report 38 out of 44 atrioventricular valve leaflets were clearly visualised by EPI, despite the study being limited, as no oblique planes could be acquired (DAVIS et al. 1995).

Cine FLASH imaging is possible but as yet no studies have reported velocity mapping across valves. This may reflect the poor temporal resolution of FLASH (80–100 ms), which has a tendency to average down the peak velocity. EPI velocity mapping in vessels is possible, but has not been reported across valves (FIRMIN et al. 1989). This probably reflects the flow-related ghosting and distortion seen with rectilinear EPI. Further, EPI is vulnerable to signal loss in the region of blood flow. Spiral velocity mapping is more robust and less prone to signal loss related to flow; however, spiral imaging is very susceptible to field inhomogeneities. Flow measurements with spiral imaging have been reported in healthy subjects (PIKE et al. 1994; GATEHOUSE et al. 1994). This technique could thus be used to calculate through-plane flow for both the aortic and pulmonary arteries. No valvular studies have been reported to date.

11.4.2
Fourier Velocity Mapping

MR Fourier velocimetry uses velocity phase-encoding, bipolar gradient waveforms to measure velocities in a single plane parallel to the gradient pulse (DUMOULIN et al. 1991). Peak velocities can thus be measured after alignment of the readout cylinder along the flow jet (Fig. 11.18). Results recently reported in healthy subjects demonstrate good correlation between Doppler echocardiography measurements and MR Fourier velocimetry for all four valves (MOHIADDIN et al. 1997). In comparison with echocardiography the jet is easily aligned without the need for a good acoustic window. The main advantages of Fourier mapping over conventional velocity mapping are that the data are not affected by partial volume averaging, the technique is less vulnerable to signal loss, and imaging time is much shorter (total imaging time of 15 min

for all valves, compared with 60 min for conventional velocity mapping). As yet no study has been performed to investigate the technique in diseased valves.

11.4.3
Velocity Vector Mapping

Velocity vector mapping is possible when 3D phase contrast cine imaging is performed. The technique has been used to define helical and retrograde flow patterns in the aortic arch of healthy subjects (KILNER et al. 1993b) and flow patterns in the left ventricles of both healthy subjects and patients with dilated ischemic cardiomyopathy (MOHIADDIN 1995). In valvular disease a potential use for this technique may be in defining the position of prosthetic valves to improve post-valvular flow characteristics. In vitro studies are ongoing, and preliminary results with tilting disc prostheses suggest that for aortic valve replacement, better flow characteristics can be achieved if the larger of the two valve orifices is positioned towards the inner aortic wall and not the outer wall (Fig. 11.19). Such simple changes in prosthesis position may result in less aortic dilatation post valve replacement and longer valve lifetimes.

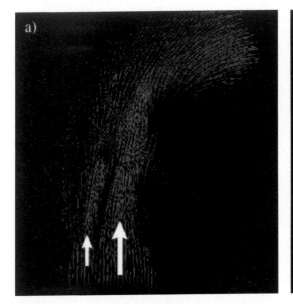
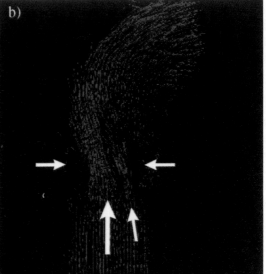

Fig. 11.19 a,b. Vector velocity mapping in an ascending aorta phantom with pulsatile flow. A tilting disc valve has been mounted within the phantom (lower edge of the images). **a** The larger orifice of the tilting valve is positioned adjacent to the inner aortic wall (*large arrow*). **b** The larger orifice is positioned adjacent to the outer wall (*larger arrow*). In the second image flow resembles that of the normal ascending aorta, with the preservation of flow in the ascending aorta and the presence of aortic sinus vortices

11.5
Conclusion

Magnetic resonance imaging can provide important information about valvular function. Both stenotic and regurgitant lesions can be quantified for all four valves. Quantification can also be performed even when multiple valves are affected. Anatomical information with regard to leaflet number, valve thickness and the presence of endocarditis is still best provided by echocardiography.

Magnetic resonance imaging offers the only noninvasive, accurate and reproducible method for quantifying valvular regurgitation, with no x-ray exposure. In combination with accurate ventricular function assessment, MRI is ideal for the long-term follow-up and evaluation of patients awaiting valvular surgery. However, long-term studies using MRI in such a role need to be performed to define the optimal timings for these interventions.

At present GE velocity mapping techniques remain time consuming, 5–6 min being required for each image. However, with the increasing availability of new MR hardware, faster imaging sequences (FLASH, EPI, spiral) will be adapted to create velocity-encoded images over ever-shorter image acquisition periods.

As cardiovascular MRI becomes more cost-effective and easily accessible, its use for the accurate assessment of valvular heart disease in clinical cardiology will increase, and enable physicians to better predict the optimal treatment for their patients with valvular heart disease.

Acknowledgements. Andrew Taylor is supported by the Coronary Artery Disease Research Association (CORDA). We thank Dr. R.H. MOHIADDIN, Dr. P. KILNER, Dr. D.N. FIRMIN, Prof. S.R. UNDERWOOD and Dr. M. KON for their help.

References

Abbasi AS, Allen MW, Decristofaro D, Ungar I (1980) Detection and estimation of the degree of mitral regurgitation by range-gated pulsed Doppler echocardiography. Circulation 61:143–149

Aurigemma G, Reichek N, Schiebler M, Axel L (1990) Evaluation of mitral regurgitation by cine MRI. Am J Cardiol 66:621–625

Aurigemma G, Reichek N, Schiebler M, Axel L (1991) Evaluation of aortic regurgitation by cardiac cine MRI: planar analysis and comparison to Doppler echocardiography. Cardiology 78:340–347

Boehrer JD, Lange RA, Willard JE, Grayburn PA, Hillis LD (1992) Advantages and limitations of methods to detect, localise and quantitate intracardiac left-to-right shunting. Am Heart J 124:448–455

Bogaert JG, Bosmans HT, Rademakers FE, et al. (1995) Left ventricular quantification with breath-hold MR imaging: comparison with echocardiography. MAGMA 3:5–12

Bogren HG, Klipstein RH, Firmin DN, Mohiaddin RH, Underwood SR, Rees RSO, Longmore DB (1989a) Quantification of antegrade and retrograde blood flow in the human aorta by magnetic resonance velocity mapping. Am Heart J 117:1214–1222

Bogren HG, Klipstein RH, Mohiaddin RH, et al. (1989b) Pulmonary artery distensibility and blood flow patterns: a magnetic resonance study of normal subjects and patients with pulmonary arterial hypertension. Am Heart J 118:990–999

Bolger AF, Eigler NL, Maurer G (1988) Quantifying valvular regurgitation: limitations and inherent assumptions of Doppler technique. Circulation 78:1316–1318

Bryan AJ, Barzilai B, Kouchoukos NT (1995) Transesophageal echocardiography and adult cardiac operations. Ann Thorac Surg 59:773–779

Caduff JH, Hernandez RJ, Ludomirsky A (1996) MR visualization of aortic valve vegetations. J Comput Assist Tomogr 20:613–615

Carroll JD (1993) Cardiac catheterisation and other imaging modalities in the evaluation of valvular heart disease. Curr Opin Cardiol 8:211–215

Chatzimavroudis GP, Walker PG, Oshinski JN, Franch RH, Pettigrew RI, Yoganathan AP (1997) Slice location dependence of aortic regurgitation measurements with MR phase velocity mapping. Magn Reson Med 37:545–551

Cohen BL (1991) Catalogue of risks extended and updated. Health Phys 61:317–335

Conway MA, Allis J, Ouwerkerk R, Niioka T, Rajagopalan B, Radda GK (1991) Detection of low phosphocreatinine to ATP ratio in failing hypertrophied human myocardium by P magnetic resonance spectroscopy. Lancet 338:973–976

Davis CP, McKinnon GC, Debatin JF, Duewell S, von Schulthess GK (1995) Single-shot versus interleaved echoplanar MR imaging: application to visualization of cardiac valve leaflets. J Magn Reson Imaging 5:107–112

Davis K, Kennedy J, Kemp H, Judkins M, Gosselin A, Killip T (1979) Complications of coronary arteriography from the collaborative study of coronary artery surgery (CASS). Circulation 59:1105–1112

DeRoos A, Reichek N, Axel L, Kressel HY (1989) Cine MR imaging in aortic stenosis. J Comput Assist Tomogr 13:421–425

Deutsch HJ, Bachmann R, Sechtem U, et al. (1992) Regurgitant flow in cardiac valve prosthesis: diagnostic value of gradient echo nuclear magnetic resonance imaging in reference to transesophageal two-dimensional color Doppler echocardiography. J Am Coll Cardiol 19:1500–1507

DiCesare E, Enrici RM, Paparoni S, et al. (1995) Low-field magnetic resonance imaging in the evaluation of mechanical and biological heart valve function. Eur J Radiol 20:224–228

Diebold B, Delouche A, Delouche P, Guglielmi J-P, Dumee P, Herment A (1996) In vitro flow mapping of regurgitant jets: systematic description of free jet with laser Doppler velocimetry. Circulation 94:158–169

Dooms G, Higgins CB (1986) MR imaging of cardiac thrombi. J Comput Assist Tomogr 10:415–420

Dulce MC, Mostbeck GH, O'Sullivan M, Cheitlin M, Caputo GR, Higgins CB (1992) Severity of aortic regurgitation: interstudy reproducibility of measurements with velocity-encoded cine MRI. Radiology 185:235–240

Dulce MC, Mostbeck GH, Friese KK, Caputo GR, Higgins CB (1993) Quantification of the left ventricular volumes and function with cine MR imaging: comparison of geometric models with three-dimensional data. Radiology 188:371–376

Dumoulin CL, Souza SP, Hardy CJ, Ash SA (1991) Quantitative measurement of blood flow using cylindrically localized Fourier velocity encoding. Magn Reson Med 21:242–250

Eichenberger AC, Jenni R, von Schulthess GK (1993) Aortic valve pressure gradients in patients with aortic valve stenosis: quantification with velocity-encoded cine MR imaging. AJR 160:971–977

Evans AJ, Blinder RA, Herfkens RJ, et al. (1988) Effects of turbulence on signal intensity in gradient echo images. Invest Radiol 23:512–518

Firmin DN, Nayler GL, Klipstein RH, Underwood SR, Longmore DB (1987) In vivo validation of MR velocity imaging. J Comput Assist Tomogr 11:751–756

Firmin DN, Klipstein RH, Hounsfield GL, Paley MP, Longmore DB (1989) Echo-planar high-resolution flow velocity mapping. Magn Reson Med 12:316–327

Fix J, Isada L, Cosgrove D, Miller DP, Savage R, Blum J, Stewart W (1993) Do patients with less than "echo-perfect" results from mitral valve repair by intraoperative echocardiography have a different outcome? Circulation 88:39–48

Fontaine AA, Heinrich RS, Walker PG, et al. (1996) Comparison of magnetic resonance imaging and laser Doppler anemometry velocity measurements downstream of replacement heart valves: implications for in vivo assessment of prosthetic valve function. J Heart Valve Dis 5:66–73

Fujita N, Chazouilleres AF, Hartiala JJ, et al. (1994) Quantification of mitral regurgitation by velocity encoded cine nuclear magnetic resonance imaging. J Am Coll Cardiol 23:951–958

Gatehouse PD, Firmin DN, Collins S, Longmore DB (1994) Real time blood flow imaging by spiral scan phase velocity mapping. Magn Reson Med 31:504–512

Globits S, Mayr H, Frank H, et al. (1991) Quantification of regurgitant lesions by MRI. Int J Card Imaging 6:109–116

Globits S, Blake L, Bourne M, et al. (1996) Assessment of haemodynamic effects of ACE inhibition therapy in chronic aortic regurgitation by using velocity-encoded cine magnetic resonance imaging. Am Heart J 131:289–293

Gorlin R, Gorlin SG (1951) Hydraulic formula for calculation of the area of the stenotic mitral valve, other valves and central circulatory shunts. Am Heart J 41:1–29

Hatle L, Angelson B (1992) Doppler ultrasound in cardiology: physical principles and clinical applications. Lea & Febiger, Philadelphia

Hausmann D, Daniel WG, Mugge A, Ziemer G, Pearlman AS (1992) Value of transesophageal color Doppler echocardiography for detection of different types of atrial septal defect in adults. J Am Soc Echocardiogr 5:481–488

Heidenreich PA, Steffens JC, Fujita N, O'Sullivan M, Caputo GR, Foster E, Higgins CB (1995) The evaluation of mitral stenosis with velocity-encoded cine MRI. Am J Cardiol 75:365–369

Hundley WG, Li HF, Willard JE, et al. (1995) Magnetic resonance imaging assessment of the severity of mitral regurgitation. Circulation 92:1151–1158

Jeang MK, Fuentes F, Gately A, Byrnes J, Lewis M (1986) Aortic root abscess – initial experience using magnetic resonance imaging. Chest 89:613–615

Kilner PJ, Firmin DN, Rees RSO, et al. (1991) Valve and great vessel stenosis: assessment with MR jet velocity mapping. Radiology 178:229–235

Kilner PJ, Manzara CC, Mohiaddin RH, et al. (1993a) Magnetic resonance jet velocity mapping in mitral and aortic valve stenosis. Circulation 87:1239–1248

Kilner PJ, Yang GZ, Mohiaddin RH, Firmin DN, Longmore DB (1993b) Helical and retrograde secondary flow patterns in the aortic arch studied by three-dimensional magnetic resonance velocity mapping. Circulation 88:2235–2247

Kondo C, Caputo GR, Semelka R, Shimakawa M, Higgins CB (1991) Right and left ventricular stroke volume measurements with velocity encoded cine NMR imaging: in vivo and in vitro evaluation. AJR 157:9–16

Laissy JP, Blanc F, Soyer P, et al. (1995) Thoracic aortic dissection: diagnosis with transesophageal echocardiography versus MR imaging. Radiology 194:331–336

Lepore V, Lamm C, Bugge M, Larsson S (1996) Magnetic resonance imaging in the follow-up of patients after aortic root reconstruction. Thorac Cardiovasc Surg 44:188–192

Manning WJ, Silverman DI, Gordon SP, Krumholz HM, Douglas PS (1993) Cardioversion from atrial fibrillation without prolonged anticoagulation with use of transesophageal echocardiography to exclude the presence of atrial thrombi. N Engl J Med 328:750–755

Meier D, Maier S, Boesiger P (1988) Quantitative flow measurements on phantoms and on blood vessels with MR. Magn Reson Med 8:25–34

Mohiaddin RH (1995) Flow patterns in the dilated ischaemic left ventricle studied by MR imaging with velocity vector mapping. J Magn Reson Imaging 5:493–498

Mohiaddin RH, Wann SL, Underwood R, Firmin DN, Rees S, Longmore DB (1990) Vena caval flow: assessment with cine MR velocity mapping. Radiology 177:537–541

Mohiaddin RH, Amanuma M, Kilner PJ, Pennell DJ, Manzara C, Longmore DB (1991a) MR phase-shift velocity mapping of mitral and pulmonary venous flow. J Comput Assist Tomogr 15:237–243

Mohiaddin RH, Paz R, Theodoropolus S, et al. (1991b) Magnetic resonance characterization of pulmonary arterial blood flow following single lung transplantation. J Thorac Cardiovasc Surg 101:1016–1023

Mohiaddin RH, Gatehouse PD, Henien M, Firmin DN (1997) Cine MR Fourier velocimetry of blood flow through cardiac valves: comparison with Doppler echocardiography. J Magn Reson Imaging 7:657–663

Nayler GL, Firmin DN, Longmore DB (1986) Blood flow imaging by cine magnetic resonance. J Comput Assist Tomogr 10:715–722

Nishimura F (1992) Oblique cine MRI for the evaluation of aortic regurgitation: comparison with cineangiography. Clin Cardiol 66:621–625

Ohnishi S, Fukui S, Kusuoka H, Kitabatake A, Inoue M, Kamada T (1992) Assessment of valvular regurgitation using cine MRI coupled with phase compensating technique: comparison with Doppler color flow mapping. Angiology 43:913–924

Pedersen WR, Walker M, Olson JD, et al. (1991) Value of transesophageal echocardiography as an adjunct to transthoracic echocardiography in evaluation of native and prosthetic valve endocarditis. Chest 100:351–356

Pike GB, Meyer CH, Brosnan TJ, Pelc NJ (1994) Magnetic resonance velocity imaging using a fast spiral phase contrast sequence. Magn Reson Med 32:476–483

Quinones MA, Young JB, Waggoner AD, Ostojic MC, Ribeiro LGT, Miller RR (1980) Assessment of pulsed Doppler echocardiography in detection and quantification of aortic and mitral regurgitation. Br Heart J 44:612–620

Randall PA, Kohman LJ, Scalzetti EM, Szeverenyi NM, Panicek DM (1988) Magnetic resonance imaging of prosthetic cardiac valves in vitro and in vivo. Am J Cardiol 62:973–976

Rebergen SA, Chin JGJ, Ottenkamp J, van der Wall, de Roos A (1993) Pulmonary regurgitation in the late postoperative follow-up of tetralogy of Fallot. Circulation 88:2257–2266

Rigo P, Alderson PO, Robertson RM, Becker LC, Wagner HN (1979) Measurement of aortic and mitral regurgitation by gated cardiac blood pool scans. Circulation 60:306–312

Rockey R, Sterling LL, Zoghbi WA, Sartori MP, Limacher MC, Kou LC, Quinones MA (1987) Determination of the regurgitant fraction in isolated mitral regurgitation by pulsed Doppler two-dimensional echocardiography. J Am Coll Cardiol 7:1273–1278

Rodriguez L, Anconina J, Flaschkampf FA, Weyman AE, Levine RA, Thomas JD (1992) Impact of finite orifice size on proximal flow convergence: implications for Doppler quantification of valvular regurgitation. Circ Res 70:923–930

Sakuma H, Fujita N, Foo TK, et al. (1993) Evaluation of left ventricular volume and mass with breath-hold cine MR imaging. Radiology 188:377–380

Sandler H, Dodge HT, Hay RE, Rackley CE (1963) Quantification of valvular insufficiency in man by angiocardiography. Am Heart J 65:501–513

Sechtem U, Pflugfelder PW, White RD, Gould RG, Holt W, Lipton MJ, Higgins CB (1987) Cine MR imaging: potential for the evaluation of cardiovascular function. AJR Am J Roentgenol 148:239–246

Sechtem U, Pflugfelder PW, Cassidy MM, White RD, Cheitlin MD, Schiller NB, Higgins CB (1988) Mitral and aortic regurgitation: quantification of regurgitant volumes with cine MR imaging. Radiology 167:425–430

Sellers RD, Levy MJ, Amplatz K, Lillehei CW (1964) Left retrograde cardioangiography in acquired cardiac disease: technique, indication and interpretation. Am J Cardiol 14:437–445

Shellock FG (1988) MR imaging of metallic implants and materials: a compilation of the literature. AJR 151:811–814

Shellock FG, Morisoli S, Kanal E (1993) MR procedures and biomedical implants, materials and devices: 1993 update. Radiology 189:587–599

Simpson IA, Maciel BC, Moises V, et al. (1993) Cine magnetic resonance imaging and color Doppler flow mapping displays of flow velocity, spatial acceleration and jet formation: a comparative in vitro study. Am Heart J 126:1165–1174

Sondergaard L, Lindvig K, Hildebrandt P, Thomsen C, Stahlberg F, Joen T, Henriksen O (1993) Quantification of aortic regurgitation by magnetic resonance velocity mapping. Am Heart J 125;1081–1090

Sorenson SG, O'Rourke RA, Chaudhuri TK (1980) Noninvasive quantification of valvular regurgitation by gated equilibrium radionuclide angiography. Circulation 62:1089–1098

Tice FD, Kisslo J (1993) Echocardiography in the diagnosis of thoracic aortic pathology. Int J Card Imaging 9 (Suppl) 2:27–38

Underwood SR, Firmin DN, Mohiaddin RH, et al. (1987a) Cine magnetic resonance imaging of valvular heart disease (abstract). Proc Soc Magn Reson Imaging 2:723

Underwood SR, Firmin DN, Klipstein RH, Rees RSO, Longmore DB (1987b) Magnetic resonance velocity mapping: clinical application of a new technique. Br Heart J 57:404–412

Utsunomiya T, Ogawa T, Doshi R, Patel D, Quan M, Henry WL, Gardin JM (1991) Doppler color flow "proximal isovelocity surface area" method for estimating volume flow rates: effects of orifice shape and machine factors. J Am Coll Cardiol 17:1103–1111

Waggoner AD, Quinones MA, Young JB, et al. (1981) Pulsed Doppler echocardiography detection of right-sided valve regurgitation. Experimental results and clinical significance. Am J Cardiol 47:279–283

Wagner S, Auffermann W, Buser P, Lim TH, Kircher B, Pflugfelder PW, Higgins CB (1989) Diagnostic accuracy and estimation of the severity of valvular regurgitation from the signal void on cine magnetic resonance imaging. Am Heart J 118:760–767

Weinmann HJ, Lanaido M, Mutzel W (1984) Pharmacokinetics of Gd-DTPA/dimeglumine after iv injection. Physiol Chem Phys Med NMR 16:167–172

Wiesmann F, Gatehouse PD, Panting JR, Taylor AM, Firmin DN, Pennell DJ (1998) Comparison of fast spiral, echo planar and FLASH magnetic resonance imaging for cardiac volumetry at 0.5T. J Magn Reson Imaging; in press.

12 Coronary Arteries: How Do I Image Them?

A.J. Duerinckx

CONTENTS

12.1 Introduction

Coronary magnetic resonance angiography (MRA) can routinely visualize the proximal and middle portions of most coronary arteries and some coronary artery branches. Coronary MRA can and should be used for noninvasive imaging in a variety of clinical situations, such as in the evaluation of congenital coronary artery anomalies, in the follow-up of proximal coronary lesions after angioplasty, and in the noninvasive determination of the patency of bypass grafts and coronary stents. The use of coronary MRA for blind prospective detection of coronary lesions is now being evaluated, and coronary MRA techniques

may become an integral part of the clinical evaluation and screening of patients with ischemic heart disease.

With the development of a new group of ultrafast imaging sequences, reliable and reproducible MRA of the coronary arteries has become possible. A first generation of coronary MRA techniques was initially described in 1991 and is now commercially available on most clinical MRI scanners. These techniques rely upon a combination of segmental acquisition in k-space of the data to minimize cardiac motion and the use of a single breath-hold to minimize respiratory motion artifacts. A second generation of techniques was described in 1993–94; these techniques, referred to as the "navigator" techniques, allow repeated breath-holding or continuous regular breathing and open the way for higher resolution coronary MRA with increased patient comfort. They are still undergoing extensive fine tuning. A third generation of breath-hold techniques was first described in 1995 and is still under development. These new techniques may provide the ultimate compromise between user-friendliness and acquisition speeds. And most recently the combination of MR contrast agents and some of the newer coronary MRA techniques seems very promising.

Many imaging tools exist to directly evaluate the coronary artery anatomy: electron-beam computed tomography (EB-CT), coronary MRA, echocardiography (both transthoracic and transesophageal), intravascular ultrasound, and invasive x-ray coronary angiography, today's gold standard. EB-CT and MRI appear very close competitors for the same market. However, unlike EB-CT, coronary MRA does not require iodinated contrast agents or x-ray radiation and has the potential to become a more widespread and easy to use cardiac screening tool.

Because only the first-generation coronary MRA techniques are now universally available on most commercial MR imagers, the bulk of our discussion will be limited to these techniques. The purpose of this chapter is to provide an understanding of these

A.J. Duerinckx, MD, PhD, Radiology Service, MRI, Bld #507, West Los Angeles VA Medical Center, 11301 Wilshire Blvd., Los Angeles, CA 90073 and Department of Radiology, UCLA Center for Health Sciences, Los Angeles, CA 90095, USA

techniques, and to discuss their use for MR imaging of normal coronary anatomy. We refer the reader to other publications for discussions of more specialized applications or detailed reviews of the newer coronary MRA techniques.

12.2
Coronary MRA Techniques

The small and tortuous nature of coronary vessels and the significant physiologic motion dictate specific requirements for coronary MRA techniques. First, there is a need for good cardiac triggering. Secondly, coronary arteries are often embedded in epicardial fat, requiring the suppression of the high MR signal from fat to increase the contrast between coronary arteries and the background. Finally, the elimination of respiratory motion is dealt with in many different ways. We will review the differences in techniques available, first from a historical perspective (first-, second-, and third-generation techniques) and then from a user perspective.

When reviewing the history of coronary MRA, there is an extensive prehistory. It was noted early on that almost any MRI pulse sequence applied to thoracic imaging, just like most CT scans of the chest, was able to occasionally show small segments of native coronary vessels and bypass grafts (PAULIN et al. 1987; GOMES et al. 1987). In the early 1990–91 period several coronary MRA techniques which were not too reliable or reproducible were experimented with and then abandoned. These techniques took advantage of averaging over multiple respiratory cycles during a very long acquisition or pseudo-respiratory gating (DUMOULIN et al. 1991; CHO et al. 1991).

The history of coronary MRA really started, at least in the published literature, in February 1991 with the article in which Dennis Atkinson and Robert Edelman (ATKINSON and EDELMAN 1991) described a new ECG-triggered k-space segmented pulse sequence for cardiac imaging. This was followed in December 1991 by a second article by Edelman et al. which described its application to coronary artery MR imaging. (EDELMAN et al. 1991). EKG-triggered k-space segmented techniques allow a significant reduction of the total acquisition time for two-dimensional (2D) imaging such that images can be acquired within a single breath-hold (ATKINSON and EDELMAN 1991; EDELMAN et al. 1991). These techniques will be referred to as the "first-generation coronary MRA techniques." They

are now available on most commercial MRI scanners. The concept of k-space segmentation is widely used in other MRI applications (MEZRICH 1995). This same technique has since been shown also to work with nonrectangular k-space sampling schemes, such as spiral scanning (MEYER et al. 1992). Spiral coronary MRA has some advantages over the traditional approach, but is not yet routinely available on most commercial MRI scanners. There are, however, several problems with these first-generation techniques. First, breath-holding, although adequate for 2D coronary MRA, cannot easily be extended to three-dimensional (3D) acquisitions (PASCHAL et al. 1992, 1993). Second, the duration of the total examination can be long because of the need to acquire many sequential 2D images, each requiring one breath-hold. Thus inconsistent breath-holding and image misregistration problems can happen (DUERINCKX et al. 1996a). Third, the technique requires a significant amount of user experience, skill, and familiarity with the cardiac and coronary anatomy to produce good results. With some training and practice, most technologists, radiologists, and/or cardiologists can learn how to perform these studies (DUERINCKX et al. 1996a; DUERINCKX 1995a, 1996). It has also been demonstrated that the first-generation techniques can provide relative good image quality for cardiac imaging, and some coronary imaging, by relying on signal averaging when patients cannot cooperate with breath-holding commands (DUERINCKX et al. 1996b). Hands-on cardiac MRI courses have been organized to teach these coronary MRA techniques. One such 2-day cardiac MRI seminar was recently offered in Leuven, Belgium on 3–4 October 1997. Several of the images shown here were acquired during this course, using participants of the course as volunteers. We hope that this chapter will further help to popularize these techniques. Initial clinical results with these techniques have been very promising, with the sensitivity for significant coronary lesion detection ranging from 56% to 100% (MANNING et al. 1993a; DUERINCKX and URMAN 1994a; PENNELL et al. 1994a,b; MOHIADDIN et al. 1996; NITATORI et al. 1995; POST et al. 1997; YOSHINO et al. 1997; DUERINCKX et al. 1997). Initial clinical results have also been very successful with regard to imaging of bypass grafts, coronary stents (DUERINCKX et al. 1995; DUERINCKX et al., to be published), and coronary artery variants, such as anomalous origin or proximal course of the coronary vessels (POST et al. 1995a; MCCONNELL et al. 1995; MANNING et al. 1995; DUERINCKX et al. 1995b) or aneurysms as in Kawasaki disease (DUERINCKX and TAKAHASHI 1996; DUERINCKX et al. 1997).

With the development of these 2D single breath-hold techniques there was also an interest in extending this to 3D imaging. 3D imaging offers the advantages of higher signal-to-noise ratio, shorter echo times, more isotropic pixel resolution, and the ability to examine the data set with a multiplanar reformatting technique. The initial attempts at using signal averaging (without breath-holding) for 3D coronary imaging did not produce very good results (PASCHAL et al. 1992, 1993; HOFMAN et al. 1995; LI et al. 1996). Another 3D coronary MRA technique, developed by SCHEIDEGGER et al., used a briefly coached breath-holding strategy that only required a 1-s breath-hold in every 4s (with the respiratory cycle typically lasting four heart beats) (SCHEIDEGGER et al. 1992, 1994; SCHEIDEGGER and BOESIGER 1994; DOYLE et al. 1993). The results were very good and have inspired others to continue in this direction. SCHEIDEGGER et al. were the first to use sophisticated 3D imaging display technology. This and other pioneering work on 3D coronary MR imaging formed the basis for the development of the second-generation techniques and has been reviewed in detail elsewhere (DUERINCKX 1996).

The second-generation techniques for coronary MRA require much less training to perform, can provide higher spatial resolution, and at least theoretically appear very promising. As mentioned above, these techniques are referred to as the "navigator" techniques. They allow higher-resolution 2D and low- or high-resolution 3D data acquisitions. These techniques were first described in 1993–94 (LIU et al. 1994; WANG et al. 1996), but because the initial proposed implementations have severe shortcomings, they are still undergoing constant improvements (DANIAS et al. 1997; MCCONNELL et al. 1997a). The initial implementations of these second-generation techniques, now available on some commercial MR scanners, use visual feedback (LIU et al. 1993, 1994; WANG et al. 1995a,b; LIU et al. 1993) or real-time or retrospective respiratory gating (BRITTAIN et al. 1994, 1995; SACHS et al. 1994, 1995) to compensate for respiratory motion. They rely upon a navigator pulse to determine motion of the diaphragm (breathing motion). Either by providing feedback to the patient (as to when to hold his/her breath) for repeated breath-holds, or by feeding information back to the MRI computer, respiratory motion and/or inconsistency in repeated breath-holding is eliminated. This allows more time to acquire image data (as one is not limited to a single breath-hold), and

thus allows for acquisition of 3D data sets (WANG et al. 1996; FU et al. 1995) or higher-resolution 2D data sets (MCCONNELL et al. 1997a; OSHINSKI et al. 1996a). The technique can also be used with a spiral data acquisition scheme (SACHS et al. 1994). The navigator pulse most often determines the motion of the diaphragm, but in some implementations it directly monitors the motion of portions of the left ventricular wall. For the repeated breath-holding versions, inconsistent breath-holding is no longer a problem, as the patient receives feedback as to when to stop breathing. For the non-breath-hold versions, the regularity of the breathing pattern during the long scan acquisition (sometimes up to 15 min) is important. It has been recommended that: the navigator echo (NE) window be placed around end-expiratory position; subjects should not sleep; and scan efficiency should be monitored and if necessary the NE window repositioned (TAYLOR et al. 1997). Because of these and similar recommendations many adaptations and improvements to this navigator scheme have been made to improve its efficacy, including adaptive windowing (to correct for upward creep of the diaphragm in the supine position after 15–20 min) and the use of three orthogonal navigator echoes (to minimize motion in all three directions) (DANIAS et al. 1997; MCCONNELL et al. 1997b; TAYLOR et al. 1997; TAYLOR et al., to be published, a). Once implemented, this technique requires less expertise and training because a 3D transaxial slab covering the top of the heart and aortic root can be acquired and images can be analyzed later. In this sense it is very similar to EB-CT acquisitions for coronary calcium determination.

There are potential problems with this second-generation coronary MRA technique, as it is now implemented on some of the commercial MRI scanners. First, each acquisition takes much longer than with first-generation techniques (up to 12–15 min in some cases, versus a single 10- to 15-s breath-hold) before the first images are generated. Second, it has been recognized that the initial implementation of the navigator techniques sometimes does not work in up to 50% of normal volunteers (for unknown reasons) (STEHLING 1996), can be very noisy and is very much a function of the regularity and type of breathing pattern.

Navigator pulse correction techniques have been used with the first-generation coronary MRA techniques to avoid slice misregistration between breath-holding (MCCONNELL et al. 1997a,b; OSHINSKI et al. 1996b). The navigator techniques have also been used to acquire small volume scan acquisitions (thin

3D slabs) oriented along the right coronary artery (OSHINSKI et al., to be published). The initial clinical results with a 3D navigator technique have shown sensitivities for coronary artery lesion detection from 65% to 87% (MÜLLER et al. 1997; KESSLER et al. 1997; ACHENBACH et al. 1997).

The third generation of coronary MRA techniques combines the user-friendliness of the second-generation techniques with the speed and reliability of the first-generation techniques. These techniques acquire the entire cardiac anatomy in a single breath-hold with isotropic resolution. A precursor of this concept was first described in 1995 by Piotr Wielopolski, using segmented echoplanar imaging (EPI) (WIELOPOLSKI et al. 1995). Wielopolski et al. have since complemented this with small volume scan acquisitions (thin 3D slabs) oriented along the coronaries or VCATS (volume coronary arteriography using targeted scans) (WIELOPOLSKI et al. 1997). Other groups have since developed similar pulse sequences (KESSLER et al., to be published, a). The small volume acquisitions use fat-suppressed 3D segmented TurboFLASH with EKG-gating and fast acquisition times to allow breath-holding. These are ECG-triggered fast implementations of the by now established dynamic contrast-enhanced MR angiographic techniques (see description in next paragraph). Hopefully more clinical research sites will get access to these new pulse sequences on their commercial scanners to start preclinical trials for this very promising approach.

Magnetic resonance contrast agents will most likely have a dramatic effect on coronary MRA techniques, just as dynamic contrast-enhanced MRA has totally changed the way thoracic and body MRA are performed today. Dynamic contrast-enhanced MRA was first described by Martin Prince in 1993; it started out with relatively long acquisition times (over a minute), but can now be used within very short breath-holding periods (PRINCE et al. 1993, 1995a,b, 1996a,b; PRINCE 1994; CLOFT et al. 1996; JOHNSON et al. 1997; MEANEY et al. 1997; FOO et al. 1997). Breath-hold periods of 7–23 s for carotid MRA and pulmonary MRA are routinely used at some centers. The same non-ECG-triggered technique can be applied for native coronary artery (Ho et al. in press) and coronary artery bypass graft (CABG) imaging (VAN ROSSUM et al. 1997; VRACHLIOTIS et al. 1996, 1997). In order to EKG-trigger these MRA pulse sequences for native coronary vessel imaging, one needs to use faster acquisition rates, k-space data segmentation, data interpolation, and other technical tricks. With such changes one has a 3D breath-

hold EKG-triggered MRA technique, as described under the "third-generation techniques" (see above).

The initial experience with extravascular MR contrast agents seemed to indicate that very high doses would be needed for first-generation techniques (Ho et al., to be published; DUERINCKX et al. 1993). With bolus arrival timing to catch the first pass of the gadolinium contrast agent, further image quality improvements have been obtained (improved signal-to-noise and contrast-to-noise ratios) for both second- and third-generation techniques (Ho et al., to be published; KESSLER et al., to be published, b). However, with the new experimental MR blood pool agents even greater image improvements are being achieved (LI et al., to be published; TAYLOR et al., to be published, b) Sequential breath-hold acquisitions as short as 5–10 s can be obtained, with relatively high resolution, to image thin 3D slabs. With several repeated short breath-holds this allows patient-friendly high-resolution coverage of large portions of the cardiac and coronary anatomy. It offers the benefit of 3D acquisitions (with the opportunity for subsequent post-processing and no misregistration) while taking advantage of the MR contrast agents. The combination of MR contrast agents with coronary MRA techniques will most likely allow coronary MRA to outperform any other noninvasive coronary imaging technique on all fronts, including spatial resolution and 3D volume coverage.

There is another way to divide the existing coronary MRA techniques based not on the generation of the technique or the complexity of the technique used, but rather on how it affects the technologist and patient set-up procedures. Based on these criteria, the techniques can be subdivided into three groups: 2D approaches using a single breath-hold (EDELMAN et al. 1991; MEYER et al. 1992; MANNING et al. 1993a,b; DUERINCKX et al. 1994a; PENNELL et al. 1993; HUNDLEY et al. 1995) or multiple breath-holds (WANG et al. 1995a; SACHS et al. 1995); 3D approaches which use averaging over multiple breath-holds (PASCHAL et al. 1992, 1993; LI et al. 1993, 1995; WANG et al. 1995c; HAACKE et al. 1995) or imaging within a breath-hold (WIELOPOLSKI et al. 1995); and projectional approaches using tagging and subtraction within a breath-hold (WANG et al. 1991; EDELMAN et al. 1994). Direct respiratory feedback (DOYLE et al. 1993; WANG et al. 1995a,b; SACHS et al. 1995) or navigator pulses with real-time (SACHS et al. 1994, 1995) or retrospective (LI et al. 1995) feedback allow performance of 2D (WANG et al. 1995a; SACHS et al. 1994) and 3D (DOYLE et al. 1993; WANG et al. 1995b; LI et al. 1995) coronary MRA without breath-holding, thus also providing the potential for higher spatial resolution and improved patient comfort. As patient set-up and scanning protocols are very different for breath-hold and non-breath-hold coronary MRA, grouping of MRA techniques should be based upon whether or not "breath-holding" is required.

12.3
Principles Underlying Coronary MRA Pulse Sequence Design

A detailed review of this topic has been provided elsewhere by Duerinckx (DUERINCKX 1995a, 1996) and others (MANNING and EDELMAN 1993; PEARLMAN and EDELMAN 1994). We will only very briefly review how the anatomy and physiology of coronary arteries is dealt with when designing coronary MRA pulse sequences.

12.3.1
Temporal Resolution

Image sharpness of coronary MRA is greatly influenced by cardiac motion and temporal resolution. Coronary MRA requires the avoidance of motion (cardiac and respiratory motion) and compensation for pulsatile blood flow, both of which degrade the image quality by causing ghosting and image blurring.

12.3.1.1
Cardiac Motion

ECG-triggering synchronizes data acquisition to the cardiac cycle, and allows better depiction of the heart and surrounding structures. The heart shows a highly variable motion pattern, most pronounced during systole and early diastole, but nearly absent during mid and late diastole. Because coronary flow decreases from early to late diastole, mid to late diastole appears optimally suited for coronary MRA.

12.3.1.2
Respiratory Motion

Breath-holding and/or respiratory compensation/feedback schemes are used to eliminate this type of motion.

12.3.2
Spatial Resolution

Temporal resolution is a key factor which indirectly determines the size of the acquisition matrix. For a given field of view (FOV), this then determines the spatial resolution. The spatial resolution and signal to noise in coronary MRA can be further improved either by switching to non-breath-hold techniques (thus eliminating some of the time constraints needed for breath-hold techniques) or by using better coil designs and faster gradients.

12.3.3
Flow-to-Background Noise Contrast Ratio

Coronary arteries are usually embedded in fat, which has high signal intensity on T1-weighted images. Suppression of the high signal from fat offers improved coronary vessel detection with MRA. This technique is called "fat saturation" and is essential in coronary MRA to suppress the signal from the peri- and epicardial fat.

12.3.4
Timing of Data Acquisition Within Each Heart Cycle

Because of the complex pattern of cardiac motion and the biphasic flow patterns in the coronary vessels, it would appear that mid to late diastole offers the best compromise when imaging coronary vessels (DUERINCKX 1995b; and MANNING and EDELMAN 1995).

12.4
Practical Aspects of Coronary MRA

Patient set-up, instruction, and image plane selection are quite different for single breath-holding, repeated breath-hold (with feedback), and non-breath-holding sequences. The non-breath-hold sequences are much simpler, as they require virtually no patient instructions besides a recommendation to breathe regularly and to keep still during the scan. Most of what follows specifically applies to single breath-hold techniques only.

12.4.1
Single Breath-Hold Instructions

Patient setup and scanning protocols for 2D breath-hold sequences have been discussed at length in a previous publication (DUERINCKX 1995a) and will only be summarized here. For the breath-hold techniques the patient should be instructed on how to hold his/her breath during a nonforced, normal end-expiration for the duration of each scan and these maneuvers should be practiced for several minutes prior to the start of the scan. It is important to work on this with the patient prior to starting the MR scan to obtain breath-holding that is as consistent as possible. Because patient cooperation is so essential it is virtually impossible to apply these techniques to children under 14 years old, because although healthy young children can easily hold their breath for 14 s they often fail to do so in a consistent way.

The question often arises as to whether or not it is best to acquire image data during end-expiration or end-inspiration. Traditionally in the cardiac imaging community many (if not most) people use end-expiration based on personal evidence that the quality of the breath-holds is better than during end-inspiration. Others, mostly in the abdominal imaging community, where breath-hold MRI has also become important, argue that it may be easier and more comfortable for sick patients to hold their breath at end-inspiration. With the development of the second-generation coronary MRA techniques, and the need for adaptive repositioning of the navigator echo window, several investigators have started to quantitate diaphragm motion during normal breathing in a supine position, during sleep periods, and even during breath-holding. HOLLAND et al. recently reported that breath-holding does not eliminate motion of the diaphragm. Based on a study of ten healthy normal volunteers (five men, five women, mean age: 31.9 years) they calculated that the average total diaphragm displacement during a 20-s breath-hold at end-inspiration was 11 mm. At end-expiration the average total diaphragm displacement was only 3 mm, with an average diaphragm velocity of 0.15 mm/s (range: 0.01–0.3 mm/s). During both end-inspiration and end-expiration there was a gradual upward creep of the diaphragm during the short 20-s period of breath-holding. It was a linear and gradual motion at end-expiration for all volunteers. But at end-inspiration it was more irregular, with time-varying velocities in some of the volunteers.

The implications for coronary artery imaging are very important. Even though these findings need to be validated in patients, they confirm what most cardiac imagers already knew from comparing end-expiration and end-inspiration. End-expiratory breath-holding is definitively better, and most patients, even very ill ones, can tolerate it just as well as end-inspiratory breath-holding.

12.4.2
Dealing with Breath-hold Difficulties

The quality of breath-holding may be confirmed by the use of posteriorly placed ECG leads (when patients are in the prone position) with loss of respiratory variation in the ECG baseline. If the patient occasionally cannot hold his/her breath, one just repeats the image acquisitions as needed. However, if this problem persists, one has to be prepared to adapt the breath-hold coronary MRA examination to each individual patient and his/her ability to cooperate. If the patient has trouble holding his/her breath for the required duration (12–16 s), one can lower the matrix size (e.g., to 126 × 254) or increase the number of views per k-space segment (e.g., increase from 9 to 11 views or phase step acquisitions per heart beat).

For sedated patients with regular breathing patterns, one can average several data sets obtained with the 2D techniques without breath-holding and sometimes still obtain diagnostic quality images, such as for aneurysm or pseudoaneurysm imaging (DUERINCKX et al. 1996b). Even in pediatric patients, in whom compliance with breath-holding is not the best, these techniques appear to produce acceptable images of larger vessels such as the aorta (HERNANDEZ et al. 1993).

12.4.3
Dealing with Poor Cardiac Triggering

The set-up for cardiac triggering was recently reviewed by Boxt in a comprehensive review article (BOXT 1996). We refer to this very good article, and will only discuss a few extra points.

In very heavy patients and patients with severe arrhythmias, it may be difficult to obtain adequate data acquisition for the following reasons. In very heavy patients whose body almost totally fills the internal diameter of the magnet, it is often difficult to obtain a relatively noise-free ECG trigger signal. In patients with arrhythmia, it is difficult to get 16 consecutive heartbeats without intervening arrhythmia.

For these reasons it is sometimes impossible to obtain good cardiac triggering in these patients.

Fortunately sometimes there are solutions for these difficult cases. The MRI system can pseudo-trigger and provide adequate image quality, although this only rarely happens. For large patients with very noisy cardiac triggering when in a prone position (lying on a surface coil), reverting to a supine position and using the body coil will reduce the noise of the cardiac trigger signal enough to make scanning possible. This will reduce the spatial resolution, but the significantly improved image quality compensates for this.

One also has to adjust the (TD) depending on the patient's heart rate. For example, if the RR interval is 1000 ms (a slow heart rate) a TD ≈ 600–700 ms would be optimal. If the heart rate is much faster, the TD should be lowered appropriately, e.g., to TD ≈ 350 ms or less. For the single breath-hold coronary MR angiograms performed at our institution the temporal resolution of 117 ms can become inadequate for patients with fast heart rates and RR intervals of less than 500 ms. Unfortunately, for most patients reducing the segmental acquisitions to six or eight views (or phase encodings) per k-space segment would increase the duration of the image acquisition too much. Even though patients may initially be able to tolerate this for a few breath-holds, they will soon tire, and not enough time will be available to complete a high-quality coronary MRA study. This compromise between somewhat suboptimal time resolution and realistic breath-holding durations needs to be made for each individual patient by the radiologist performing the procedure.

12.4.4
Typical Image Acquisition Sequences

The image acquisition sequence for 2D techniques is typically as follows. Beginning at the level of the aortic sinus, transaxial images are obtained along the aortic root over a vertical distance from 2 to 3 cm with an overlap of 2–3 mm. Subsequently, single and double oblique images are obtained in planes positioned in the right atrioventricular and interventricular grooves to visualize the right coronary artery (RCA) and the left anterior descending (LAD) coronary artery. No systematic attempt is made to visualize the circumflex coronary artery, as it is located too posteriorly in the chest wall to be well visualized with a surface coil. Total imaging time ranges from 45 min to 1 h 30 min per patient.

For the 3D techniques the approach is different as a 3D slab covering the proximal portions of the coronary arteries is acquired in one sitting. Subsequent data processing (multiplanar reconstruction, segmentation, etc.) can then be used to visualize the vessels. Total imaging times range from one breath-hold for 3D segmented EPI to 12–15 min for 3D techniques with retrospective respiratory gating.

12.4.5
Surface Coils

There is still no final word on which surface coils are best to use. The circular polarized body array coils, which are available on most MRI scanners, allow more homogeneous coverage of the heart and coronary vessels. They also increase patient comfort, as the patient can be in a supine position. The early work on coronary MRA using the first-generation techniques was almost all performed with the patient in a supine position on a spine surface coil, with the heart positioned close to the coil (MANNING et al. 1993a,b; MANNING and EDELMAN 1993, 1995; DUERINCKX and URMAN 1994a; PENNELL et al. 1993; DUERINCKX 1995b). It is important to realize that occasionally this still may be the best approach, as the fat suppression algorithms do not always provide homogeneous fat suppression with the body array coils. Fat suppression is essential for good coronary artery contrast, and whenever inhomogeneous fat suppression becomes a problem it is often more efficient to reposition the patient in a prone position and continue the study with a different surface coil (such as a spine phased-array coil).

12.5
Optimal Selection of Imaging Planes

For 3D transaxial plane acquisitions with navigator echo techniques, optimal selection of imaging planes is not an issue, and one should follow the same guidelines as given for coronary calcium screening protocols using EB-CT. But for 2D breath-hold acquisitions or the newer targeted thin-slab 3D breath-hold techniques it is an important issue. One has to find the main axis of the heart. This is well known to cardiologists and people performing echocardiography, but it does not always seem so easy to radiologists starting out in this field.

For 2D breath-hold coronary MRA, several approaches have been described to select the best imaging planes to visualize the coronary arteries (DUERINCKX and URMAN 1994b; SAKUMA et al. 1993; POST et al. 1995b; GATES et al. 1994). There are basically two approaches: the iterative approach and the direct anatomic approach. We will briefly describe both.

The iterative approach works as follows. One can first localize the aortic root and then acquire sequential transaxial images throughout the lowest portion of the aortic root. This usually allows visualization of the left main coronary artery, the proximal left anterior descending and circumflex coronary arteries, and – on the lowest cuts – the origin of the RCA. Using this approach, one can then interactively try to find the right atrioventricular groove, and continue imaging the RCA. A similar approach with multiangle double-obliqued imaging planes can be used to image the more distal LAD (SAKUMA et al. 1994).

DUERINCKX et al. (1994a) have suggested an anatomic approach. Their approach is based on a priori knowledge of the cardiac anatomy and course of the coronary vessels. Imaging planes are selected comparable to those obtained with conventional x-ray coronary angiography and echocardiography. Imaging plane selection for cardiac MRI can be relatively easy and fast for some of the coronary vessels, and has been previously described (AXEL 1992; BURBANK et al. 1988). A quick start for RCA imaging is to use a transverse image at the level of the left ventricle (short-axis view) to prescribe a sagittal oblique slice through the middle of the left ventricle (long-axis view). From this, one can then easily acquire images along the atrioventricular groove. Us-

ing this anatomic approach, imaging of the RCA can be easily and reliably performed (Fig. 12.1). SAKUMA et al. reported a similar anatomic approach to LAD imaging where they used multiangle epicardial tangential views for better visualization of the distal LAD (SAKUMA et al. 1994). Furthermore the use of cine-display can improve recognition of the continuity of the coronary artery tree (SAKUMA et al. 1993).

New interactive MR image plane selection techniques are being developed to facilitate the selection of optimal section orientations (HANGIANDREOU et al. 1995). When they become commercially available they may have a dramatic effect on the total duration of coronary MRA and cardiac MR examinations.

12.6
Typical Coronary MR Angiograms

Typical 2D coronary MR angiograms are shown in Figs. 12.2, 12.3, and 12.4. In most volunteers and a significant number of patients who can cooperate with breath-holding commands, large portions of the proximal coronary arterial tree can be imaged.

Coronary MRA studies done mostly in normal volunteers (PASCHAL et al. 1993; HOFMAN et al. 1995; MANNING et al. 1993b; PENNELL et al. 1993; SAKUMA et al. 1994; DUERINCKX et al. 1994b) and several studies done in patients only (DUERINCKX and URMAN 1994a; POST et al. 1995c) have measured the length of the coronary arteries typically visualized with the coronary MRA technique. These findings are summarized in Table 12.1. For comparison

Table 12.1. Comparison of the length of coronary arteries visualized by coronary MRA (data from 1992–1995) (from DUERINCKX 1996)

	No.	RCA	LM	LAD	LCx
2D: MANNING et al. (1993b)	25	58 (24–122)	10 (8–14)	44 (28–93)	25 (9–42)
2D: PENNELL et al. (1993)	26	53.7 ± 27.9	10.4 ± 5.2	46.7 ± 22.8	26.3 ± 17.5
2D: DUERINCKX and URMAN (1994a)	21	65 ± 23	12 ± 3	53 ± 19	19 ± 12
2D: SAKUMA et al. (1994)	18	65 ± 23	n/a	62 ± 10	23 ± 11
2D: DUERINCKX et al. (1994b)	15	78.4	13.9	54.9	14.7
2D: HOFMAN et al. (1995)[a]	10	55 ± 11	8 ± 2	42 ± 14	16 ± 12
3D: LI et al. (1993)	?	3–7[b]	n/a	5–50[b]	5–50[b]
3D: PASCHAL et al. (1993)[a]	7	34 (12–50)	5 (4–14)	24 (5–47)	24 (8–64)
3D: HOFMAN et al. (1995)[a]	10	37 ± 14	7 ± 3	37 ± 9	11 ± 12
3D gated: HOFMAN et al. (1995)[a]	10	46 ± 10	8 ± 4	37 ± 11	17 ± 14
2D: POST et al. (1997)	35	89 ± 32	9 ± 4	62 ± 16	21 ± 9
TEE: SAMDARSHI et al. (1992)	111	7 ± 2	9.3 ± 1	8.2 ± 8	6.7 ± 9

Results are expressed in millimeters, and depending on the study, as: mean ± standard deviation or mean (range: min–max). No., Number of subjects; RCA, right coronary artery; LM, left main stem artery; LAD, left anterior descending artery; LCx, left circumflex artery; n/a, not available.
[a] Not all vessels could be visualized in each subject.
[b] Range reflects the most frequently measured lengths, not the full range.

we have included data from a transesophageal (TEE) study of proximal coronary artery lesions (SAMDARSHI et al. 1992). The difference in measured lengths between the different studies may be explained by a different approach to the selection of imaging planes.

Flow in the diagonal branches of the LAD was visible in 80% of the subjects in a study by MANNING et al. (1993b). In a study of 15 patients by DUERINCKX et al. (1994b), however, the branch vessels were seldom visualized except for the acute marginal and diagonal branches. Moreover, the proximal circumflex artery was poorly visualized, due to the use of a surface coil and prone positioning.

The frequency of significant lesions in the left circumflex artery (LCx) is relatively low. Because of this 2D coronary MRA, even with its limitation of poor visualization of the LCx, may still be a valuable noninvasive screening tool for coronary artery disease.

12.7
Artifacts and Limitations of First-Generation Techniques

The most important limitation of today's coronary MRA is the great variation in the appearance of significant (>50%) coronary lesions and the large

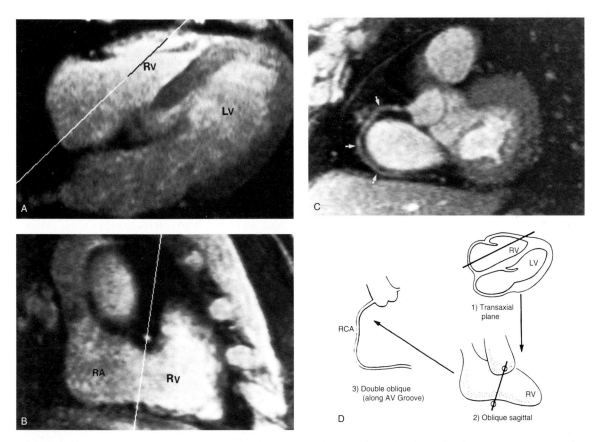

Fig. 12.1 a–d. Optimal image plane selection sequence to image the RCA. **A** Transaxial view through the left ventricle. This image is used to determine the orientation of the long axis of the heart projected onto a transaxial plane. It is then used to select the orientation of the next imaging plane (as indicated by the line). **B** Oblique coronal plane through the right ventricle which transects the RCA in two points (*arrows*). This image is used to select a plane located in the anterior atrioventricular groove which contains the RCA (indicated by *line*). It also gives an idea as to the orientation of the cardiac long axis in an oblique coronal plane. *RA*, right atrium; *RV*, right ventricle. **C** Plane located in the anterior atrioventricular groove shows a large segment of the RCA (*arrows*). This plane corresponds to a conventional angiogram, left anterior oblique view with caudal angulation. **D** Schematic drawing of the method used for optimal selection of imaging planes for coronary MRA depiction of RCA. *RV*, right ventricle; *LV*, left ventricle. [**b, c** from DUERINCKX (1995) MR angiography of the coronary arteries. Topics MRI 7:267–285, with permission; **a, d** from DUERINCKX (1996) Coronary MR angiography, MRI Clin North Am 4:361–418, with permission]

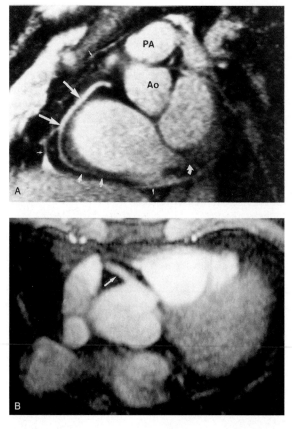

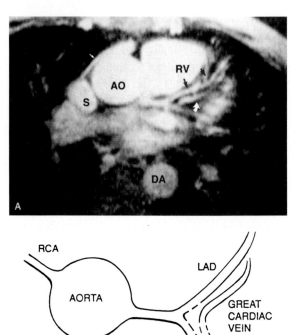

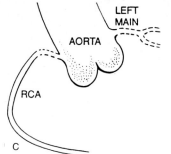

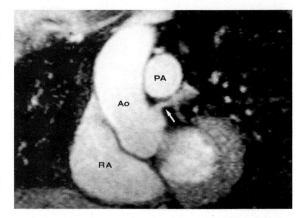

Fig. 12.3 a,b. Left coronary artery system. The left coronary artery system is relatively complex and requires multiple imaging planes to visualize its proximal course. **A** Oblique transaxial plane showing the proximal and middle LAD (*black arrows*) and the great cardiac vein (*curved arrow*). Also shown are the pericardial sac (*thin arrow*), ascending aorta (*Ao*), right ventricle (*RV*), left ventricle (*LV*), left atrium (*LA*), descending aorta (*DA*), and superior vena cava (*s*). **B** Schematic drawing of a typical appearance of the left main, LAD, and proximal circumflex arteries and great cardiac vein on oblique transaxial planes. The origin of the LAD and circumflex artery are shown in *dashed (thin) lines* to emphasize the point that often these origins are better seen in another plane. [From Duerinckx (1995) MR angiography of the coronary arteries. Topics MRI 7:267–285, with permission]

Fig. 12.2 a–c. The right coronary artery. The RCA lies in the anterior atrioventricular groove. A large portion of the RCA (*arrows*) can usually be visualized with a single imaging plane through the anterior atrioventricular groove (**a**) Often one additional transaxial plane is needed to clearly show the ostium of the RCA (**b**). A schematic drawing of the typical appearance of the RCA on coronary MR angiograms is shown (**c**). **A** The proximal and middle RCA shown (*long white arrows*); the distal RCA (*short white arrows*) is slightly out-of-plane and better seen on an image obtained in a parallel imaging plane. The origin of the RCA is out-of-plane. Also shown are: the pericardial sac (*thin arrows*); the ascending aorta (*Ao*), the main pulmonary artery (*PA*) and the coronary sinus (*curved arrow*). **B** Origin of the RCA is best seen on an oblique transaxial plane. **C** Schematic drawing of a typical appearance of the proximal and mid-RCA on coronary angiograms. The origin is shown in *dashed (thin) lines* to emphasize the point that often the origin is better seen in an additional plane. [**a, c** from Duerinckx (1995) MR angiography of the coronary arteries. Topics MRI 7:267–285, with permission; **b, d** from Duerinckx (1996) Coronary MR angiography. MRI Clin North Am 4:361–418, with permission]

Fig. 12.4. Left main coronary artery (*arrow*). The optimal plane for imaging of the left main coronary artery is often an oblique coronal plane, as shown here. This corresponds to a left anterior oblique orientation in conventional coronary angiography. *Ao*, Ascending aorta; *PA*, pulmonary artery; *RA*, right atrium. [From Duerinckx (1996) Coronary MR angiography. MRI Clin North Am 4:361–418, with permission]

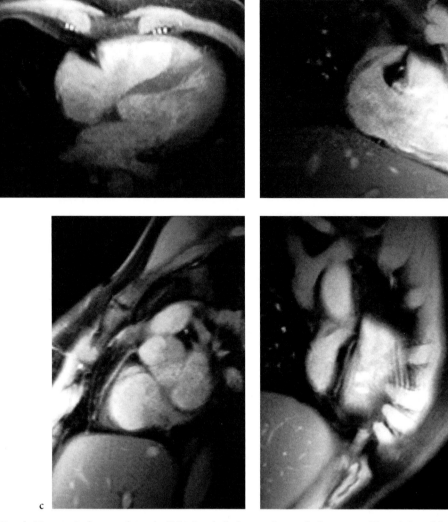

Fig. 12.5 a–d. Most typical case, where the RCA is relatively straight in its middle course. **a** The initial transaxial image visualizes a cross-section of the RCA. **b** Oblique coronal plane through the right ventricle intersects the RCA in two points. The cross-section of the proximal right coronary artery in this particular case has the shape of a comma. This comma shape most likely presents a cross-section of the RCA and either partial voluming of the more distal portion of the RCA and/or the beginning of a side branch. **c** Plane located in the anterior atrioventricular groove. The origins of the RCA and proximal RCA are clearly shown. **d** One additional imaging plane was obtained perpendicular to the atrioventricular groove plane. The mid RCA is also shown, providing an orthogonal view of the vessel (when compared to image **c**). [From DUERINCKX A., Two-dimensional coronary MR angiography: How do I do it? In: Coronary MR Angiography, Duerinckx A J, Ed., Springer-Verlag, New York, 1999 (In Press)]

number of image artifacts which can be misinterpreted as representing lesions. It can be very tempting to interpret an artifactual change in the signal intensity of flow in a vessel as representing a lesion, especially if the artifact just happens to be located in the vicinity of the real lesion. Such erroneous over-interpretation of artifacts as lesions will increase the sensitivity for lesion detection, as will be explained and illustrated in the next section. Unfortunately if done consistently, it would also significantly reduce the specificity of the technique, thus ultimately reducing its clinical impact. Issues relating to "lesion" appearance on MR will be discussed in the next section. The discussion here will be limited to general artifacts and limitations as seen in healthy normal volunteers without coronary lesions.

12.8
The Anatomic Approach to Imaging of the Right Coronary Artery

As most clinical users only have access to the first-generation coronary MRA techniques, I shall spend

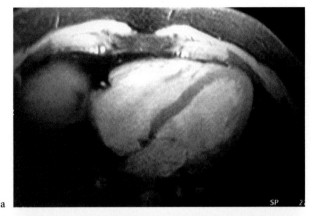

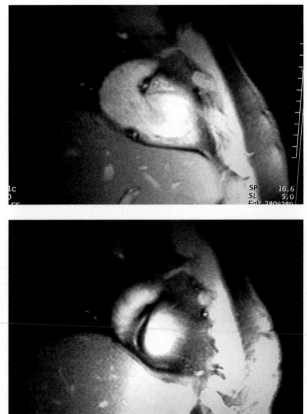

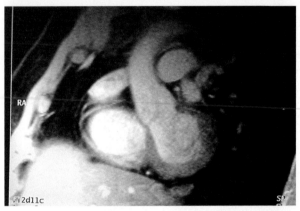

Fig. 12.6 a–d. Mild out-of-plane tortuosity of the RCA. **a** Transaxial image shows dot-like cross-section of the RCA. **b** Oblique coronal plane through the right ventricle intersects the RCA in two dot-like points. **c** Plane located in the right atrioventricular (*V*) groove only shows portions of the RCA. A small fragment of the mid RCA is not seen. **d** plane providing 90° view (perpendicular to image plane shown in **c**). The mid RCA courses posteriorly over a short segment. This explains the interrupted appearance of the RCA as seen on the AV groove plane; it was due to mild tortuosity of the RCA. [From DUERINCKX A., Two-dimensional coronary MR angiography: How do I do it? In: Coronary MR Angiography, Duerinckx A J, Ed., Springer-Verlag, New York, 1999 (In Press)]

some more time discussing practical aspects of the use of these techniques, specifically as they relate to RCA imaging.

The anatomic approach to imaging of the RCA was already shown in Fig. 12.1 and can be very easily applied. The learning curve for this technique is relatively reasonable. The key requirement to performing this type of study is the ability to be able to determine quickly the direction of the long axis of the right ventricle and/or left ventricle. One starts off with the transaxial image for the left ventricle followed by an oblique sagittal image to get the second component of the axis of the heart. Using that information a short-axis view can be obtained which is positioned at the level of the anterior atrioventricular groove, and, therefore, visualizes the right coronary artery. This is the equivalent of a caudal LAO view in conventional x-ray coronary angiography.

Because of the necessity to recognize the cardiac axis and be able to determine the orientation of the heart, specialized training of and/or practice by the MR technologist or the presence of a physician familiar with cardiac anatomy is required. This is unlike the three-dimensional coronary MRA techniques using navigator pulses, where minimal training is required.

I shall now illustrate in detail variations encountered when imaging the proximal and middle RCA with a single breath-hold 2-s technique. The images shown are from real volunteers scanned during the 2-day cardiac MRI seminar held in Leuven, Belgium on 3–4 October 1997. MRI studies were performed on volunteers within a small class group of five to ten radiologists. Each of these acquisitions was performed in 4–7 min.

Figure 12.5 shows a straightforward case where the RCA is relatively straight in its middle course.

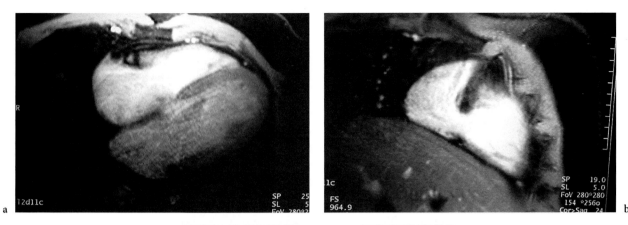

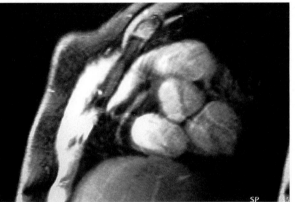

Fig. 12.7 a–c. Image degradation due to suboptimal breath-holding. **a** Transaxial image shows dot-like cross-section of the RCA. **b** Oblique coronal plane through the right ventricle should normally intersect the RCA in two dot-like points; this is not the case here. In this particular case the atrioventricular groove is clearly seen as an area of low signal intensity. The coronary MRA sequences rely on fat suppression. The low-signal area seen is the pericardial fat and subpericardial fat surrounding the RCA. The cross-sections of the RCA on this oblique coronal image are not clearly seen, but the orientation of the atrioventricular groove can be easily determined. By selecting the imaging plane through this right atrioventricular groove (as done in Figs. 12.1, 12.5, and 12.6) one still obtains the usual image of the RCA. **c** Plane located in the right atrioventricular (*V*) groove shows the RCA. The RCA image is somewhat blurred again due to lack of complete breath-holding or other slight motion artifact. [From Duerinckx A., Two-dimensional coronary MR angiography: How do I do it? In: Coronary MR Angiography, Duerinckx A J, Ed., Springer-Verlag, New York, 1999 (In Press)]

Figure 12.6 illustrates what happens when there is mild out-of-plane tortuosity of the RCA. During mid and late diastole, due to dilatation of the heart, the RCA is stretched out and almost completely lies within a single plane (the anterior or right atrioventricular groove), as illustrated in Fig. 12.1 and 12.5. Figure 12.7 illustrates a moderate amount of image degradation due to very slight motion artifacts. Even when there is perfect breath-holding, there could be up to 3 mm of upward creep of the diaphragm during a 20-s breath-hold (see earlier discussion). Figure 12.8 illustrates what happens when there is severe out-of-plane tortuosity of the RCA. This case clearly illustrates how, for a very tortuous RCA, additional image acquisitions need to be obtained in order to follow that vessel with the two-dimensional coronary MRA techniques. If not done correctly, one could easily misinterpret these gaps and areas of low signal as representing coronary lesions. Figure 12.9 illustrates what happens when there is mild in-plane tortuosity of the RCA. Figure 12.10 illustrates what happens when there is a combination of mild in-plane and mild out-of-plane tortuosity of the RCA.

These techniques can also be used to image the left coronary artery system. However, imaging of the left coronary artery system requires a much more sophisticated level of interactivity. Many different schemes have been developed. Basically the idea is to start with a semitransaxial plane through the aortic root to localize the left main coronary artery and then follow the LAD. Different approaches to

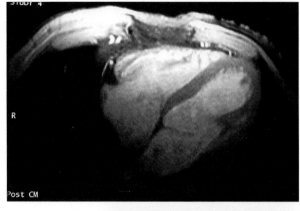

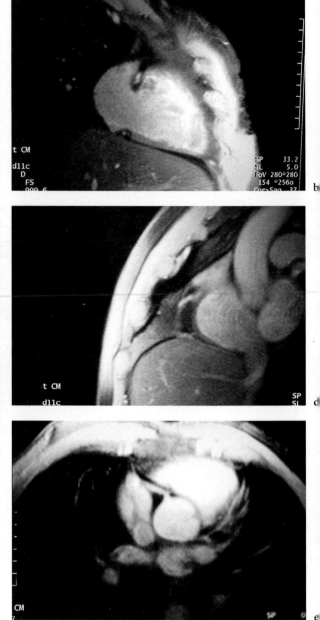

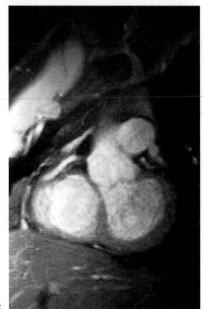

Fig. 12.8 a–e. Severe out-of-plane tortuosity of the RCA. **a** Transaxial image shows dot-like cross-section of the RCA. Portions of the mitral valve are shown. **b** Oblique coronal plane through the right ventricle intersects the RCA in two dot-like points **c** Plane located in the right atrioventricular (*V*) groove only shows portions of the RCA. A small fragment of the mid RCA is not seen. Only a small portion of the proximal RCA is shown. **d** Plane parallel to the right artrioventricular (*V*) groove plane in **c**, but displaced posteriorly. The missing portion of the RCA is now shown. **e** Oblique transaxial image through the aortic root, which shows the origin of the RCA. [From Duerinckx A., Two-dimensional coronary MR angiography: How do I do it? In: Coronary MR Angiography, Duerinckx A J, Ed., Springer-Verlag, New York, 1999 (In Press)]

this can be used. One consists in tracking down the LAD along the interventricular groove and obtaining planes transaxial to the cardiac surface which contain both the LAD and the great cardiac vein.

12.9
The Need for Post-processing

Representation of three-dimensional vascular structures is a complex task, often requiring significant

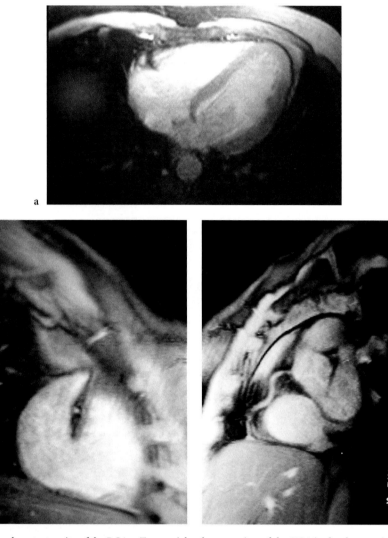

Fig 12.9 a–c. Mild in-plane tortuosity of the RCA. **a** Transaxial image shows dot-like cross-section of the RCA. **b** Oblique coronal plane through the right ventricle intersects the RCA in two points. The proximal cross-section of the RCA is clearly shown, but the distal one is only faintly seen. However, the right atrioventricular groove is clearly visible and allows selection of the plane through this groove. **c** Plane located in the right atrioventricular (*V*) groove shows a tortuous RCA. A long portion of the RCA is clearly seen; it is very tortuous but almost totally lies within a single plane with no anterior or posterior displacement. In this particular description, anterior and posterior refer to displacement towards the base or apex of the heart. [From DUERINCKX A., Two-dimensional coronary MR angiography: How do I do it? In: Coronary MR Angiography, Duerinckx A J, Ed., Springer-Verlag, New York, 1999 (In Press)]

post-processing not routinely available at clinical sites. The best known techniques are: maximum intensity projection (MIP) as used with traditional MRA acquisitions; surface rendering after segmentation, which has become very popular with helical CT angiography; and multiplanar reconstruction from 3D data sets. We will not discuss these options in detail given their limited availability at the present time.

Three-dimensional rendering of coronary arteries is one type of post-processing which requires seg-

mentation of the data (DOYLE et al. 1993; BÖRNERT and JENSEN 1995). To execute this 3D rendering routine, "seeds" are placed in both the left and right coronary vessels, and thresholds are set to discriminate individual coronary vessels from adjacent structures (DOYLE et al. 1993). Segmentation of the left coronary system with its many branches is much more involved than the RCA segmentation.

EDELMAN et al. (1993) have also described a technique to render projection MR angiograms depicting a substantial length of human coronary arteries from

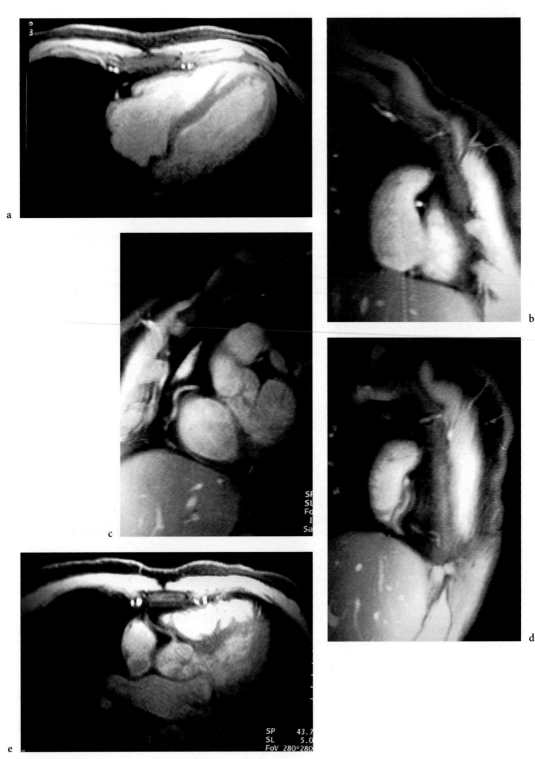

Fig. 12.10 a–e. Mild in-plane and out-of-plane tortuosity of the RCA. **a** Transaxial image shows dot-like cross-section of the RCA. **b** Oblique coronal plane through the right ventricle intersects the RCA in two points. **c** Plane located in the right atrioventricular (*V*) groove shows a tortuous RCA (in-plane) with missing segments more distally (due to out-of-plane tortuosity). There is also no signal seen in the proximal RCA ostium. **d** An image plane perpendicular to **c**. The mid to distal RCA is clearly seen, as is a right ventricular branch. **e** An oblique transaxial plane clearly shows the ostium (see also Fig. 12.1). [From DUERINCKX A., Two-dimensional coronary MR angiography: How do I do it? In: Coronary MR Angiography, Duerinckx A J, Ed., Springer-Verlag, New York, 1999 (In Press)]

sequential 2D breath-hold images. They applied the technique to five normal volunteers and ten patients.

Most recently other aspects of post-processing were discussed by several authors in the April 1998 issue of the *American Journal of Roentgenology* (ROGERS 1998; DUERINCKX and LIPTON 1998; ACHENBACH et al. 1998; WOODARD et al. 1998; SHIMAMOTA et al. 1998).

12.10
The Future of Coronary MRA

Some of the questions we asked in 1996 relating to future technical developments in coronary MRA (DUERINCKX 1996) are still unanswered. In 1996 the questions were as follows: Will the best coronary MRA technique require a 2D, a 3D, or a projectional approach? Will an echoplanar approach (which allows almost real-time imaging) or spiral approach really make a difference? Will MR contrast agents be needed to better visualize certain lesions? Given that coronary MRA will probably never become as good as the existing "gold standard," are there specific clinical problems where it would be good enough to be able to replace or complement conventional coronary angiography?

Over the last 2 years many of these questions are beginning to be answered. The first-generation techniques have now reached a level of stability and commercial implementation such that most MR users can use them. The distinction between 2D and 3D techniques may no longer be so great, as both approaches can now benefit from second- and third-generation technical improvements (navigator echoes and breath-hold acquisitions of thin 3D slabs). MR contrast agents do indeed appear to have a major future role, and with their use the need for EB-CT of coronary artery anatomy (not coronary calcium screening) may disappear. The new targeted breath-hold thin-slab techniques recently developed show great promise. Changes in technique have been and continue to occur so rapidly that there has been no time or interest for in-depth large-scale clinical testing of any of the coronary MRA techniques.

Both the second- and third-generation improvements to coronary MRA techniques are continuously evolving. This and the use of contrast agents will make coronary MRA an important component of a comprehensive MR-based noninvasive evaluation of patients with ischemic heart disease. Coronary flow reserve assessment by MRI, which was not discussed here, can be added to the evaluation of such patients. Such combined noninvasive MR study of anatomy and flow may become the ultimate cost-effective coronary screening tool. Despite their current limitations, first- and second-generation MRA techniques can help in many clinical applications, such as in the identification of congenital coronary anatomy variants and in the noninvasive follow-up of patients who have undergone coronary angioplasty, coronary stent placement, or bypass grafting.

References

Achenbach S, Kessler W, Moshage WE, et al. (1997) Visualization of the coronary arteries in three-dimensional reconstructions using respiratory gated magnetic resonance imaging. Coronary Artery Dis 8:441–448

Achenbach S, Moshage W, Ropers D, Bachmann K (1998) Curved multiplanar reconstructions for the evaluation of contrast-enhanced electron beam CT of the coronary arteries. AJR 170:895–899

Atkinson D, Edelman R (1991) Cineangiography of the heart in a single breathhold with a segmented TurboFLASH sequence. Radiology 178:359–362

Axel L (1992) Efficient methods for selecting cardiac magnetic resonance image locations. Invest Radiol 27:91–93

Börnert P, Jensen D (1995) Coronary artery imaging at 0.5 T using segmented 3D echo planar imaging. Magn Reson Med 34:779–785

Boxt LM (1996) How to perform Cardiac MR Imaging. In: Boxt LM (guest ed) Cardiac MR imaging. MRI Clinics of North America. Saunders, Philadelphia, 4 (2):191–216

Brittain JH, Hu BS, Wright GA, Meyer CH, Macovski A, Nishimura DG (1994) Multislice coronary angiography with muscle and venous suppression (#367) (abstract). In: Printed program of the second meeting of the Society of Magnetic Resonance (SMR). San Francisco, California, 7–12 August 7–12 1994

Brittain JH, Hu BS, Wright GA, Meyer CH, Macovski A, Nishimura DG (1995) Coronary angiography with magnetization-prepared T2 contrast. Mag Reson Med 33:689–696

Burbank F, Parish D, Wexler L (1988) Echocardiographic-like angled views of the heart by MR imaging. J Comput Assist Tomogr 12:181–195

Cho Z, Mun C, Friedenberg R (1991) NMR angiography of coronary vessels with 2-D planar image scanning. Magn Res Med 20:134–143

Cloft HJ, Murphy KJ, Prince MR, Brunberg JA (1996) 3D gadolinium-enhanced MR angiography of the carotid arteries. Magn Reson Imag 14:593–600

Danias PG, McConnell MV, Khasgiwala VC, Chuang ML, Edelman RR, Manning WJ (1997) Prospective navigator correction of image position for coronary. Radiology 203:733–736

Doyle M, Scheidegger MB, DeGraaf RG, Vermeulen J, Pohost GM (1993) Coronary artery imaging in multiple 1-sec breath holds. Magn Reson Imaging 11:3–6

Duerinckx AJ (1995a) Review: MR angiography of the coronary arteries. Topics Magn Reson Imaging 7:267–285

Duerinckx AJ (1995b) Coronary MR angiography (response to letter to the editor). Radiology 195:876

Duerinckx AJ (1996) Coronary MR angiography. In: Boxt Lm (guest ed) Cardiac MR imaging. MRI Clinics of North America. Saunders, Philadelphia, 4 (2):361–418

Duerinckx AJ (1997) MRI of coronary arteries. Int J Card Imaging 1997; 13:191–197

Duerinckx AJ, Lipton MJ (1998) Noninvasive coronary artery imaging using CT and MR imaging (an invited commentary). AJR 170:900–902

Duerinckx AJ, Takahashi M. (1996) Coronary MR angiography in Kawasaki disease (abstract). Radiology 201(P): 274

Duerinckx AJ, Urman M (1994a) Two-dimensional coronary MR angiography: analysis of initial clinical results. Radiology 193:731–738

Duerinckx AJ, Urman M (1994b) Optimal imaging planes for MR coronary angiography (abstract). In: Book of Abstracts of the 11th Annual Scientific Meeting of the European Society for Magnetic Resonance in Medicine and Biology. Vienna, Austria, 20–24 April 1994:83

Duerinckx AJ, Urman M, Sinha U, Atkinson D, Simonetti O (1993) Evaluation of gadolinium-enhanced MR coronary angiography (abstract). In: 79th Scientific Assembly and Annual Meeting of the Radiological Society of North America (RSNA). Chicago, 28 November-3 December 1993; Radiology 189(P):278

Duerinckx AJ, Urman MK, Atkinson DJ, Simonetti OP, Sinha U (1994a) Optimal imaging planes for coronary MR angiography (abstract). In: Printed Program of the First Meeting of the Society of Magnetic Resonance (SMR). Dallas, Texas. J Magn Reson Imaging P(4):123

Duerinckx AJ, Urman MK, Atkinson DJ, Simonetti OP, Sinha U, Lewis B (1994b) Limitations of MR coronary angiography (abstract). In: Printed Program of the First Meeting of the Society of Magnetic Resonance (SMR). Dallas, Texas, 5–9 March 1994; J Magn Reson Imaging 4:81

Duerinckx AJ, Atkinson D, Hurwitz R, Mintorovitch J, Whitney W (1995a) Coronary MR angiography after coronary stent placement (case report). AJR 165:662–664

Duerinckx AJ, Bogaert J, Jiang H, Lewis BS (1995b) Anomalous origin of the left coronary artery: diagnosis by coronary MR angiography (case report). AJR 164:1095–1097.

Duerinckx AJ, Atkinson DP, Mintorovitch J, Simonetti OP, Urman MK (1996a) Two-dimensional coronary MR angiography: limitations and artifacts. Eur Radiol 6:312–325

Duerinckx AJ, Lewis BS, Louie HW, Urman MK (1996b) MRI of pseudoaneurysm of a brachial venous coronary bypass graft. Cathet Cardiovasc Diagn 37:281–286

Duerinckx AJ, Troutman B, Allada V, Kim D (1997) Coronary MR angiography in Kawasaki disease. A case report. AJR 168:114–116

Duerinckx AJ, Atkinson D, Hurwitz R (to be published) Coronary stent imaging with coronary MR angiography. J Magn Reson Med

Dumoulin C, Souza S, Darrow R, Adams W (1991) A method of coronary MR angiography (technical note). J Comput Assist Tomogr 15:705–710

Edelman R, Manning W, Burstein D, Paulin S (1991) Coronary arteries: breath-hold MR angiography. Radiology 1991; 181:641–643

Edelman RR, Manning WJ, Pearlman J, Wei L (1993) Human coronary arteries: projection angiograms reconstructed from breath-hold two-dimensional MR images. Radiology 187:719–722

Edelman RR, Siewert B, Adamis M, Gaa J, Laub G, Wielopolski P (1994) Signal targeting with alternating radiofrequency (STAR) sequences: application to MR angiography. Magn Reson Med 31:233–238

Foo TK, Saranathan M, Prince MR, Chenevert TL (1997) Automated detection of bolus arrival and initiation of data acquisition in fast, three-dimensional, gadolinium-enhanced MR angiography. Radiology 203:275–280

Fu Z, Wang Y, Grimm RC, et al. (1995) Orbital navigator echoes for motion measurement in magnetic resonance imaging. Magn Reson Med 34:746–753

Gates ARC, Huang CL-H, Crowley JJ, et al. (1994) Magnetic resonance imaging planes for the 3-dimensional characterization of human coronary arteries. J Anat 185:335–346

Gomes A, Lois J, Drinkwater D, Corday S (1987) Coronary artery bypass grafts: visualization with MR imaging. Radiology 162:175–179

Haacke EM, Li D, Kaushikkar S (1995) Cardiac MR imaging: principles and techniques. Topics Magn Reson Imaging 7:200–217

Hangiandreou NJ, Debbins JP, Rossman PJ, Riederer SJ (1995) Interactive selection of optimal section orientations using real-time MRI. J Magn Reson Imaging 34:114–119

Hernandez RJ, Aisen AM, Foo TKF, Beekman RH (1993) Thoracic cardiovascular anomalies in children: evaluation with a fast gradient-recalled-echo sequence with cardiac-triggered segmented acquisition. Radiology 188:75–780

Holland A, Goldfarb JW, Barentsz JO, Edelman, RR. Diaphragm motion during suspended breathing: implications for MR imaging of the heart (abstr). In: Proceedings of the Sixth Scientific Meeting of the International Society for Magnetic Resonance in Medicine (ISMRM), April 18–24, 1998. Sydney, Australia

Ho VB, Foo TKF, Arai AE, Wolff SD (to be published) Gadolinium-enhanced two-dimensional coronary MR angiography using an automated contrast bolus detection algorithm (MR smartprep) (abstract). In: Proceedings of the Sixth Scientific Meeting of the International Society for Magnetic Resonance in Medicine (ISMRM), 18–24 April 1998. Sydney, Australia

Hofman MBM, Paschal CB, Li D, Haacke M, van Rossum AC, Sprenger M (1995) MRI of coronary arteries: 2D breath-hold vs 3D respiratory-gated acquisition. J Comput Assist Tomogr 19:56–62

Hundley WG, Clarke GD, Landau C, et al. (1995) Noninvasive determination of infarct artery patency by cine magnetic resonance angiography. Circulation 91:1347–1353

Johnson DB, Lerner CA, Prince MR, et al. (1997) Gadolinium-enhanced magnetic resonance angiography of renal transplants. Magn Reson Imaging 15:13–20

Kessler W, Achenbach S, Moshage W, et al. (1997) Usefulness of respiratory gated magnetic resonance coronary angiography in assessing narrowings >50% in diameter in native coronary arteries and in aortocoronary bypass conduits. Am J Cardiol 80:989–993

Kessler W, Achenbach S, Moshage W, Ropers D, Laub G (to be published, a) Coronary arteries: three-dimensional breath-hold MR angiography using a gadolinium-enhanced ultrafast gradient-echo technique (abstract). In:Proceedings of the Sixth Scientific Meeting of the International Society for Magnetic Resonance in Medicine (ISMRM), 18–24 April 1998 Sydney, Australia

Kessler W, Laub G, Ropers D, Achenbach S, Moshage W, Bachmann K (to be published, b) Contrast-enhanced 3D breath-hold MRA for the visualization of the coronary arteries in oblique projection angiograms (abstract). In: Proceedings of the Sixth Scientific Meeting of the International Society for Magnetic Resonance in Medicine (ISMRM), 18–24 April 1998 Sydney, Australia

Li D, Paschal CB, Haacke EM, Adler LP (1993) Coronary arteries: three-dimensional MR imaging with fat saturation and magnetization transfer contrast. Radiology 187:401–406

Li D, Kaushikkar S, Woodard P, Dhawale P, Haacke EM (1995) Three-dimensional MRI of coronary arteries (abstract). In: Book of Abstracts of VII International Workshop on Magnetic Resonance Angiography. Matsuyama, Japan

Li D, Kaushikkar S, Haacke EM, et al. (1996) Coronary arteries: three-dimensional MR imaging with retrospective respiratory gating (technical development and instrumentation). Radiology 201:857–863

Li D, Zheng J, Weinmann H-J, et al. (to be bpublished) Comparison of intravascular and extravascular contrast agents in coronary artery imaging (abstract). In: Proceedings of the Sixth Scientific Meeting of the International Society for Magnetic Resonance in Medicine (ISMRM), 18–24 April 1998. Sydney, Australia

Liu YL, Riederer SJ, Rossman PJ, Grimm RG, Debbins JF, Ehman RL (1993) A monitoring, feedback, and triggering system for reproducible breath-hold MR imaging. Magn Reson Med 30:507–511

Liu YL, Rossman PJ, Grimm RC, Debbins JP, Ehman RL, Riederer SJ (1994) Comparison of two breath-hold feedback techniques for reproducible breath holds in MRI (abstract). In: Printed Program of the First Meeting of the Society of Magnetic Resonance (SMR). Dallas, Texas, 5–9 March 1994; J Magn Reson Imaging 4(P):61

Manning W, Edelman R (1993) Magnetic resonance coronary angiography. Magn Reson Q 1993; 9:131–151

Manning WJ, Edelman RR (1995) Coronary MR angiography (letter to the editor). Radiology 195:875

Manning WJ, Li W, Edelman RR (1993a) A preliminary report comparing magnetic resonance coronary angiography with conventional angiography. N Engl J Med 328:828–832

Manning WJ, Li W, Boyle NG, Edelman RE (1993b) Fat-suppressed breath-hold magnetic resonance coronary angiography. Circulation 1993; 87:94–104

Manning WJ, Li W, Cohen SI, Johnson RG, Edelman RR (1995) Improved definition of anomalous left coronary artery by magnetic resonance coronary angiography. Am Heart J 130:615–617

McConnell MV, Ganz P, Selwyn AP, Li W, Edelman RR, Manning WJ (1995) Identification of anomalous coronary arteries and their anatomic course by magnetic resonance coronary angiography. Circulation 92:3158–3162

McConnell MV, Khasgiwala VC, Savord BJ, et al. (1997a) Prospective adaptive navigator correction for breath-hold MR coronary angiography. Magn Reson Med 1997; 37:148–152

McConnell MV, Khasgiwala VC, Savord BJ, et al. (1997b) Comparison of respiratory suppression methods and navigator locations for MR coronary angiography. AJR 168:1369–1375

Meaney JF, Prince MR, Nostrant TT, Stanley JC (1997) Gadolinium-enhanced MR angiography of visceral arteries in patients with suspected chronic mesenteric ischemia. J Magn Reson Imaging 7:171–176

Meyer CH, Hu BS, Nishimura DG, Macovski A (1992) Fast spiral coronary artery imaging. Magn Reson Med 28:401–406

Mezrich R (1995). A perspective on k-space. Radiology 195:297–315

Mohiaddin RH, Bogren HG, Lazim F, et al. (1996) Magnetic resonance coronary angiography in heart transplant recipients. Coronary Artery Dis 7:591–597

Müller MF, Fleisch M, Kroeker R, Chatterjee T, Meier B, Vock P (1997) Proximal coronary artery stenosis: three-dimensional MRI with fat saturation and navigator echo. J Magn Reson Imaging 7:644–651

Nitatori T, Hanaoka H, Yoshino A, et al. (1995) Clinical application of magnetic resonance angiography for coronary arteries: correlation with conventional angiography and evaluation of imaging time. Nippon Acta Radiol 55:670–676

Oshinski JN, Hofland L, Dixon WT, Parks WJ, Pettigrew RI (1996a) Magnetic resonance coronary angiography without breathholding using navigator echoes (abstract). In: Book of Abstracts of the 4th Meeting of the International Society of Magnetic Resonance in Medicine (ISMRM). New York, 27 April 3 May 1996; vol 1:449.

Oshinski JN, Hofland L, Mukundan S, Dixon WT, James WJ, Pettigrew RI (1996b) Two-dimensional MR coronary angiography without breath holding. Radiology 201:737–743

Oshinski JN, Dixon WT, Pettigrew R (to be published) Magnetic resonance coronary angiography with navigator echo gated real-time slice following. Int J Card Imaging

Paschal C, Haacke E, Adler L, Finelli DA (1992) Magnetic resonance coronary artery imaging. Cardiovasc Intervent Radiol 15:23–31

Paschal CB, Haacke EM, Adler LP (1993) Three-dimensional MR imaging of the coronary arteries: preliminary clinical experience. J Magn Reson Imaging 3:491–501.

Paulin S, von Schulthess GK, Fossel E, Krayenbuehl HP (1987) MR imaging of the aortic root and proximal coronary arteries. AJR 148:665–670

Pearlman JD, Edelman RE (1994) Ultrafast magnetic resonance imaging: segmented TurboFLASH, echo-planar, and real-time nuclear magnetic resonance. Radiol Clin North Am 32:593–612

Pennell DJ, Keegan J, Firmin DN, Gatehouse PD, Underwood SR, Longmore DB (1993) Magnetic resonance imaging of coronary arteries: technique and preliminary results. Br Heart J 70:315–326

Pennell DJ, Bogren HG, Keegan J, Firmin DW, Underwood SR (1994a) Coronary artery stenosis: assessment by magnetic resonance imaging (abstract). In: Book of Abstracts of the 11th Annual Scientific Meeting of the European Society for Magnetic Resonance in Medicine and Biology. Vienna, Austria, 20–24 April 1994:374

Pennell DJ, Bogren HG, Keegan J, Firmin DN, Underwood SR (1994b) Detection, localization and assessment of coronary artery stenosis by magnetic resonance imaging (abstract). In: Printed program of the second meeting of the Society of Magnetic Resonance (SMR). San Francisco, California, 6–12 August 1994

Post JC, van Rossum AC, Bronzwaer JGF, et al. (1995a) Magnetic resonance angiography of anomalous coronary arteries. A new gold standard for delineating the proximal course? Circulation 92:3163–3171

Post JC, vanRossum AC, Hofman MB, Valk J, Visser CA (1995b) A protocol for two-dimensional magnetic resonance coronary angiography, studied in three-dimensional magnetic resonance data sets. Am Heart J 1995; 130:167–173

Post JC, vanRossum AC, Hofman MBM, Valk J, Visser CA (1995c) Clinical utility of two dimensional breathhold MR angiography in coronary artery disease (abstract). In: Book of Abstracts of the 3rd Meeting of the Society of Magnetic Resonance (SMR) and the 12th Annual Scientific Meeting of the European Society for Magnetic Resonance in Medicine and Biology (ESMRMB). Nice, France, 20–25 August 1995

Post JC, van Rossum AC, Hofman MB, de Cock CC, Valk J, Visser CA (1997) Clinical utility of two-dimensional magnetic resonance angiography in detecting coronary artery disease. Eur Heart J 18:426–433.

Prince MR (1994) Gadolinium-enhanced MR aortography. Radiology 191:155–164

Prince MR, Yucel EK, Kaufman JA, Harrison DC, Geller SC (1993) Dynamic gadolinium-enhanced three-dimensional abdominal MR Arteriography. J Magn Reson Imaging 3:877–881.

Prince MR, Narasimham DL, Stanley JC, et al. (1995a) Breath-hold gadolinium-enhanced MR angiography of the abdominal aorta and its major branches. Radiology 197:785–792

Prince MR, Narasimham DL, Stanley JC, et al. (1995b) Gadolinium-enhanced magnetic resonance angiography of abdominal aortic aneurysms. J Vasc Surg 21:656–669.

Prince MR, Narisimham DL, Stanley JC, et al. (1995c) Breath-hold gadolinium-enhanced MR angiography of the abdominal aorta and its major branches. Radiology 197:785–792

Prince MR, Narasimham DL, Jacoby WT, et al. (1996a) Three-dimensional gadolinium-enhanced MR angiography of the thoracic aorta. AJR 166:1387–1397

Prince MR, Arnoldus C, Frisoli JK (1996b) Nephrotoxicity of high-dose gadolinium compared with iodinated contrast. J Magn Reson Imaging 1:162–166.

Rogers LF (1998) The heart of the matter: noninvasive coronary artery imaging (editorial). AJR 170:841

Sachs TS, Meyer CH, Hu BS, Kohli J, Nishimura DG, Macovski A (1994) Real-time motion detection in spiral MRI using navigators. Magn Reson Med 32:639–645

Sachs TS, Meyer CH, Irazzabal P, Hu BS, Nishimura DG, Macovski A (1995) The diminishing variance algorithm for real-time reduction of motion artifacts in MRI. Magn Reson Med 34:412–422

Sakuma H, Caputo GR, Steffens J, Shimakawa A, Foo TKF, Higgins CB (1993) Breath-hold MR angiography of coronary arteries with optimal double-oblique imaging planes and cine display (abstract). In: 79th Scientific Assembly and Annual Meeting of the Radiological Society of North America (RSNA). Chicago, Illinois, 28 November–3 December 1993; Radiology 189(P):278

Sakuma H, Caputo GR, Steffens JC, et al. (1994) Breath-hold MR cine angiography of coronary arteries in healthy volunteers: value of multiangle oblique imaging planes. AJR 163:533–537

Samdarshi T, Nanda N, Gatewood R, et al. (1992) Usefulness and limitations of transesophageal echocardiography in the assessment of proximal coronary artery stenosis. J Am Coll Cardiol 19:572–580

Scheidegger M, deGraaf R, Doyle M, Vermeulen J, vanDijk P, Pohost G (1992) Coronary artery MR imaging during multiple brief (1 sec) expiratory breath-holds (abstract). In: Proceedings of the Eleventh Annual Scientific Meeting of the Society of Magnetic Resonance Imaging (SMRM). Berlin, Germany, 8–14 August 1992:602

Scheidegger MB, Boesiger P (1994) Coronary MR imaging. In: Lanzer P, Rösch J (eds) Vascular diagnosis. Springer, Berlin Heidelberg New York, pp 415–420.

Scheidegger MB, Müller R, Boesiger P (1994) Magnetic resonance angiography: methods and its applications to the coroanry arteries. Technol Health Care 2:255–265

Scheidegger MB, Stuber M, Boesiger P, Hess OM (1996) Coronary artery imaging by magnetic resonance. Herz 21:90–96

Shimamota R, Suzuki J-I, Nishikawa J-I, et al. (1998) Measuring the diameter of coronary arteries on MR angiograms using spatial profile curves. AJR 170:889–893

Stehling M (1996) Coronary arteries: experience with navigator echoes (abstract). In: VIII International Workshop on Magnetic Resonance Angiography. Rome, Italy; 16–19 October 1996

Stuber M, Botnar RM, McConnell MV, et al. (to be published) Coronary artery imaging with the intravascular contrast agent MS-325 (abstract). In: Proceedings of the Sixth Scientific Meeting of the International Society for Magnetic Resonance in Medicine (ISMRM), 18–24 April 1998. Sydney, Australia

Taylor AM, Jhooti P, Wiesmann F, Keegan J, Firmin DN, Pennell DJ (1997) MR navigator-echo monitoring of temporal changes in diaphragm position: implications for MR coronary angiography. J Magn Reson Imaging 7:629–636

Taylor AM, Jhooti P, Firmin DN, Pennell DJ (to be published, a) Automated monitoring of diaphragm end-expiratory position for real-time navigator echo MR coronary angiography (abstract). In: Proceedings of the Sixth Scientific Meeting of the International Society for Magnetic Resonance in Medicine (ISMRM), 18–24 April 1998. Sydney, Australia

Taylor AM, Panting JR, Gatehouse PD, et al. (to be published, b) Safety and preliminary findings with an intravascular contrast agent, NC100150 for MR coronary angiography (abstract). In: Proceedings of the Sixth Scientific Meeting of the International Society for Magnetic Resonance in Medicine (ISMRM), 18–24 April 1998. Sydney, Australia

van Rossum AC, Galjee MA, Post JC, Visser CA (1997) A practical approach to MRI of coronary artery bypass graft patency and flow. Int J Cardiac Imaging 13:199–204

Vrachliotis TG, Aliabadi D, Bis KG, Shetty AN, London J, Farah J (1996) Breath-hold electrocardiogram-triggered, contrast-enhanced, 3D MR angiography to evaluate patency of coronary artery bypass graft. Radiology 201(P):273

Vrachliotis TG, Bis KG, Aliabadi D, Shetty AN, Safian R, Simonetti O (1997) Contrast-enhanced breath-hold MR angiography for evaluating patency of coronary artery bypass grafts. AJR 168:1073–1080

Wang S, Hu B, Macovski A, Nishimura D (1991) Coronary angiography using fast selective inversion recovery. Magn Res Med 18:417–423

Wang Y, Christy PS, Korosec FR, et al. (1995a) Coronary MRI with a respiratory feedback monitor: the 2D imaging case. Magn Reson Med 33:116–121

Wang Y, Grimm RC, Rossman PJ, Debbins JP, Riederer SJ, Ehman RL (1995b) 3D coronary MR angiography in multiple breath-holds using a respiratory feedback monitor. Magn Res Med 34:11–16

Wang Y, Grist TM, Korosec FR, et al. (1995c) Respiratory blur in 3D coronary MR imaging. Magn Reson Med 33:541–548.

Wang Y, Rossman PJ, Grimm RC, Riederer SJ, Ehman RL (1996) Navigator-echo-based real-time respiratory gating and triggering for reduction of respiration effects in three-dimensional coronary MR angiography. Radiology 198:55–60

Wielopolski PA, Manning WJ, Edelman RE (1995) Single breath-hold volumetric imaging of the heart using magnetization-prepared 3-dimensional segmented echo-planar imaging. J Magn Res Imaging 5:403–409

Wielopolski PA, VanGeuns RJ, DeFeijter PJ, DeBruin HG, Bongaerts AH, Oudkerk M (1997) Comparison of breath-hold 3D and retrospectively respiratory gated 3D MR coronary angiography with conventional coronary angiography (abstract). In: 1997 Scientific Program of the 83rd Scientific Assembly and Annual Meeting of the Radiological Society of North America (RSNA). 30 November–5 December 1997, Chicago, Ill.: Radiology 205(P):154

Woodard PK, Li D, Haacke EM, et al. (1998) Detection of coronary stenosis on source and projection images using three-dimensional MR angiography with retrospective respiratory gating: preliminary experience. AJR 170:883–888

Yoshino H, Nitatori T, Kachi E, et al. (1997) Directed proximal magnetic resonance coronary angiography compared with conventional contrast coronary angiography. Am J Cardiol 80:514–518

13 Great Vessels of the Chest

G.G. HARTNELL

13.1 Introduction

Among some of the earliest accepted cardiovascular applications for MRI was the evaluation of the great vessels of the chest (GAMSU et al. 1983; GEISINGER et al. 1985). In particular, examination of the thoracic aorta was one of the first uses of conventional ECG-gated spin-echo magnetic resonance imaging (SE MRI). This allowed accurate diagnosis of aortic aneurysms, aortic dissection, and other acquired and congenital aortic diseases (AMPARO et al. 1985; WHITE et al. 1988). SE MRI with ECG gating remains the mainstay of many imaging algorithms for diagnosing thoracic aortic disease (LINK and LESKO 1992; NIENABER et al. 1993).

Although imaging of the other great vessels of the chest (pulmonary arteries and systemic and pulmonary veins) can be performed adequately with SE (WHITE et al. 1997), the results can be less satisfactory

G.G. HARTNELL, FRCR, FACC, Department of Radiology, Beth Israel Deaconess Medical Center, West Campus, and Associate Professor of Radiology, Harvard Medical School, One Deaconess Road, Boston, MA 02215, USA

than when imaging the aorta. This is partly related to more complicated three-dimensional (3D) anatomy, limitations due to the smaller caliber of the major veins, and artifacts related to signal from slow flow or in-plane flow signal (ARRIVÉ et al. 1991). With the development of magnetic resonance angiography (MRA) the application of MRI techniques to the diagnosis of great vessel disease advanced rapidly.

More recent developments, such as rapid breath-hold MRI, turbo-spin echo (TSE), breath-hold MRA, and contrast-enhanced MRA allow fast, comprehensive, and accurate examination of the great vessels in a cost-effective manner (Fig. 13.1). Many traditional reservations concerning MRI (PETASNIK 1991) have been answered and MRI and MRA should be regarded as stand-alone definitive diagnostic methods for the diagnosis of great vessel disease.

In many instances with chest MRA, no contrast medium needs to be given and complicated 3D anatomy can be evaluated in a completely non-invasive manner which is not possible with any other diagnostic technique (LEWIN et al. 1991; WHITE et al. 1997). The relationship of vascular abnormalities to surrounding soft tissue structures is well shown. When branch vessel anatomy is unclear, for whatever reason, contrast-enhanced 3D MRA allows accurate definition of branch vessel anatomy (Fig. 13.1d) with an accuracy which is essentially the same as for conventional contrast angiography (PRINCE 1994; KRINSKY et al. 1997). In addition to defining great vessel anatomy, simultaneous imaging of intracardiac abnormalities (including valve lesions and congenital abnormalities) and the complications of great vessel disease (i.e., hemopericardium, left ventricular dysfunction, valvular regurgitation) is possible during the same examination.

The advantages of MRI for vascular diagnosis are well known and include safety, its completely noninvasive nature (unless contrast needs to be given), wide field of view, multiplanar imaging, and the ability to show complicated 3D relationships in a way which is not possible with conventional angiography. Although similar information may be

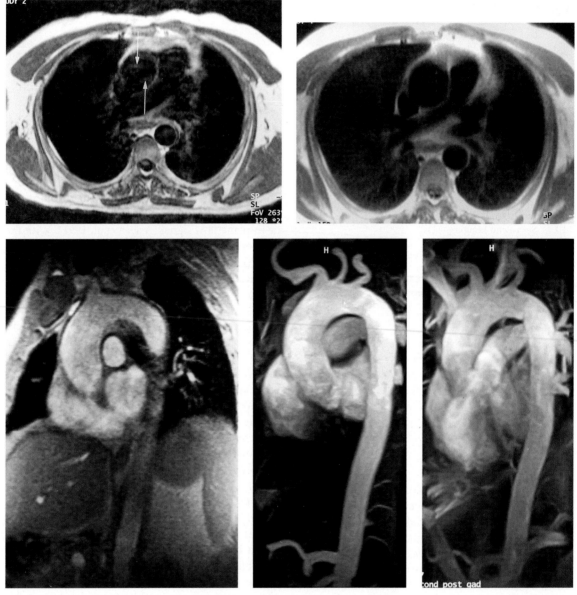

Fig. 13.1. a Axial SE image at level of right pulmonary artery in patient with dilated ascending aorta and suspected aortic dissection. The aorta is mildly dilated but there is no flap. Respiratory artifact (*arrows*) could possible obscure a small flap. **b** Axial HASTE image at level shown in **a** shows dilated aorta with no obscuring respiratory artifact. **c** Oblique ECG-triggered MRA from patient in **a** and **b** shows dilated ascending aorta with no evidence of a flap. Notice limited definition of the origin of the branches of aortic arch. Complete anatomi-cal coverage requires multiple breath-hold acquisitions. **d** Breath-hold, contrast-enhanced 3D MRA (first acquisition, MIP left anterior oblique perspective) shows the full extent of the thoracic aorta and the origin of the head and neck vessels. **e** Breath-hold, contrast-enhanced 3D MRA (second acquisition, MIP left anterior oblique perspective) now shows enhancement of the chest veins which obscures some of the arterial anatomy

acquired using CT angiography (CTA), this uses large volumes of iodinated contrast medium, can require more complicated image processing, and is subject to inflow dilution effects which may mimic or obscure disease. Compared with echocardiography, MRI of the great vessels has a major advantage in that large parts of the aorta and the systemic veins are obscured by overlying lung or bone and are inaccessible to echocardiography. Only the most proximal pulmonary arteries are visible by trans-esophageal echocardiography (TEE) and these are almost invisible to transthoracic echocardiography (TTE). MRI suffers from none of these limitations and of course does not involve some of the, admittedly uncommon, risks associated with TEE (GEIBEL et al. 1988).

13.2
Available Techniques for Great Vessel Imaging by MRI and MRA

13.2.1
Spin-Echo Imaging

Conventional ECG-gated SE is in many respects the reference standard for great vessel imaging. This is the technique which has been most widely evaluated in the assessment of acquired and congenital aortic disease and venous abnormalities complicating congenital heart disease. SE MRI provides good spatial resolution for defining great vessel anatomy and relationships to adjacent tissues. There are limitations in that it can be time consuming, particularly if multiplanar imaging is required, and complicated 3D anatomy may be difficult to elucidate. There are a variety of sources of error which may mislead the novice (SOLOMON et al. 1990). Conventional SE (i.e., non-breath-hold) is susceptible to respiratory artifacts, but this can be overcome by using TSE (SIMONETTI et al. 1996). In addition, with SE there are artifacts related to slow flow or flow within the imaging plane which may mimic thrombus or obscure intravascular pathology.

13.2.2
Fast Anatomical Imaging

In addition to TSE, there are other breath-hold, anatomical imaging methods available for imaging the great vessels. These have the advantage of even greater speed but may lack the spatial resolution required for making confident anatomical diagnosis. Techniques such as HASTE and turboFLASH may provide adequate information in some cases but are susceptible to unpredictable variations in image quality. In particular, most turboFLASH sequences used without gadolinium enhancement do not provide adequate signal-to-noise ratios and spatial resolution to allow confident anatomical diagnosis in the chest (HARTNELL et al. 1994). With contrast enhancement the performance of turboFLASH is adequate for diagnosing aneurysms and dissections (LOUBEYRE et al. 1996).

13.2.3
Magnetic Resonance Angiography

Numerous variations on a theme of MRA are useful for great vessel imaging. They can be divided into several basic categories.

13.2.3.1
Non-breath-hold Time-of-Flight MRA

Respiratory movement limits the use of non-breath-hold MRA for great vessel imaging. Non-breath-hold cine MRA is useful for assessment of flow abnormalities; for instance identifying true and false lumens in patients with aortic dissection, as well as assessing cardiac anatomy and cardiac function (SONNABEND et al. 1990). Non-breath-hold 3D techniques have been used by some to examine the origins of the head and neck vessels, but these images are too frequently affected by respiratory and other artifacts obscuring disease or producing pseudolesions.

13.2.3.2
Breath-hold Time-of-Flight MRA

Early versions of breath-hold time-of-flight (TOF) MRA were not gated to the patient's ECG and therefore had limited value for imaging the heart and the aorta, due to pulsation artifacts. There is relatively little artifact when imaging the systemic veins, and one of the earliest validated applications for ungated breath-hold MRA was the accurate 3D demonstration of systemic and pulmonary chest vein anatomy (LEWIN et al. 1991; COHEN et al. 1994; FINN et al. 1993). Subsequently ECG-gated MRA, which reduces pulsatility effects and allows clearer definition of 3D anatomy, has allowed more extensive evaluation of the aorta and pulmonary arteries as well as the heart (HARTNELL and MEIER 1995). Segmented k-space or ECG-gated MRA also produces higher signal than ungated MRA by ensuring image acquisition takes advantage of the highest flow rates during systole. Lack of pulsatility artifacts improves imaging of smaller branch vessels. Breath-hold MRA can be easily manipulated to produce 3D projectional angiograms using selective presaturation (FELMLEE and EHMAN 1987) and the maximum intensity projection (MIP) algorithm (LEWIN et al. 1991). Artifacts on MIP may suppress signal from small branch vessels and adjacent high signal from fluid may also obscure detail (ANDERSON et al. 1990). This type of error can be avoided by reviewing the two-dimensional (2D) source images, as should be the case whenever performing 3D reconstructions from 2D images.

Breath-hold cine MRA is a variation of segmented k-space or ECG-gated MRA which allows 15 or more images to be acquired per R-R interval, depending on heart rate, during a single breath-hold period (up to 20 s depending on heart rate). Although temporal resolution remains slightly inferior to conventional non-breath-hold cine MRA, in most patients breath-hold cine MRA improves image quality by reducing respiratory artifacts, which can mimic lesions or obscure anatomical details. Although cine MRA has limited additional value in the direct evaluation of the great vessels, it is valuable for the assessment of some lesions, e.g., dissection, coarctation, and compressive lesions such as tumor invading the pulmonary artery. Cine MRA provides accurate additional information, when required, on cardiac function.

13.2.3.3
Phase Contrast Imaging

Phase contrast MRA (PC) has numerous applications, including assessment of the thoracic aorta and congenital heart disease (DINSMORE et al. 1986, 1987). However, PC techniques generally require a higher degree of technical performance from the imaging system, as they are more sensitive to eddy currents, gradient instabilities, and field inhomogeneity. Although PC can be used as both a non-breath-hold and breath-hold method for identifying other great vessel abnormalities, the longer time for acquisition and greater difficulty with implementing this technique make this still a rather limited approach. In spite of this, PC evaluation of aortic dissection and differentiating true from false lumens (Fig. 13.2) may be valuable (DINSMORE et al. 1986; LEUNG and DEBATIN 1997). Quantification of shunts and determination of flow direction and volume is valuable in congenital heart disease.

13.2.3.4
Contrast-Enhanced 3D MRA

Although conventional and breath-hold SE and MRA accurately define most great vessel abnormalities (HARTNELL et al. 1994), there are some situations where branch vessel anatomy is not seen with sufficient clarity or respiratory or other artifacts obscure

detail. In addition, some patients are unable to tolerate the time required for an unenhanced MRA study. In these situations, contrast (gadolinium) enhancement with non-breath-hold or breath-hold 3D acquisition is valuable (PRINCE 1994; KRINSKY et al. 1997). Contrast-enhanced 3D MRA is very accurate for defining thoracic aortic and pulmonary artery anatomy and is particularly good for defining branch vessel abnormality (Fig. 13.1). The high signal provided by vascular contrast enhancement makes 3D image processing easier than with unenhanced images. The requirement for very short TR and TE means that the availability of 3D contrast-enhanced MRA is still limited, especially for breath-hold MRA (LEUNG and DEBATIN 1997). Some skill is required when timing the injection to prevent anatomy being obscured by adjacent veins (Fig. 13.1e).

Contrast-enhanced MRA seems to be substantially more accurate in defining pulmonary artery anatomy than unenhanced techniques (LEUNG and DEBATIN 1997). There is less experience and probably less need for contrast enhancement when evaluating the systemic and pulmonary veins, where unenhanced techniques already show almost 100% accuracy (COHEN et al. 1994; HARTNELL et al. 1995). Contrast enhancement is useful for defining abnormalities which may be obscured or mimicked by slow flow or turbulent flow, or where complicated small vessel anatomy needs to be evaluated (LEUNG and DEBATIN 1997).

13.3
MRI and MRA of the Great Veins

Demonstrating abnormalities of the great veins of the chest with methods other than MRI may be difficult. Until recently, contrast venography was regarded as the "gold standard" for defining systemic venous anatomy, but this has significant limitations. These include the requirement to inject contrast agents, failure to opacify all of the venous anatomy, and the inability to clearly define 3D relationships, which may be important when planning venous access or bypass surgery. For the same reason, contrast-enhanced CT or CTA is also somewhat limited. Contrast medium needs to be injected (appropriate venous access may be difficult) and wash-in effects from unopacified vessels and other artifacts can mimic occlusions or thrombus (GODWIN and WEBB 1982). A complete examination may require multiple contrast injections from several sites, which may not be possible. In addition, difficulty in sepa-

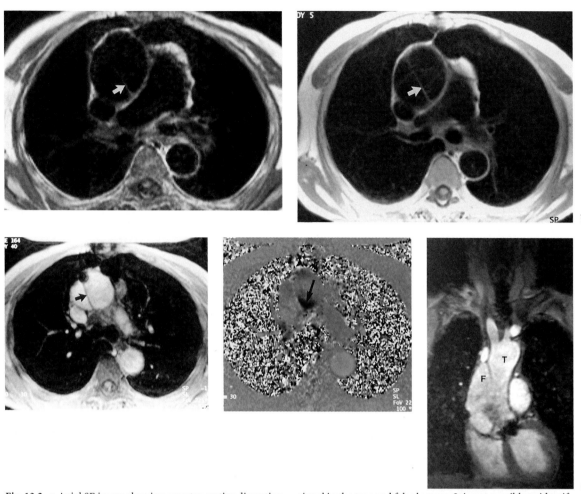

Fig. 13.2. **a** Axial SE image showing a postoperative dissection flap in the ascending aorta (*arrow*). Due to respiratory movement not all of the flap is visible. **b** Axial TSE image at same level as **a**, showing the dissection flap extending across the full diameter of the ascending aorta (*arrow*). Note the absence of respiratory artifact. **c** Axial PC magnitude image just cranial to **a** and **b**, showing the dissection flap extending across the full diameter of the ascending aorta (*arrow*), surrounded by high signal in the true and false lumens. It is not possible to identify the true lumen from this image. **d** Axial PC velocity map image from same sequence as in **c**, showing the dissection flap and cranially directed flow signal (*black arrow*) in the true lumen. **e** Coronal ECG-triggered MRA from patient shown in **a–d**, showing the extent of the dissection flap in the ascending aorta with a large communication between the true (*T*) and false (*F*) lumens

rating arterial from venous structures and more difficult 3D image reconstruction limit the use of CTA.

Duplex Doppler ultrasound is well established in the assessment of lower extremity venous disease. Unfortunately, disadvantages related to restricted acoustic access to the great veins seriously limit the use of this modality for investigating both the systemic thoracic and pulmonary veins.

Early experience showed that although SE can show major systemic and some pulmonary venous abnormalities (GEISINGER et al. 1985; VESELY et al. 1991; MASUI et al. 1991; HANSEN et al. 1990), there are important potential errors. These may be related to in-plane signal saturation effects, respiratory arti-facts, and difficulty in distinguishing between signal in slow-flowing blood and thrombus (ARRIVÉ et al. 1991; HAIRE et al. 1991). In particular, evaluation of complicated 3D anatomy, an important consideration when assessing the great veins, is difficult with the tomographic images provided by SE. For this reason, the more widespread application of MRI to evaluating the great veins had to await the development of MRA.

Time-of-flight techniques have proved to be sufficiently robust to assess great vein anatomy (HARTNELL et al. 1995). Chest veins are less affected by respiratory and cardiac motion than are the arteries; hence ungated MRA techniques provide good quality 3D images which are almost always of diagnostic quality. Venous imaging using TOF is also easier, when compared to imaging of arteries, because venous flow has lower peak velocity, the veins have a larger lumen, and the technique is less prone to the complex motion which causes signal loss when assessing arterial disease. Arteries and veins frequently run together and separating the two may be difficult. Because arterial flow tends to diverge from a single source, whereas venous flow converges, it is easier to implement selective presaturation to suppress arterial flow signal when imaging the venous system (LEWIN et al. 1991; EDELMAN et al. 1989). Although 3D MRA, with and without contrast enhancement, may be suitable for great vein imaging, in most situations 2D TOF techniques are more than adequate for most diagnostic purposes (Fig. 13.3).

Congenital anomalies of the systemic veins (Table 13.1) are relatively uncommon and seldom of importance, except when patients undergo cardio pulmonary bypass or require central venous access, although they are well shown by MRA (HARTNELL et al. 1996). More commonly it is necessary to demonstrate systemic venous anatomy to determine pa-

tency in association with one of the causes of acquired venous abnormality listed in Table 13.2. Long-term central venous cannulation for hemodynamic monitoring, dialysis, hyperalimentation, or chemotherapy has a high incidence of central venous stenosis or occlusion, as may mediastinal tumors. All these abnormalities are well demonstrated by 2D TOF MRA (HARTNELL et al. 1995), which accurately demonstrates occlusion and stenosis and relates these lesions to adjacent soft tissue abnormalities. Of particular importance, in patients who require long-term central venous access, MR shows not only the area of abnormality but also normal veins which

Table 13.1. Causes of pulmonary venous abnormalities

Congenital
Partial anomalous pulmonary venous drainage
Total anomalous pulmonary venous drainage
Hypoplastic lung syndrome (Scimitar vein)

Surgical
Complicating atrial baffle procedures

Hypercoagulable states

Cor triatriatum

Table 13.2. Causes of systemic central venous abnormalities

Neoplastic
Direct invasion
Extrinsic compression
Secondary thrombosis
Intravascular tumor (rare)

Inflammatory
(i.e., fibrosing mediastinitis)

Infective
Spread of peripheral thrombophlebitis
Iatrogenic
Infective mediastinitis

Congenital
Duplicated superior vena cava
Atresia/hypoplasia
Aberrant course
Persistent anomalous veins (systemic or pulmonary)

Trauma/surgical
Motor vehicle accident
Central venous catheterization
Pacemaker
Ligation/filter insertion
Arteriovenous fistulae

Hypercoagulable states

Compression by nonmalignant masses
Arterial aneurysms
Fractures
Benign tumors
Effort syndrome (Paget-von Schrötter syndrome)

Veno-occlusive Behçet's disease

Radiotherapy

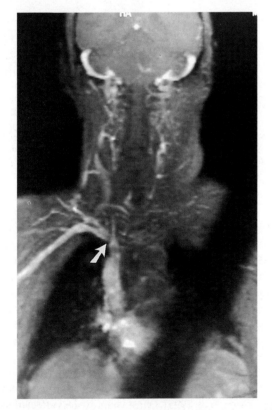

Fig. 13.3. Breath-hold, coronal 2D TOF MRA with arterial presaturation (MIP anterior perspective) shows stenosis of the lower right brachiocephalic vein (*arrow*) and occlusion of both internal jugular veins

maybe suitable alternative sites for central venous cannulation. In this last respect, MRA has substantial advantages when compared with venography, CTA, and ultrasound.

Congenital pulmonary abnormalities of clinical significance are relatively uncommon, and usually present in early childhood (i.e., Tapvd). In these patients TTE is usually adequate for defining the pulmonary veins. If echocardiography is inadequate, even in the neonate, SE or non-breath-hold MRA can define pulmonary venous drainage (White et al. 1997; Cohen et al. 1994; Masui et al. 1991). Rarely congenital abnormalities of pulmonary venous drainage are detected in adults and are best defined using MRA (Fig. 13.4). In postoperative patients, particularly those with intra-atrial baffles, MRI reliably shows the patency of the intra-atrial structures (Fig. 13.5) (see also Fig. 10.27).

13.4
Diseases of the Thoracic Aorta

Classically, assessment of thoracic aortic disease has required contrast aortography. This has obvious disadvantages related to the risks of arterial catheterization and the use of large amounts of iodi-

nated contrast medium. In addition, aortography provides only limited information on complicated anatomy and may fail to fully demonstrate the size of thrombosed aneurysms or partly thrombosed dissections. For this reason, aortography has been largely, if not completely, replaced in most applications by cross-sectional imaging. TTE and TEE are the usual initial methods for investigating aortic disease. Because of their limited field of view (particularly with TTE), and inability to demonstrate much branch vessel anatomy, it is often necessary also to perform imaging with CTA or MRI. The disadvantages of CTA have already been discussed. MRI with SE is accurate for diagnosing aortic disease, and improved definition of complicated 3D structures, and in particular branch vessel anatomy, is provided by ECG-gated unenhanced MRA and contrast-enhanced 3D sequences (Prince 1994; Leung and Debatin 1997). The applications of different techniques of MRI and MRA to the diagnosis of aortic disease should be considered in relation to each of the different diagnostic entities.

13.4.1
Thoracic Aortic Aneurysms

In most patients, MRI and MRA are appropriate methods for investigating thoracic aortic aneurysms.

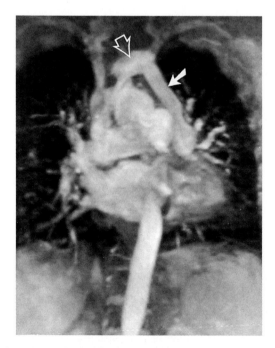

Fig. 13.4. Projectional angiogram (MIP coronal perspective from ECG-triggered 2D TOF) showing partial anomalous pulmonary venous drainage from the left lung via an ascending cardinal vein (*arrow*) into the left brachiocephalic vein (*open arrow*)

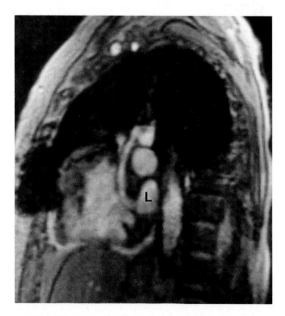

Fig. 13.5. Oblique breath-hold MRA (PC magnitude image) showing intra-atrial conduit following correction of partial anomalous pulmonary venous drainage from the right upper lobe, and confirming good flow into the left atrium (*L*). Flow was measured using a PC velocity map (not shown)

However, when considering whether to use an alternative test, the information that is required in the management of aortic aneurysms needs to be considered. The basic diagnosis needs to be made, although this is often made on the basis of the chest radiograph or other cross-sectional imaging before the patient is referred for MRI. Diagnostic accuracy is necessary and is provided by the ability not only to define clearly the full diameter of the aortic aneurysm but also to assess the amount of thrombus within it and its craniocaudal extent. Many thoracic aneurysms extend into the abdomen and hence the ability to image the entire aorta (which may not be available with TEE or TTE) is important.

The precise relationship of the aneurysm to major branch arteries, particularly the head and neck vessels, is crucial when planning the surgical approach and site of cross-clamping. Definition of branch vessel anatomy, including congenital variations of anatomy and proximal stenotic or aneurysmal disease, is essential prior to surgery (Fig. 13.6). In ascending aortic disease, assessment of aortic valve morphology, aortic regurgitation, and the relationship of aneurysmal disease to the coronary arteries is required. MRI and MRA can provide all of this

information relatively rapidly and reliably, although it may be necessary to use a combination of imaging protocols to provide all this information. For instance, a combination of SE and cine MRA is suitable for defining the size of the aneurysm and assessing branch vessel involvement and aortic regurgitation. If contrast-enhanced 3D MRA is used to define branch vessel anatomy, an unenhanced sequence may also be required to more precisely define the true diameter of the thrombosed part of the aneurysm, as well as assess aortic valve abnormalities.

Numerous studies have shown that SE is accurate for assessing aortic aneurysms dimensions. Combination with cine MRA allows definition of aortic valve disease while the ability to use contrast enhancement, if branch vessel anatomy is unclear, provides an extra degree of reliability (Prince 1994; Krinsky et al. 1997). The accuracy of this combined approach using MRI is such that the role of aortography is now extremely limited, mainly to those patients who are unable to undergo MRI because of metal implants. There is some dispute about the relative merits of CTA and MRA is evaluating the thoracic aorta. Both are extremely accurate and versatile (Fig. 13.7). CTA requires the use of more toxic

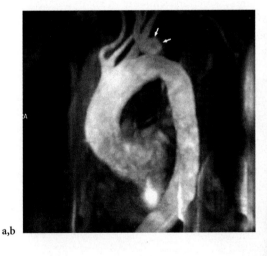

a,b

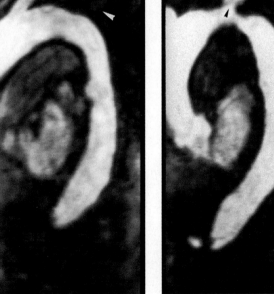

c

Fig. 13.6. a Breath-hold, contrast-enhanced 3D MRA (MIP left anterior oblique perspective) shows a partially thrombosed aneurysm at the origin of an aberrant right subclavian artery (*small arrows*). Note the common origin of the right and left carotid artery. **b,c** Breath-hold, contrast-enhanced 3D MRA (MPR oblique views). The full extent of the aneurysm, which is partially thrombosed, can be better evaluated on the MPR images than on the MIP image (*white arrowheads*). The origin of the aberrant right subclavian artery is indicated (*small black arrow*)

iodinated contrast agents, when compared with gadolinium-based agents, and at the moment is unable to assess aortic regurgitation. In addition, some branch vessel anatomy may be obscured by calcifications in the vessel wall.

13.4.2
Aortic Ulceration and Intramural Hematoma

Aortic ulceration occurs less commonly than aortic aneurysms, although ulceration frequently progresses to aneurysm. Aortic ulcers are seen as focal outpouchings from the lumen of the aorta which may be filled with thrombus or high signal from static blood on T1 imaging (Fig. 13.8). Increased signal from ulcers (on T1- and T2-weighted images) can mimic the variable high signal from intramural hematoma (Sonnabend et al. 1990; Murray et al. 1997) or from a thrombosed false lumen in aortic dissection (Yucel et al. 1990). Differentiation between slow flow in a false lumen and thrombus can be made using cine, PC, selective presaturation, or contrast-enhanced MRA (Fig. 13.9). Occasionally the wall of the hematoma, with the chemical shift artifact from the surface of the luminal thrombus, may simulate a dissection (Solomon et al. 1990). Administration of contrast or conventional cine MRA should allow accurate distinction between the two (Sonnabend et al. 1990). Differentiation of intramural hematoma from frank aortic dissection is important as distal (type B) hematoma may resolve without surgical treatment, while proximal (type A) hematoma usually progresses to dissection and

requires surgical treatment (Murray et al. 1997). Changes in signal intensity may help to identify healing hematomas which do not require intervention (Murray et al. 1997; Bluemke 1997).

13.4.3
Dissection of the Thoracic Aorta

The diagnosis of aortic dissection is a high profile application for cardiovascular MR, although the diagnosis is relatively uncommon. Because patients frequently present acutely, the imaging technique used is often determined more by what is most readily available, rather than by what is theoretically the best possible technique. Patients frequently present out of normal working hours, when the appropriate expertise for TEE or MRI may not be readily to hand. In addition, patients with acute thoracic aortic dissection are medical emergencies, are in pain, and may be hemodynamically unstable. The need for intensive hemodynamic monitoring and hypotensive medication may make imaging by MRI impossible. In these circumstances, TEE or CTA is more appropriate (Erbel et al. 1989; Mast et al. 1991; Cigarroa et al. 1993). MRI is suitable for patients with acute dissection who are hemodynamically stable (Nienaber et al. 1993) or patients with chronic dissection or requiring postoperative evaluation following repair of dissection (White et al. 1988; Loubeyre et al. 1996; Laissy et al. 1995; Mendelson et al. 1991).

In patients who are suitable for MRI, there are extensive data that this is the most accurate tech-

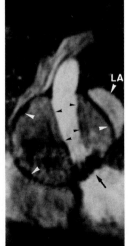

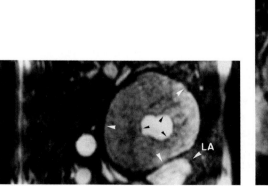

Fig. 13.7 a,b. Breath-hold, contrast-enhanced 3D MRA [MPR axial view (a) and oblique view (b)] in a patient with previous Bentall surgery for a huge aneurysm of the aneurysm aorta. The metallic aortic valve prosthesis is visible as an area devoid of signal (*arrow*). There is dehiscence of the graft (*black arrowheads*) at its insertion on the valve prosthesis with filling of the "old" aortic aneurysm (*white arrowheads*). Compression of the aneurysm on the left atrium (*LA*) is present

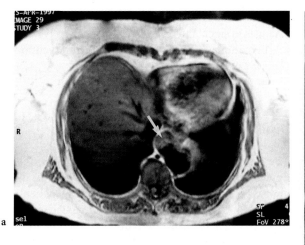
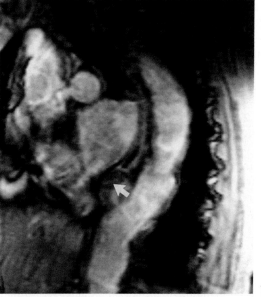

Fig. 13.8. a Axial SE image showing anterior outpouching from the descending aorta, representing a large aortic ulcer. A rim of intermediate signal (*arrow*) could represent slow- flowing blood or thrombus. **b** Coronal breath-hold ECG-trig- gered 2D TOF MRA image showing intermediate signal (*ar- row*) in ulcer, confirming the presence of thrombus

Table 13.3. Accuracy (sensitivity/specificity) of methods for diagnosing aortic dissection

Reference	Type of dissection	TEE	CT/CTA	MRI (SE)
NIENABER et al. (1993)	Acute	97%/77% (TTE 59%/83%)	94%/87%	98%/98%
	Stable suspected	86%/90%		95%/95%
LAISSY et al. (1995)	Postoperative	86%/67%		100%/100%
SOMMER et al. (1996)	Symptomatic	100%/94%	100%/100%	100%/94%
PANTING et al. (1995)	Acute			96%/100%

nique for diagnosing acute and chronic aortic dissec- tion (NIENABER et al. 1993; LAISSY et al. 1995) (Table 13.3), provided the images are interpreted by an ex- perienced reader (WHITE et al. 1988). The high speci- ficity of MRI as well as its noninvasive nature are major advantages over TEE, as is the ability to image the aorta below the diaphragm, should dissection extend into the abdomen. Conventional ECG-gated SE (Fig. 13.2a) accurately demonstrates acute and chronic dissections and postoperative complications such as extensive dissection, increasing diameter of the residual aorta, development of false channels, and anastomotic aneurysms (HARTNELL et al. 1994; MENDELSON et al. 1991; DI CESARE et al. 1991). Contrast-enhanced 3D MRA aids in understanding the relationship of false lumens and branch vessels to the aorta (PRINCE 1994; KRINSKY et al. 1997; LOUBEYRE et al. 1996), where CTA has been reported to be supe- rior to MRI, although the appropriate MRA ap-

proach was not used for this comparison (SOMMER et al. 1996). Using SE, errors of diagnosis can occur related to slow flow mimicking thrombus, chemical shift artifacts, respiratory artifacts, signal from adja- cent veins (i.e., the superior vena cava), tumors, aor- tic ulcers, etc. (PETASNIK 1991; SOLOMON et al. 1990; LOTAN et al. 1989). The use of MRA, contrast-en- hanced MRA, or PC (Fig. 13.2c,d) has largely abol- ished these errors. Occasionally, early dissection may appear as an intramural hematoma without a distinct flap or tear when MRI will just show wall thickening (WOLFF et al. 1991). In this situation, high signal within the wall usually indicates the diagnosis (MURRAY et al. 1997).

Postoperatively, MRI is probably the most reliable method for detecting complications such as anasto- motic aneurysms, extension of false lumens into branch vessels (Fig. 13.10), and further dilatation (WHITE et al. 1988; LOUBEYRE et al. 1996; LAISSY et al.

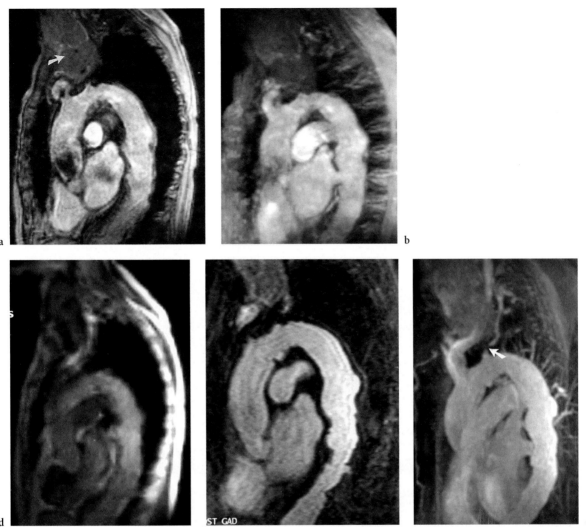

Fig. 13.9. a Oblique sagittal ECG-triggered 2D TOF MRA showing extensive ulceration in the descending aorta. There is an incidental mass in the thyroid (*arrow*). **b** Projectional angiogram (MIP from ECG-triggered 2D TOF parallel to **a**), showing ulceration of the descending aorta but poor definition of branches. **c** Oblique sagittal TurboFLASH image acquired 22 s after injection of 1 ml of gadolinium-DTPA shows high signal in the descending aorta, indicating the appropriate timing for 3D acquisition. **d** Source image from 3D MRA acquired in the same orientation as **a–c** shows better definition of ulceration of the descending aorta. **e** Projectional angiogram following injection of 0.2 mmol/kg body weight gadolinium-DTPA (MIP from 3D contrast-enhanced MRA parallel to **d**) provides excellent definition of branches, including a bovine left common carotid and stenosis of left subclavian artery (*arrow*)

1995; DI CESARE et al. 1991; BOGAERT et al. 1997). It is the most appropriate way for routinely following patients with chronic or progressive aortic abnormalities which require frequent surveillance, such as patients with Marfan syndrome (SOULEN et al. 1987; KAWAMOTO et al. 1997).

13.4.4
Aortic Infections and Inflammation

Infection of the aorta may complicate a number of conditions, including bacterial endocarditis, aortic surgery, and mediastinal sepsis. Infection can also occur in a severely atherosclerotic aorta. MRI will show the abnormalities associated with any coexistent mediastinitis, and perivalvar abscesses (Fig. 13.11) or mycotic aneurysms (GUINET et al. 1992). In postoperative patients clear differentiation from postoperative changes may be difficult (ROFSKY et al. 1993; RANDALL et al. 1993). Although MRI is not recommended as a first-line imaging technique in patients with endocarditis, it provides useful information outside the field of view of echocardiography. However, the improved spatial resolution and ability to show valvar regurgitation more accurately by echocardiography means that TTE and TEE remain the initial investigations of choice in patients with aortic infection or endocarditis. MRI is also useful for assessing complications of inflammatory aortitis syndromes (such as Takayasu's arteritis) where contrast angiography may be particularly hazardous (Fig. 13.12).

13.4.5
Congenital Abnormalities of the Aorta

Both MRI and MRA have extensive potential applications in the assessment of congenital heart disease (FELLOWS et al. 1992). As has already been discussed, congenital lesions affecting the systemic and pulmonary veins are well demonstrated by MRI (WHITE et al. 1997). In infants, good views of most of the aorta can be obtained by transthoracic routes. In adolescents and adults echocardiography can evaluate most intracardiac aspects of congenital heart disease, but as children grow older, and particularly in adults, limited acoustic access severely limits evalua-

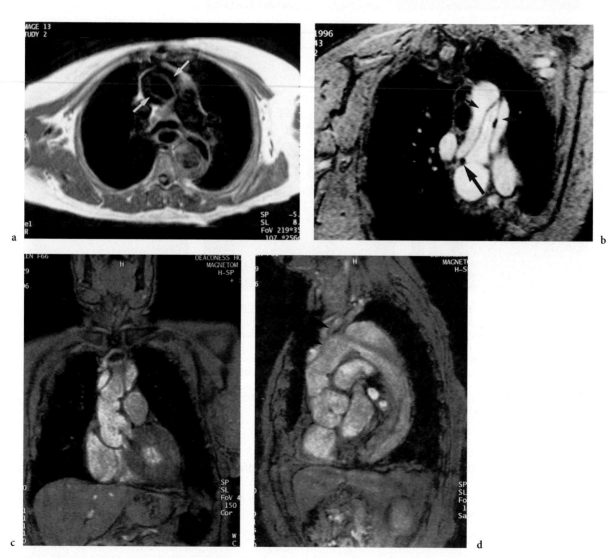

Fig. 13.10. a Axial SE image showing persistent false lumens (*arrows*) following tube graft of the ascending aorta for acute proximal aortic dissection. **b** Oblique axial ECG-triggered 2D TOF MRA showing anastomosis (*large arrow*) between aortic replacement and upper ascending aorta with residual false lumens (*small arrows*) surrounding true lumen. **c** Coronal ECG-triggered 2D TOF MRA showing mild aortic regurgitation, aortic replacement, and dissection extending into the base of the neck. **d** Oblique axial ECG-triggered 2D TOF MRA showing dissection flap at various levels. Note involvement of the origin of the brachiocephalic artery (*arrows*). The dissection extended into the right internal carotid artery

tion of the aorta and great veins. MRI with MRA usually provides all the information required about aortic anatomy, its relationships to adjacent structures, and branch vessel anatomy (MIROWITZ et al. 1990; AKINS et al. 1987). In this regard, MRI is as accurate as angiography in defining anatomy, although it cannot provide pressure data (PARSONS et al.

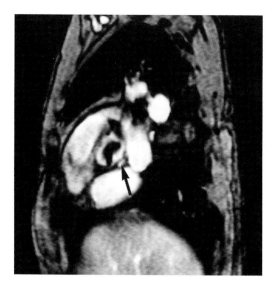

Fig. 13.11. Systolic image from short-axis cine MRA of bicuspid aortic valve showing the elongated signal void due to turbulent flow through the distorted valve orifice. There is a paravalvar abscess (*arrow*) complicating bacterial endocarditis

1990). Coarctation (Fig. 13.13), vascular rings and the results of surgery are well defined, along with their relationships to major branch vessels (AZAROW et al. 1992) (Fig. 13.14). Coarctation can be differentiated from pseudocoarctation (Fig. 13.15). Although SE may be susceptible to some artifacts related to partial volume effects (MIROWITZ et al. 1990) or slow flow, MRA, particularly with contrast enhancement, has essentially overcome these limitations.

13.5
Mediastinal Tumors

Primary tumors of the great vessels are rare but secondary involvement by mediastinal and lung tumors is common. Although such tumors often are initially diagnosed by echocardiography or CT, MRI and MRA provide excellent demonstration of relationships between tumors and the great vessels (KAUCZOR et al. 1991). The 3D relationships of tumors to great vessels is easier to appreciate with the multiplanar imaging available with MRI and separation of tumor from slow flow signal in the vessel lumen is possible with MRA. It may be possible to differentiate postoperative or postradiotherapy changes from tumor with some sequences, although this is not a universally accepted application. Visualization of vessels in the tumor or prominent contrast enhancement may occasionally

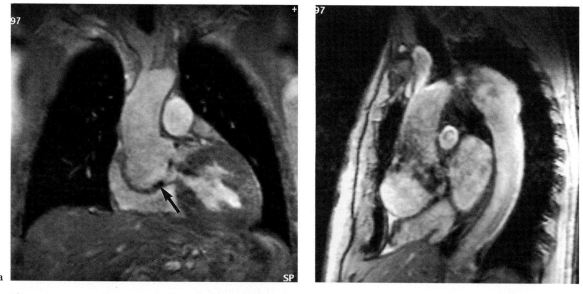

a   b

Fig. 13.12. a Coronal ECG-triggered 2D TOF MRA showing mild aortic regurgitation and dilatation of the right coronary artery sinus of Valsalva. Note low signal (*arrow*) due to calcification in the wall of the dilated sinus of Valsalva. **b** Oblique

sagittal ECG-triggered 2D TOF MRA again showing dilatation of the right coronary artery sinus of Valsalva but also showing aneurysmal dilatation distal to the origin of the subclavian artery

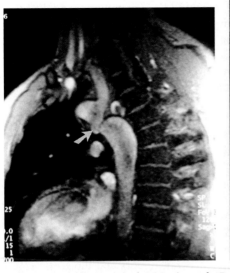

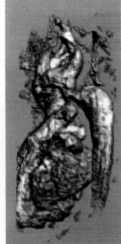

Fig. 13.13. a Oblique sagittal ECG-triggered 2D TOF MRA showing true coarctation (*arrow*) distal to the left subclavian artery. **b** Projectional angiogram (MIP from coronal ECG-triggered 2D TOF MRA) showing true coarctation, dilated left subclavian artery, and numerous dilated collateral arteries (*arrows*). **c** Projectional angiogram (surface shaded rendering oblique sagittal perspective from coronal ECG-triggered 2D TOF MRA) showing true coarctation and dilated left subclavian artery

suggest a more limited pathological differential diagnosis such as Castleman disease or angiosarcoma (MADER et al. 1997; ECKLUND and HARTNELL 1994).

13.6
Conclusion

In many areas, MRI with MRA is established as a "gold" or reference standard for imaging of the great vessels. In adults with congenital heart disease or acquired disease involving the aorta and systemic veins, MRI is as accurate or more accurate than any alternative technique. Using an appropriate combination of SE and MRA, comprehensive imaging of all aspects of systemic venous and thoracic aortic disease is possible. The main limitation on using MR in these situation is either cost or lack of understanding of how to best use MRI and MRA to diagnose and fully evaluate the lesions under investigation. The development of faster, more robust imaging, particularly based on contrast-enhanced sequences, will aid the acceptance of MRI for diagnosing diseases of the great vessels.

Appendix. Typical Sequence Parameters used for Great Vessel MRI and MRA

Protocols for MRI and MRA Using Siemens Equipment (Vision at 1.5 T; Expert at 1 T)
These sequences are implemented on Siemens equipment (Siemens Medical Systems, Iselin, N.J.) and are used for the Vision MR imager operating at 1.5 T and the Impact (Expert) MR imager operating at 1 T.

ECG-Gated Spin Echo. TE 25 ms, TR R-R interval, matrix 160–192 × 256, NSA 3, slice thickness 5 mm. Respiratory compensation is not used. Typical acquisition time for a set of SE images is 4–5 min, depending on the R-R interval.

Breath-hold Turbo Spin Echo. TE 30 ms for T1, 57–76 ms for T2 weighting; TR (T1) R-R interval or (T2) twice R-R interval, matrix 160–192 × 256, NSA 1, slice thickness 6–8 mm. Parameters can be varied to produce T1- or T2-weighted images.

Black-Blood Single Shot (TurboFLASH). TE 2.3 ms, TR 5 or 12 ms, flip angle 15° or 25°, matrix 128 × 256, NSA 1, slice thickness 10 mm, one image/heart beat, acquisition window 640 ms at end of R-R interval (hence diastolic image). Non-selective 90° inversion preparation pulse.

HASTE. TE 4.3 ms, TI varied to push acquisition window to late diastole, TR infinity. Trigger alternate

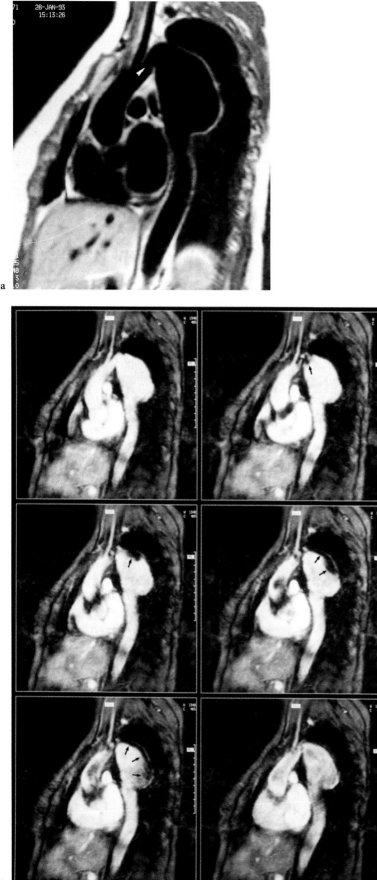

Fig. 13.14. a Oblique sagittal SE in a patient with previous patch angioplasty for coarctation of the aorta. Huge - aneurysmal dilation of the proximal descending thoracic aorta. Note the presence of concomitant hypoplasia of the transverse aortic arch (*arrowhead*). **b** Oblique sagittal MRA (PC magnitude image at six different time points during the cardiac cycle). Hypointense jet originating in the hypoplastic aortic arch and extending along the postero-lateral side of the aneurysm (small arrows). [**a, b** from BOGAERT et al. (1995) J Am Coll Cardiol 26:521–527. Reprinted with permission of the Journal of the American College of Cardiologists]

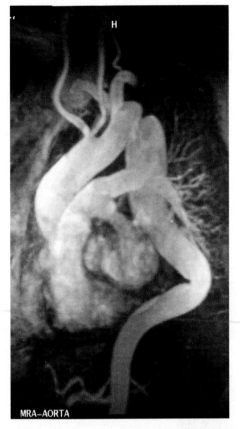

Fig. 13.15. Projectional angiogram following injection of 0.2 mmol/kg body weight gadolinium-DTPA (MIP oblique sagittal perspective from 3D contrast-enhanced MRA) showing tortuous aorta with pseudocoarctation (*arrow*) distal to the left subclavian artery. No collateral vessels are visible

heart beats, matrix 128 × 256, NSA 1, slice thickness 6 mm. Black-blood preparation pulse, a longer echo train (300 ms), and a medium effective TE every other cardiac cycle produce weakly T2-weighted images. Each slice is acquired during a single heart beat, with a 320 ms acquisition window, acquired every other heart beat to give seven sections per breath-hold.

Non-breath-hold ECG-Gated Cine MRA. TE 10 ms, TR 30 ms, flip angle 30°, matrix 160 × 256, NSA 2, slice thickness 5 mm. Typical acquisition time for non-breath-hold cine MRA 4–5 min, depending on the R-R interval.

Conventional Breath-hold 2D Time-of-flight MRA (FLASH). TE 9 ms, TR 27 ms, flip angle 30°, matrix 160–192 × 256, NSA 1, section thickness 5 mm, 20% overlap to facilitate 3D reconstruction. Up to three images can be acquired in a 14-s breath-hold, although the longer breath-hold required for this may degrade image quality. A presaturation pulse is placed through the heart to suppress aortic and branch artery signal. Appropriately positioned axial, coronal, and sagittal images are acquired.

Bolus tracking. Flow direction is determined using bolus tracking rather than phase contrast MRA, being quicker and more robust on this equipment. Typical sequence parameters for bolus-tracking venous flow are TR = 80 ms; flip angle = 25°, NSA = 1, with gradient-echo images acquired at Δt 20 ms/ 40 ms/60 ms/±80 ms (Δt = interval between the center of the presaturation radiofrequency pulse and the gradient echo). Imaging matrix 128 × 256, breath-hold 11 s.

Gadolinium-Enhanced 3D MRA (3D FISP). TE 1.4 ms, TR 3.5 ms, flip angle 25°, matrix 128 × 256, NSA 1, field of view 300–350 mm, 40 partitions. Typical image acquisition time 25 s per 3D data set, two acquisitions during two breath-holds 5 s apart. A double dose (0.2 mmol/kg body weight) of gadolinium-DTPA (Magnevist, Berlex Laboratories, Wayne, N.J.) is given after a patient-specific delay (mean 19 s). The imaging delay is determined by giving a 1 ml injection of gadolinium-DTPA followed by a saline bolus (10 ml) with continuous imaging of the aorta using turboFLASH at 1–2 images/s to calculate time of arrival of the contrast in the area of interest (EARLS et al. 1996).

Breath-hold MRA ECG-Gated Segmented k-Space. TR 20 ms (320-ms acquisition window within the R-R interval for collection of 16 lines of k-space), TE 10 ms flip angle 30°, matrix 160 × 256, slice thickness 5 mm, 2 NSA.

Extracranial Carotid Arteries – Unenhanced MRA Evaluation of cervical carotid arteries uses axial 2D and 3D time-of-flight (TOF) MRA centered at the carotid bifurcation with a dedicated surface coil.

Axial Cervical 2D TOF. TR 30 ms, TE 9 ms, flip angle 45°, matrix 160 × 256, slice thickness 3 mm, 1 NSA. A slice thickness for the 2D sequence allows coverage of the entire field of view of the neck coil with a single set of acquisitions.

Axial Cervical 3D TOF. TR 35 ms, TE 10 ms, flip angle 20°, matrix 160 × 256, slice thickness 1 mm, 1 NSA.

Aortic Arch – Carotid Origins. Sagittal segmented k-space (ECG-gated) 2D TOF (TR 20 ms with 320-ms acquisition window within the R-R interval to collect 16 lines of k-space data, TE 10 ms, flip angle 30°, matrix 160 × 256, slice thickness 5 mm, 2 NSA) or axial 3D TOF (TR 35 ms, TE 10 ms, flip angle 20°, matrix 160 × 256, slice thickness 1 mm, 1 NSA).

References

Akins EW, Carmichael MJ, Hill JA, et al. (1987) Preoperative evaluation of the thoracic aorta using MRI and angiography. Ann Thorac Surg 44:499–507

Amparo EG, Higgins CB, Hricak H, et al. (1985) Aortic dissection: magnetic resonance imaging. Radiology 55:399–406

Anderson CM, Saloner D, Tsuruda JS, et al. (1990) Artefacts in maximum-intensity projection display of MR angiograms. AJR 154:623–629

Arrivé L, Menu Y, Dessarts I, et al. (1991) Diagnosis of abdominal venous thrombosis by means of spin echo and gradient echo MR imaging: analysis with receiver operating characteristic curves. Radiology 181:661–668

Azarow KS, Pearl RH, Hoffman MA, et al. (1992) Vascular ring: does magnetic resonance imaging replace angiography? Ann Thorac Surg 53:882–885

Bluemke DA (1997) Definitive diagnosis of intramural hematoma of the thoracic aorta with MR imaging. Radiology 204:319–321

Bogaert J, Meyns B, Rademakers FE, et al. (1997) Follow-up of aortic dissection: contribution of MR angiography for evaluation of the abdominal aorta and its branches. Eur Radiol 7:695–702

Chang J-M, Friese K, Caputo GR, et al. (1991) MR measurement of blood flow in the true and false channel in chronic aortic dissection. J Comput Assist Tomogr 15:418–423

Cigarroa JE, Isselbacher EM, DeSanctis RW, et al. (1993) Diagnostic imaging in the evaluation of suspected aortic dissection: old and new standards. N Engl J Med 328:35–43

Cohen MC, Hartnell GG, Finn JP (1994) Magnetic resonance angiography of congenital pulmonary vein anomalies. Am Heart J 127:954–955

Di Cesare E, Dorenzi P, Pavone P, et al. (1991) Postsurgical follow-up of aortic dissections by MRI. Eur J Radiol 13:27–30

Dinsmore RE, Wedeen VJ, Miller SW, et al. (1986) MRI of dissection of the aorta: recognition of the intimal tear and differential flow velocities. AJR 146:1286–1288

Dinsmore RE, Van Weeden VJ, Rosen B, et al. (1987) Phase-offset technique to distinguish slow blood flow and thrombus on MRI images. AJR 148:634–636

Earls JP, Rofsky NM, DeCorato DR, Krinsky GA, Weinreb JC (1996) Breath-hold single-dose gadolinium-enhanced three-dimensional MR aortography: usefulness of a timing examination and MR power injector. Radiology 201:705–710

Ecklund KE, Hartnell GG (1994) Mediastinal Castleman disease: MR and MRA features. J Thorac Imaging 9:156–159

Edelman RR, Mattle HP, Kleefield J, et al. (1989) Quantification of blood flow with dynamic MR imaging and presaturation bolus tracking. Radiology 171:551–556

Erbel R, Engberding R, Daniel W, et al. (1989) Echocardiography in diagnosis of aortic dissection. Lancet I:457–461

Fellows KE, Weinberg PM, Baffa JM, et al. (1992) Evaluation of congenital heart disease with MR imaging: current and coming attractions. AJR 159:925–931

Felmlee JP, Ehman RL (1987) Spatial presaturation: a method for suppressing flow artefacts and improved depiction of vascular anatomy on MRI. Radiology 64:559–564

Finn JP, Zisk J, Edelman RR, et al. (1993) MR angiography in central venous occlusions. Radiology 187:245–250

Gamsu G, Webb WR, Sheldon P, et al. (1983) Nuclear magnetic resonance imaging of the thorax. Radiology 147:473–480

Geibel A, Kasper W, Behrox A, Przewolka U, Meinertz T, Just H (1988) Risk of transesophageal echocardiography in awake patients with cardiac diseases. Am J Cardiol 62:337–339

Geisinger MA, Risius B, O'Donnell JA, et al. (1985) Thoracic aortic dissections: magnetic resonance imaging. Radiology 155:407–412

Godwin JD, Webb WR (1982) Contrast related flow phenomena mimicking pathology on thoracic computed tomography. J Comput Assist Tomogr 6:460–464

Guinet C, Buy J-N, Ghossain MA, et al. (1992) Aortic anastomotic pseudoaneurysms: US, CT, MR and angiography. J Comput Assist Tomogr 16:182–188

Haire WD, Lynch TG, Lund GB, et al. (1991) Limitations of magnetic resonance imaging and ultrasound directed (duplex) scanning in the diagnosis of subclavian vein thrombosis. J Vasc Surg 13:391–397

Hansen ME, Spritzer CE, Sostman HD (1990) Assessing the patency of mediastinal and thoracic inlet veins; value of MR imaging. AJR 155:1177–1182

Hartnell GG, Meier RA (1995) MR angiography of congenital heart disease in adults. Radiographics 15:781–794

Hartnell GG, Finn JP, Zenni M, et al. (1994) Magnetic resonance imaging of the thoracic aorta: a comparison of spin echo, angiographic and breathhold techniques. Radiology 191:697–704

Hartnell GG, Hughes LA, Finn JP, Longmaid HE (1995) Magnetic resonance angiography of the central chest veins: a new gold standard? Chest 107:1053–1057

Hartnell GG, Cohen MC, Meier RA, Finn JP (1996) Magnetic resonance angiography demonstration of congenital heart disease in adults. Clin Radiol 51:851–857

Kauczor HU, Layer G, Schad LR, et al. (1991) Clinical applications of MR angiography in intrathoracic masses. J Comput Assist Tomog 15:409–417

Kawamoto S, Bluemke DA, Traill TA, Zerhouni EA (1997) Thoracoabdominal aorta in Marfan syndrome: MR imaging findings of progression of vasculopathy after surgical repair. Radiology 203:727–732

Krinsky GA, Rofsky NM, DeCorato DR, et al. (1997) Thoracic aorta: gadolinium-enhanced three-dimensional MR angiograhy with conventional MR imaging. Radiology 202:183–193

Laissy JP, Blanc F, Soyer P, et al. (1995) Thoracic aortic dissection: diagnosis with transesophageal echocardiography versus MR imaging. Radiology 194:331–336

Leung DA, Debatin JF (1997) Three-dimensional contrast-enhanced magnetic resonance angiography of the thoracic vasculature. Eur Radiol 7:981–989

Lewin JS, Laub G, Hausmann R (1991) Three dimensional time-of-flight MR angiography: applications in the abdomen and thorax. Radiology 179:261–264

Link KM, Lesko NJ (1992) The role of MR imaging in the evaluation of acquired diseases of the thoracic aorta. AJR 158:1115–1125

Lotan CS, Cranney GB, Doyle M, et al. (1989) Fat-shift artifact simulating aortic dissection on MR images. AJR 152:385–386

Loubeyre P, Delignette A, Bonefoy L, Douek P, Amiel M, Revel D (1996) Magnetic resonance imaging evaluation of the ascending aorta after graft inclusion surgery: comparison between an ultrafast contrast-enhanced MR sequence and conventional cine-MRI. J Magn Reson Imaging 6:478–483

Mader MT, Poulton TB, White RD (1997) Malignant tumors of the heart and great vessels: MR imaging appearance. Radiographics 17:145–153

Mast HL, Gordon DH, Kantor AM (1991) Pitfalls in diagnosis of aortic dissection by angiography: algorithmic approach utilizing CT and MRI. Comput Med Imaging Graph 15:431–440

Masui T, Seelos KC, Kersting-Sommerhof BA, Higgins CB (1991) Abnormalities of the pulmonary veins: evaluation with MR imaging and comparison with cardiac angiography and echocardiography. Radiology 181: 645–649

Mendelson DS, Apter S, Mitty HA, et al. (1991) Residual dissection of the thoracic aorta after repair: MRI-angiographic correlation. Comput Med Imaging Graph 15:31–35

Mirowitz SA, Lee JKT, Gutierrez FR, et al. (1990) "Pseudocoarctation" of the aorta: pitfall on cine MR imaging. J Comput Assist Tomogr 14:753–755

Murray JG, Manisali M, Flamm SD, et al. (1997) Intramural hematoma of the thoracic aorta: MR image findings and their prognostic implications. Radiology 204:349–355

Nienaber CA, von Kodolitsch Y, Nicolas V, et al. (1993) The diagnosis of thoracic aortic dissection by noninvasive imaging procedures. N Engl J Med 328:1–9

Panting JR, Norell MS, Baker C, Nicholson AA (1995) Feasibility, accuracy and safety of magnetic resonance imaging in acute aortic dissection. Clin Radiol 50:455–458

Parsons JM, Baker EJ, Hayes A, et al. (1990) Magnetic resonance imaging of the great arteries in infants. Int J Cardiol 28:73–85

Petasnik JP (1991) Radiologic evaluation of aortic dissection. Radiology 180:297–305

Prince MR (1994) Gadolinium-enhanced MR aortography. Radiology 191:155–164

Randall PA, Trasolini NC, Kohman LJ, et al. (1993) MR imaging in the evaluation of the chest after uncomplicated median sternotomy. Radiographics 13:329–340

Rofsky NM, Weinreb JC, Grossi EA, et al. (1993) Aortic aneurysm and dissection: normal MR imaging and CT findings after surgical repair with the continuous-suture graft-inclusion technique. Radiology 186:195–201

Simonetti OP, Finn JP, White RD, Laub G, Henry DA (1996) "Black blood" T2-weighted inversion-recovery MR imaging of the heart. Radiology 199:49–57

Solomon SL, Brown JJ, Glazer HS, et al. (1990) Thoracic aortic dissection; pitfalls and artifacts in MR imaging. Radiology 177:223–228

Sommer BW, Fehske W, Holznecht N, et al. (1996) Aortic dissection: a comparative study of diagnosis with spiral CT, multiplanar transesophageal echocardiography, and MR imaging. Radiology 199:347–352

Sonnabend SB, Colletti PM, Pentecost M (1990) Demonstration of aortic lesions via cine magnetic resonance imaging. Magn Reson Imaging 8:613–618

Soulen RL, Fishman EK, Pyeritz RE, et al. (1987) Marfan syndrome: evaluation with MR imaging versus CT. Radiology 165:697–701

Vesely TM, Julsrud PR, Brown JJ, et al. (1991) MR imaging of partial anomalous pulmonary venous connections. J Comput Assist Tomogr 15:752–756

White CS, Baffa JM, Haney PJ, Pace ME, Campbell AB (1997) MR imaging of congenital anomalies of the thoracic veins. Radiographics 17:595–608

White RD, Ullyot DJ, Higgins CB (1988) MR imaging of the aorta after surgery for aortic dissection. AJR 150: 87–92

Wolff KA, Herold CJ, Tempany CM, et al. (1991) Aortic dissection: atypical patterns seen at MR imaging. Radiology 181:489–495

Yucel EK, Steinberg FL, Egglin TK, et al. (1990) Penetrating aortic ulcers: diagnosis with MR imaging. Radiology 177:779–781

14 Interventional Cardiovascular MRI

S. Wildermuth, T. Pfammatter, and J.F. Debatin

14.1
Introduction

Central to the success and safety of any image-guided interventional procedure such as embolization or percutaneous transluminal angioplasty (PTA) is the accurate visualization of the interventional instruments relative to the surrounding morphology. To date this has been achieved with x-ray fluoroscopy; however, the exposure to ionizing radiation, the limited soft tissue contrast, and the inability to image in cross-section have led to the exploration of alternative imaging strategies. Ideally, the instruments should be easily identifiable in the image, and the imaging system should provide high positional accuracy, along with near real-time imaging for good maneuverability.

Magnetic resonance imaging (MRI) seems well suited for monitoring vascular interventions. MRI causes no radiation exposure, is capable of combining high temporal and spatial resolution (Edelman 1993), and provides cross-sectional images in any desired plane. The influence of flow on both amplitude and phase of spins provides the basis for "time-of-flight" and "phase contrast" MR angiography (MRA), though their dependence on flow effects makes these techniques vulnerable to pulsatility and saturation artifacts. These limitations can be overcome by contrast-enhanced three-dimensional (3D) MRA – a technique based on the use of intravenously administered paramagnetic contrast agents in combination with ultrafast 3D acquisition strategies (Leung et al. 1996).

Among the further advantages of MRI is the fact that the soft tissue contrast is vastly superior to that of fluoroscopy, permitting the concurrent evaluation of tissues surrounding the vessel of interest. In addition, quantitative velocity and flow volume characterization can be integrated in the same noninvasive vascular evaluation (Pelc et al. 1991a).

Patient access remains a significant problem for any scenario involving MR guidance and control of intravascular interventions. The "ideal" interventional MRA scanner has yet to be designed. At this time, high field strength and fast gradient systems seem incompatible with an open scanner design. Recent hardware developements have provided more patient access by shortening the bore, whilst maintaining field strength and gradient performance. Further progress will need to be made in this respect for the concept of interventional MRA to evolve into clinical practice.

A difficult challenge with regard to MR-guided intravascular interventions pertains to the actual visualization of the catheter or guide wire within the

S. Wildermuth, MD, Department of Diagnostic Radiology, Zurich University Hospital, Rämistrasse 100, CH-8091 Zurich, Switzerland
T. Pfammatter, MD, Department of Diagnostic Radiology, Zurich University Hospital, Rämistrasse 100, CH-8091 Zurich, Switzerland
J.F. Debatin, MD, Department of Diagnostic Radiology, Zurich University Hospital, Rämistrasse 100, CH-8091 Zurich, Switzerland

vascular system. There are two fundamental approaches to device localization with MRI: electrically passive techniques based on visualization of the susceptibility-induced signal void caused by the instrument (DUMOULIN et al. 1991; LEUNG et al. 1995a), and electrically active techniques, first suggested by ACKERMAN et al. (1986). Both techniques are described in detail in this book.

This chapter will focus on MR-guided intravascular interventions based on active visualization of catheters and guide wires.

14.2
Active MR Visualization of Catheters and Guide Wires

14.2.1
MR-tracking: The Technique

MR-tracking was developed by DUMOULIN et al. (1993) for active monitoring of devices under real-time conditions. As first suggested by ACKERMAN et al. (1986), a small receive-only coil is incorporated into the tip of the device. Following nonselective RF excitation of a volume defined in size by the dimensions of the field of view, a gradient echo (GE) is generated by the miniature receive coil. Following Fourier transformation, a signal peak is obtained, the frequency of which corresponds to the position of the coil on a particular axis. Using a Hadamard multiplexed pulse sequence, the 3D position of the coil is encoded with only four excitations (DUMOULIN et al. 1991). Thus, with a short TR, the coil's position can be computed up to 16 times per second. The coil position is displayed by graphic overlay as a cursor on any previously acquired MR "roadmap" image. Ultrafast data links and a powerful processor limit the delay between the end of data acquisition and display of the coil position to less than 10 ms, assuring truly real-time tracking.

By separating the positional information from the data contained within the image, MR-tracking of a device is possible without having to update images. The real-time position of the coil within the catheter or guide wire is simply superimposed on previously acquired MR images. This strategy works only as long as the area of interest has remained unchanged in position. As soon as patient motion occurs, updated images need to be obtained to provide a new basis for tracking of the device. Periodic motion processes, such as respiration-induced motion in the craniocaudad plane, may be compensated for by in-

corporation of some sort of gating or "navigator" sequence. The latter provides an adaptive correction system based on specially encoded navigator echoes, which may be interleaved into the tracking sequence and thus compensate for gross patient motion (see Chap. 1).

For real-time control, update images can, however, be easily obtained. The actively available positional information of the coil can be used to guide the imaging plane, so that new images are acquired in a position always corresponding to the position of the coil, integrated into the tip of the catheter or guide wire. For this purpose the acquisition of fast GE images is most useful. The images can be acquired in any plane relative to the tip of the device. The center of the image will always correspond to the position of the tracking coil. In this mode the scanner intermittently switches between image acquisition and tracking. Hence, the position of the coil is updated discontinuously and its movement is not displayed as smoothly as in the continuous tracking mode. Data acquisition and subsequent reconstruction for GE "update" images takes several seconds and is clearly not performed in real time. Improving the temporal resolution of update images would require the implementation of ultrafast EPI data acquisition strategies, mandating improved hardware.

14.2.2
Multiplanar MR-tracking

The coil position can be projected onto multiple images simultaneously without loss in temporal resolution. For multiplanar tracking, the coil position is projected onto two or more images covering the same imaging volume in different planes (LEUNG et al. 1995a). Biplanar tracking vastly enhances the ability to target any desired area, provided the area under consideration is contained within the imaging volume. The simultaneous display of the catheter tip on a coronal and a sagittal roadmap image of the aorta greatly facilitates positional determinations relative to the celiac trunk and the superior mesenteric artery as well as both renal arteries.

14.2.3
Multicoil MR-tracking

Simultaneous tracking of multiple coils has recently become possible. This is accomplished by attaching each of the four coils to separate receivers. Separate tracking symbols and colors are assigned to the four different receivers, permitting easy separation of the tracking devices. The number of coils that can be tracked simultaneously is dependent on the number of receivers available.

14.2.4
Active Visualization of Guide Wires

Several techniques for active visualization of thin and flexible devices have been introduced, attempting to use electrically coupled antennas to outline instruments such as vascular catheters and especially guide wires (McKINNON et al. 1996; OCALI and ATALAR 1997). These techniques show promise, but generally generate an outline which has a spatial extent significantly greater than the size of the device itself.

A new technique is to use a magnetically coupled antenna which is very thin but extends over a length of several centimeters (LADD et al. 1997). These antennas generate a device outline of limited extent, which sharply delineates the device. In this chapter the use of such an antenna to visualize a 0.035-in. vascular guide wire in an in vivo environment is described.

14.3
Materials and Methods

14.3.1
Animal Experiments

In vivo animal experiments were performed on fully anesthetized swine with a body weight ranging between 40 and 55 kg. All experiments had been approved by the appropriate governmental regulatory bodies.

The swine were fully anesthetized and ventilated at all times during the experiments. The arterial system of the animals was accessed by arteriotomy of the carotid arteries; the venous system by cut-down to the jugular veins. Under fluoroscopic guidance an introducer sheath was passed over a conventional 0.035-in. guide wire made out of MR-compatible Nitinol into either the carotid artery or the jugular vein. Through the indwelling introducer, MR-tracking catheters and guide wires were advanced into the aorta or the superior vena cava.

The animals were placed into the bore of the magnet system in the supine position. Experiments were performed on either a 1.5-T MR system (SIGNA, General Electric, Milwaukee, Wis.) or an open configuration 0.5-T system (SIGNA SP, General Electric, Milwaukee, Wis.), interfaced via a high-speed data link with a Sparc 20 as well as a Sparc 10 (Sun Microsystems, Palo Alto, Calif.) workstation. Two-dimensional time-of-flight (TOF) angiograms (TR/TE 30/8 ms, 30° flip angle, 36–40 cm FOV, 256 × 192 matrix, 1 excitation) of the abdominal vascular systems were acquired in the coronal and axial planes using 5-mm sections. Maximum intensity projection (MIP) images containing different regions of vascular anatomy were obtained and used as "roadmaps" for the positional display of the tracked intravascular devices. Depending on the number of 5-mm images required for a particular MIP projection, time for data acquisition in one plane ranged between 1 and 3 min. Acquisition times were broken up into 20- to 30-s packages, so that the data could be collected during breath-hold (the respirator was stopped) in end-expiration. Based on these images, the MR-tracking catheters and guide wires were manipulated under active MR guidance.

Continuous MR-tracking was based on nonselective RF excitation of a volume defined by the dimensions of the field of view (36–40 cm), using the following parameters: TR 15–30 ms, TE 8 ms, flip angle 60°. Depending on the TR length, the coil position was sampled every 60–120 ms or 8–16 times/second.

To compensate for motion, TOF roadmaps were updated every 15 min. In addition, fast GE updates were acquired during the catheter tracking process using the following parameters: TR 20 ms, TE 4 ms, flip angle 20°, 10 mm sections, FOV 36–40 cm, 256 × 128 matrix, 1 NEX. The tracking information was used to assure that each acquired update image, regardless of the chosen imaging plane, was centered on the most recent coil position. The update images were fed into one of the two displays on a "need basis," defined by the interventionalist.

14.3.2
MR-tracking Catheter Design

Prototype MR-tracking catheters were constructed by Schneider Europe AG, Bulach, Switzerland. An untuned, receive-only copper RF coil consisting of 8–16 loops with an outer diameter of 1.1 mm is integrated into the catheter tip (LEUNG et al. 1995b) (Fig. 14.1). These coils are incorporated into the catheter material itself and connected to a plug at the base of

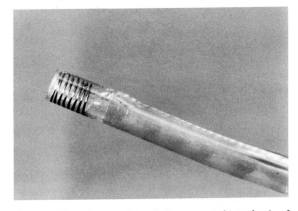

Fig. 14.1. The miniature RF coil is incorporated into the tip of a 5-F catheter. The coaxial cable, embedded in the catheter wall, is also seen

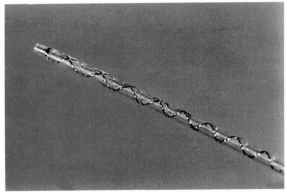

Fig. 14.2. Close-up of guide wire tip showing a loosely wound solenoidal coil

the catheter via a fully insulated coaxial cable with a diameter of 0.38 mm, embedded in the catheter wall.

MR-tracking catheters were manufactured in a length of 120 cm and were made of a polyamide (PM 200, Schneider AG, Bulach, Switzerland), a flexible material providing optimum force transmission and covered with softglide coating. The material is approved for human use and found in commercially available catheters. The catheters contained a standard 0.035-in. lumen for placement of a guide wire, or application of contrast or other materials.

Catheter force transmission (trackability) was assessed for a 5-F coil-tipped catheter in comparison to a standard 5-F catheter in a guidance system (inside diameter of 2.5 mm) with several preformed bends. Force transmission, monitored continuously over distance as the catheters were mechanically advanced for 140 mm around a 90° bend with a 12 mm radius, was 18% poorer for the coil-tipped catheter than for a standard catheter (WILDERMUTH et al. 1998).

14.3.3
MR-tracking Guide Wire Design

An MR-tracking guide wire was constructed with a 0.6-mm-diameter solenoid coil integrated into the tip (Schneider Europe AG, Bulach, Switzerland). The solenoid coil consisted of 16 windings in two layers. The coil was attached to a coaxial cable. The distal 10 cm, including the coil itself, was coated by a sheath of fluoroethylenepropylene (FEP) (Fig. 14.2). The remainder of the 1.8-m-long wire was sheathed with a polyamide to lend some mechanical stability. FEP, a less rigid polymer, provided a very flexible tip. The outer diameter of the guide wire was 0.75 mm,

small enough to fit into the standard 0.035-in. (0.89 mm) lumen of a 5-F catheter.

14.4
Positional Accuracy and Robustness of MR-Tracking

In vitro phantom experiments demonstrated the MR-tracking technique to be highly accurate with regard to positioning of the tracking coil (LEUNG et al. 1995b).

For the in vivo evaluation of the positional accuracy inherent to MR-tracking, a 5-F MR-tracking catheter was advanced into the descending aorta of a swine via an introducer placed in the carotid artery. Based on TOF MIP projection images depicting the abdominal aorta with its branch vessels in the coronal projection, the catheter was maneuvered under MR guidance into the splenic artery as well as both renal arteries (Fig. 14.3). After each placement, a radiograph was obtained to confirm the position of the catheter, following the administration of an iodinated contrast material through the catheter. These radiographs confirmed the correct positions in the respective vessels as had been indicated by the MR-tracking position on the roadmap MIP images.

14.5
MR-Guided Intravascular Procedures

14.5.1
Embolization

A 5-F MR-tracking catheter was tracked into the right renal artery based on previously acquired TOF MIP roadmap images. Following secure positioning

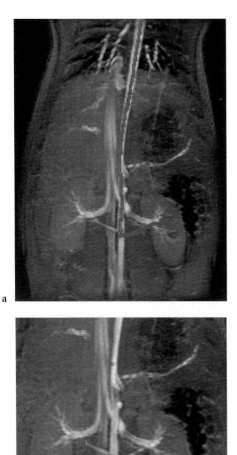

Fig. 14.3 a,b. Coronal MR TOF angiographic "roadmap" images (computer screen shots) of the swine's abdominal arterial system. With the cursor in continuous mode, the path of the catheter tip into the left renal artery is displayed. Generally the catheter tip is displayed as a single dot (**b**)

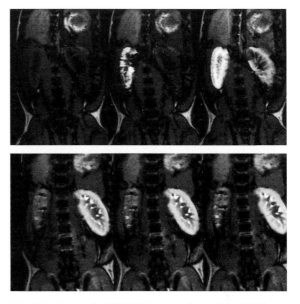

Fig. 14.4. Coronal FMPSPGR images through both kidneys acquired before (*top row*) and following embolization (*bottom row*). Images were collected prior to (*left*), 10 s after (*middle*), and 30 s after contrast administration through the MR-tracking catheter, which remained lodged in the right renal artery throughout the procedure. Before embolization, enhancement of the right kidney is seen at 10 s with enhancement of the contralateral kidney at 30 s. Following embolization, there is enhancement only of the contralateral kidney due to backflow after contrast administration

of the catheter tip in the proximal right renal artery, MR contrast (Gd-DTPA, Schering AG, Berlin, Germany) was injected through the catheter lumen at a concentration of 0.01 mmol/kg. Prior to, and at 10-s intervals following contrast administration, eight contiguous 10-mm coronal sections were acquired through the kidneys using a fast, multiplanar spoiled GE sequence (FMPSPGR: TR/TE 90/2.1, flip 60°, 1 NEX). These dynamically acquired images revealed isolated early enhancement of the right kidney with subsequent enhancement of the contralateral kidney 30 s after contrast administration (Fig. 14.4).

Subsequently the right renal artery was embolized by injecting Ethibloc (Ethicon, Germany) embolization material through the lumen of the catheter with

its tip lodged in the right renal artery. Dynamic FMPSPGR imaging was repeated. The images now demonstrated isolated enhancement of the contralateral kidney commencing 10 s after contrast application due to backflow out of the occluded right renal arterial system.

14.5.2
In Vivo Animal Balloon Occlusion

The design of the PTA MR-tracking catheter, 5.3 F in diameter, was based on the commercially available SMASH model (Schneider Europe AG, Bulach, Switzerland). The cylindrical balloon portion extends over 40 mm from 10 to 50 mm proximal to the tracking coil at the catheter's tip (Fig. 14.5). The balloon is made out of a special polyamide (PM 300, Schneider AG, Switzerland). The inflated balloon is 6 mm in diameter, and has a recommended pressure range of 5–10 atm (burst pressure 14–18 atm).

The function of the MR-tracking PTA catheter was assessed in vivo in a fully anesthetized 45-kg swine. Coronal TOF images of the abdominal aorta and pelvic arterial system were acquired. Based on

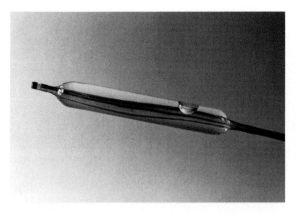

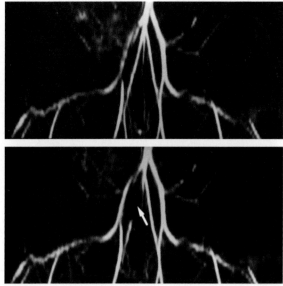

Fig. 14.5. Proximal portion of the 5.3-F PTA MR-tracking catheter contains the cylindrical balloon, which extends over 40 mm and can be inflated to a diameter of 6 mm. The coaxial cable, embedded in the catheter wall, is also seen. The coil is positioned at the catheter's tip, 10 mm distal to the balloon

Fig. 14.6. Coronal reprojections of axially acquired MR angiography TOF-images (TR/TE 33/8 ms) of the pelvis of a swine. Based on MRA roadmap images, a PTA catheter was placed into the right sacral artery. MRA images were acquired before (*top*) and during balloon inflation (*bottom*). The balloon inflation caused a signal void in the right sacral artery (*arrow*)

these MIP roadmap images the PTA catheter was tracked into the right sacral artery of the swine (Fig. 14.6). To evaluate the functioning of the PTA balloon, it was inflated with water whilst the catheter was positioned in the sacral artery. To demonstrate the effect of balloon inflation in the sacral artery, the MRA acquisition of the pelvic arterial system was repeated whilst the balloon remained inflated. Over the entire 40 mm length of the balloon, the vessel was in effect occluded, as shown by the total lack of intravascular signal. Tracking remained possible throughout the in vivo experiment, even while the balloon was inflated.

14.5.3
Human PTA of Common Iliac Artery Stenosis

The feasibility and safety of MR-guided percutaneous arterial angioplasty of a focal common iliac artery stenosis was demonstrated in a patient with an isolated, concentric stenosis. Following conventional angiography the stenosis was crossed under fluoroscopic guidance with an MR-compatible guide wire. The patient was subsequently moved into the open MR system (0.5-T, Signa SP, General Electrics) with the guide wire remaining in place. A flexible transmit/receive coil was placed over the area of interest. TOF MRA was used as a roadmap to position the MR-tracking balloon catheter. For position verification during the PTA procedure, the balloon was fully expanded with a $0.5 M$ solution of Gd-DTPA (Fig. 14.7). Based on the signal void caused by the para-

magnetic contrast, the balloon location was easily confirmed. The angioplasty result was evaluated on repeated postinterventional MR and conventional angiograms. Beyond the usual local discomfort at dilatation, the procedure was tolerated well. Although the MRA image quality obtained on the open MR scanner was limited, the lesion as well as the morphologic angioplasty results could be visualized.

14.5.4
Transjugular Intrahepatic Puncture of the Portal System

For this procedure a modified MReye transjugular intrahepatic portosystemic shunt (TIPS) set (William Cook Europe A/S, Bjaeverskov Denmark) was used. It consisted of the following components: a 41-cm-long 10-F introducer; a curved 10-F TFE catheter; a 51.5-cm-long, 14-gauge curved MRI-compatible MReye cannula; a 5-F, 59.5-cm-long TFE catheter, equipped at its tip with a tracking coil (Schneider Europe AG, Bulach, Switzerland); and a 60-cm-long, 20-gauge flexible MRI-compatible MReye puncture needle (Fig.14.8). The puncture needle was contained within the 5-F tracking catheter. Since

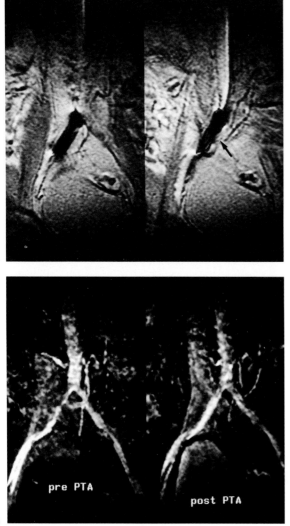

a

b,c

Fig. 14.7 a–c. PTA in a human. After ascertaining the correct catheter tip position, the balloon was fully expanded with a 0.5 *M* solution of Gd-DTPA. Based on the signal void caused by the paramagnetic contrast (*arrow*), the balloon location was confirmed on fast GE images (**a**). The angioplasty result was documented on repeated conventional angiograms and MR angiograms before (**b**) the PTA and following intervention (**c**)

hepatic vein was mapped. The actual puncture was performed with the swine in suspended respiration using biplanar tracking of the coil-tipped catheter covering the puncture needle. The intraportal position of the 5-F catheter was subsequently verified fluoroscopically. A stent was not placed.

Transjugular intrahepatic puncture of the portal system was possible in both of two animals. The procedures lasted around 90 min. Based on the MIP roadmaps acquired in both the axial and the coronal plane, the parenchymal puncture was in effect guided in real time from the middle hepatic vein into the right portal vein (Fig. 14.10). Tracking remained robust, as the puncture unit consisting of the needle and tracking catheter was maneuvered from the hepatic vein into the portal vein.

14.5.5
MR-tracking of Guide Wire-Catheter Composition

In order to perform any vascular intervention, catheters as well as guide wires need to be visible to the interventionist. An MR-tracking guide wire with an outer diameter of 0.75 mm, compatible with a standard 5-F catheter, was built. The guide wire-catheter composition was also assessed in an in vivo swine experiment. Based on coronal and sagittal TOF MIP roadmaps, the combined guide wire-catheter composition was maneuvered through the thoracic and abdominal aorta into the superior mesenteric artery as well as both renal arteries with ease. Tracking of both the catheter tip and the guide wire tip remained robust in the presence of pulsatile flow throughout the in vivo experiment. MR-tracking of the guide wire was possible inside as well as outside the catheter. The relationship of the catheter and guide wire tip to each another was visible at all times. Even superimposition of the two receive coils did not result in any interruption of the tracking process.

14.6
Discussion

The described experiments demonstrate that robust MR-tracking and precise positioning of catheters and guide wires equipped with small RF coils at their tip can be achieved under in vivo conditions on standard as well as "open configuration" MR scanning systems. The high precision of the MR-tracking technique with regard to positional accuracy was docu-

both components are advanced at the same time for the puncture, the needle tip could in effect be tracked by virtue of its position 5 mm distal to the tracking coil integrated in the tip of the catheter (Fig. 14.9).

The procedure was performed with biplanar MR-tracking, based on axial and coronal roadmap images depicting the inferior vena cava, the hepatic veins, and the portal venous system. Based on the axial and coronal roadmap images, a course for puncturing the right portal vein from the middle

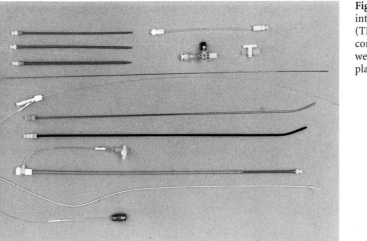

Fig. 14.8. The complete transjugular intrahepatic portosystemic shunt (TIPS) set is shown. To achieve MR compatability, all metallic components were replaced with titanium or hard plastics

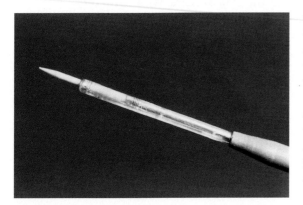

Fig. 14.9. A small RF coil is integrated into the catheter tip draping the puncture needle

mented in phantom experiments (LEUNG et al. 1995a,b).

There are several unique characteristics of the MR-based active tracking technique. The technique is virtually independent of device orientation and provides maximal flexibility with regard to the characteristics of the underlying MR image on which MR-tracking is based. A position update of 16 updates per second with a display delay of under 10 ms ensures real-time tracking of the instrument (LEUNG et al. 1995a,b). A great advantage, compared with passive visualization, lies in the electronic availability of the position of the interventional device, in this case the catheter or guide wire. It can therefore be used to automatically control image acquisition at a location corresponding to the updated position of the coil. Another characteristic inherent to MRI is that the position of the coil can be determined in any desired plane. With biplanar display implementation, it is possible to track any instrument in real time simultaneously in any two planes (LEUNG et al. 1995a). Thus the catheter position may be continuously tracked on a coronal or sagittal roadmap image while its progress is monitored on serially updated axial images traversing the tip of the catheter. This feature was found to be particularly helpful in cannulating the renal arteries.

The concept of active tracking has been extended to the guidance of up to four devices. The availability of active multidevice MR-tracking must be considered a significant step towards the clinical realization of interventional MRA. Considerable challenges, however, still need to be overcome. Visualization of the guide wire and possibly also the catheter must extend beyond the mere tip. This could be accomplished by use of multiple coils or the integration of other active device visualization techniques as described elsewhere (LUFKIN et al. 1987; LADD et al. 1997).

Based on active, biplanar MR-tracking, various intravascular procedures were successfully performed (WILDERMUTH et al. 1997). Arterial and venous vessels in the abdomen and pelvis were selectively cannulated with specially manufactured MR-tracking catheters. The course of the catheter tips was monitored in real time simultaneously in two planes, permitting active steering into the vessels of interest. Catheters were successfully steered even into small vessels, as illustrated by balloon occlusion

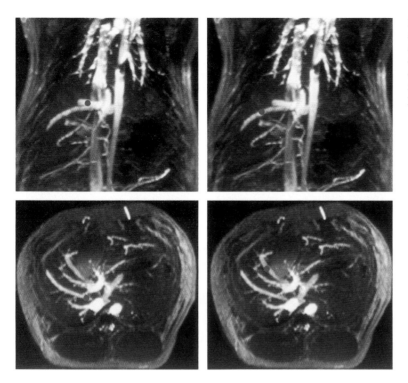

Fig. 14.10. Based on the roadmap MR angiograms acquired in the axial (*top*) and coronal (*bottom*) planes, the parenchymal transhepatic puncture was in effect guided in real time from the middle hepatic vein (*left*) into the right portal vein (*right*)

of the right sacral artery, where the functioning of the balloon catheter was confirmed. The favorable result of a first MR-guided PTA in a human must be considered encouraging. Clearly more work is required prior to any serious clinical implementation of this technique.

The ability to track catheters was not limited to the confines of vessels, as shown by the transhepatic puncture of the portal system. MR-tracking permitted active monitoring of the puncture needle, enclosed by the tracking catheter, as it was advanced through the hepatic parenchyma into the portal vein. The availability of both vascular and parenchymal information was shown to be useful in assessing the extent of embolization of the right kidney. While the tracking was guided on roadmap images sensitive to flow, the embolization results were documented on images sensitive to changes in T1-relaxation times induced by the application of paramagnetic contrast agents. The combination of vascular and parenchymal data was also helpful in guiding the transhepatic puncture of the portal system from the hepatic vein, which represents the most critical step in the placement of a transjugular intrahepatic portosystemic shunt (SKEENS et al. 1995; ROIZENTAL et al. 1995). While ultrasound can provide some guidance, the puncture is generally performed with the interventionalist more or less blinded to the exact posi-

tion of the portal vein. With MRA, the perihepatic vascular anatomy is easily displayed in any desired plane. Based on these images, the puncture may be accurately targeted and monitored in real time with MR-tracking. By bridging the blind spot between hepatic and portal vein, the procedure is greatly facilitated. The real-time monitoring ability in two planes allows for the interactive correction of the needle's course.

Tracking of the catheters is possible on the MRA TOF roadmap images. However, their acquisition remains time consuming, and as with angiographic roadmap techniques, the tracking process on roadmap images is sensitive to patient motion. Motion should thus be avoided if at all possible. Once motion does occur, the roadmap image needs to be updated, or at least modified to avoid localization errors. In fully anesthetized and relaxed animals used for experiments, motion has proved less of a problem. The development of ultrafast imaging techniques (MANSFIELD 1977, WETTER et al. 1995) will reduce the time required to update such roadmaps. In addition, cyclical motion such as breathing could be compensated for by the use of "navigator sequences" (PELC et al. 1991b; HAUSMANN et al. 1991), obviating the need for the acquisition of a totally new roadmap image. The spatial tracking coordinates of the instrument's tip could be displayed on the roadmap image relative to the concurrent position of the diaphragm. The latter would be continuously updated in real time by means of the "navigator sequence." Until the implementation of these techniques in an interventional MRA environment, however, the motion-induced need for time-consuming roadmap updates will remain a significant hurdle.

The concept of interventional MRA may be further enhanced by the application of intravascular receiver coils for high-resolution imaging of blood vessels. Together with conventional MRA and non-invasive flow quantitation, the possibilities of MR-tracking of catheters and guide wires outlined in this chapter constitute a fascinating, integrative MR-based approach to intravascular interventions.

References

Ackerman JL, Offut MC, Buxton RB, Brady TJ (1986) Rapid 3D tracking of small RF coils. In: Book of abstracts: Society of Magnetic Resonance in Medicine. Society of Magnetic Resonance in Medicine, Berkeley, Calif., p 1131

Dumoulin CL, Souza SP, Darrow RD, Pelc NJ, Adams WJ, Ash SA (1991) Simultaneous acquisition of phase contrast angiograms and stationary tissue images with Hadamard encoding of flow-induced phase shifts. J Magn Reson Imaging 1:399–404

Dumoulin CL, Souza SP, Darrow RD (1993) Real-time position monitoring of invasive devices using magnetic resonance. Magn Reson Med 29:411–415

Edelman RR (1993) MR angiography: present and future. AJR 161:1–11

Hausmann R, Lewin JS, Laub G (1991) Phase-contrast MR angiography with reduced acquisition time: new concepts in sequence design. J Magn Reson Imaging 1:415–422

Ladd ME, Erhart P, Debatin JF, et al. (1997) Guide wire antennas for MR fluoroscopy. Magn Reson Med 37:891–897

Leung DA, Debatin JF, Wildermuth S, et al. (1995a) Real-time biplanar needle tracking for interventional MR imaging procedures. Radiology 197:485–488

Leung DA, Debatin JF, Wildermuth S, et al. (1995b) Intra-vascular MR-tracking catheter: preliminary experimental evaluation. AJR 164:1265–1270

Leung DA, McKinnon GC, Davis CP, Pfammatter T, Krestin GP, Debatin JF (1996) Breath-hold, contrast-enhanced, three-dimensional MR angiography. Radiology 201:569–571

Lufkin RB, Teresi L, Hanafee WN (1987) New needle for MR-guided aspiration cytology of the head and neck. AJR 149:380–382

Mansfield P (1977) Multiplanar image formation using NMR spin-echoes. J Phys C 10:L55-L58

McKinnon GC, Debatin JF, Leung DA, Wildermuth S, Holtz DJ, von Schulthess GK (1996) Toward active guide wire visualization in interventional magnetic resonance imaging. MAGMA 4:13–18

Ocali O, Atalar E (1997) Intravascular magnetic resonance imaging using a loopless catheter antenna. Magn Reson Med 37:112–118

Pelc NJ, Herfkens RJ, Shimakawa A, Enzmann DR (1991a) Phase contrast cine magnetic resonance imaging. Magn Reson Q 7:229–254

Pelc NJ, Bernstein MA, Shimakawa A, Glover GH (1991b) Encoding strategies for three-direction phase-contrast MR imaging of flow. J Magn Reson Imaging 1:405–413

Roizental M, Kane RA, Takahashi J, et al. (1995) Portal vein: US-guided localization prior to transjugular intrahepatic portosystemic shunt placement. Radiology 196:868–870

Skeens J, Semba C, Dake M (1995) Transjugular intrahepatic portosystemic shunts. Annu Rev Med 46:95–102

Wetter DR, McKinnon GC, Debatin JF, von Schulthess GK (1995) Cardiac echo-planar MR imaging: comparison of single- and multiple-shot techniques. Radiology 194:765–770

Wildermuth S, Debatin JF, Leung DA, Dumoulin CE, Darrow R, Uhlschmidt U, von Schulthess GK (1997) MR-guided intravascular prodedures: initial demonstration in a pig model. Radiology 202:578–583

Wildermuth S, Dumoulin CL, Pfammatter T, et al. (1998) MR guided angioplasty: assessment of tracking safety, catheter handling and functionality. CVIR, to be published

15 General Conclusions and Future Perspectives

J. Bogaert, A.J. Duerinckx, and F.E. Rademakers

In preceding chapters, a detailed description was given of the current role of magnetic resonance (MR) in the study of the heart and great vessels by recognized authorities in the field. MR is not just an imaging technique but combines many facets to investigate the cardiovascular system and comes close to the goal of a complete examination with a single technical modality. This property of MR is not matched by any other technique. Whereas in the early years of MR in medicine, the heart was unquestionably the most difficult organ to investigate, improvements in MR hardware (e.g., fast gradients, coil design), MR software (e.g., MR sequence design, navigator echoes), and postprocessing techniques have made cardiac MR into a clinically useful technique. Relevant information on all aspects of the heart, including structure, global and regional ventricular function, valve function, flow patterns, myocardial perfusion, myocardial viability, and myocardial metabolism, can be obtained in a totally noninvasive manner. Introduction of new techniques, such as ultrafast three-dimensional contrast-enhanced MR angiography techniques, have opened new avenues in the noninvasive visualization of the thoracic vasculature including the coronaries. Moreover, the beginning of the third millennium will probably coincide with a breakthrough in interventional MR in the cardiovascular domain.

In the current climate of rising health care costs, assessment of the cost-effectiveness of cardiac imaging techniques and their effect on diagnosis, diagnostic certainty, and patient management and outcome, will be of utmost importance in the coming years. A description of the actual cost of each cardiac imaging is beyond the scope of this chapter because of the great differences in cost and reimbursement between countries. The cost efficiency of MR as a cardiac imaging technique is under active evaluation, and will determine whether MR may result in significant economic benefits in diagnosing cardiac disease.

Although debatable, the current clinical position of MR among the cardiac imaging techniques is shown in Table 15.1. This table can be considered as a short résumé of all previous chapters, and may serve as a guideline for the clinician in choosing the most appropriate diagnostic imaging modality for a particular cardiovascular problem. It is obvious that MR is the only imaging technique that achieves a satisfactory score for nearly all aspects of the heart and great vessels. Moreover, for several issues it can even be considered as the gold standard. However, despite these excellent scores the present clinical utilization of MR is still too often restricted to case studies in which other (i.e., more accustomed) techniques fail to identify the cardiac or cardiovascular abnormalities.

Several explanations for this situation can be identified. First, whereas in the early 1980s the introduction of MR caused a real revolution in the imaging of other parts of the body such as the brain and musculoskeletal system, this "revolution" was absent or certainly much less pronounced for the heart. This was due to the difficulties in imaging the heart with MR, as discussed in Chap. 1, and to the availability of other excellent cardiac imaging techniques, such as echocardiography and x-ray angiography. In the last decade several technical innovations have gradually surmounted the problems with which cardiac MR struggled in its "infancy." Unfortunately, these stepwise innovations have not effectively impacted on the choice of diagnostic imaging modalities by the cardiologist. Next, cardiologists are still not very familiar with the huge possibilities of cardiovascular MR, while most radiologists are not familiar with imaging the heart,

J. Bogaert, MD, PhD, Department of Radiology, University Hospitals Gasthuisberg, Catholic University of Leuven, Herestraat 49, B-3000 Leuven, Belgium

A.J. Duerinckx, MD, PhD, Radiology Service (mail route: W114), MRI-Bld# 507, West Los Angeles Veterans Affairs Medical Center (VAMC)-Wadsworth, 11301 Wilshire Blvd, Los Angeles, CA 90073, USA

F.E. Rademakers, MD, PhD, Department of Cardiology, University Hospitals Gasthuisberg, Catholic University of Leuven, Herestraat 49, B-3000 Leuven, Belgium

Table 15.1. Current clinical position of MR among the cardiac imaging modalities

	MR	Echocardiography		(UF)CT	Nuclear cardiology	X-ray angiography
		TTE	TEE			
Cardiac anatomy						
Pericardium						
Thickness	+++	+	++	++	0	−
Effusion	+++	++	+++	+++	0	−/+
Calcifications	+	−	−	+++	0	+
Myocardium						
Thickness	+++	+	++	++	−	+
Mass	+++	+	+	++	0	0
Tissue characterization	++	+	+	+	+	−
Cardiac cavities						
Endoluminal masses	+++	++	+++	++	0	++
Volume quantification	+++	++	++	++	++	+(+)
Cardiac valves						
Number of leaflets	+(+)	++	+++	−	0	++
Valve integrity	+	++	+++	−	0	+
Perivalvular masses	++	++	+++	+	0	+
Intra-and extracardiac communications						
Patent foramen ovale	+	+	+++	−	0	0
Patent ductus arteriosus	+(+)	++	++	−	0	++
Atrial septal defect	++	++	+++	+	0	++
Ventricular septal defect	++	++	+++	+	0	+++
Extracardiac spaces	+++	+(+)	+(+)	+++	0	0
Cardiac function						
Systolic function						
Global	+++	++	++	++	++(+)	++
Regional	+++	++	++	+	++	+(+)
Stress imaging	++	+++	+++	+	++	++
Diastolic function	+	+++	+++	0	+	+
Valvular function						
Valve stenosis	++	+++	++(+)	0	0	++(+)
Valve regurgitation	++(+)	++	+++	0	+	++
Myocardial perfusion	++(+)	+(+)	+(+)	0	++(+)	−
Myocardial viability						
Myocardial ischemia	++(+)	++	++	0	++(+)	+
Myocardial stunning	++	++	++	0	++	+
Myocardial hibernation	++	++	++	0	++(+)	+
Myocardial infarction	+++	+	+	0	++	+
Myocardial metabolism	+	0	0	0	+(+)	0
Coronary arteries						
Anatomy	+(+)	−	−	+	0	+++
Patency	+	−	−	+	0	+++
Calcifications	−	−	−	+++	0	+
Flow and flow reserve	+	−	−(+++)[a]	−	+	+
Great vessels						
Anatomy	+++	+(+)	++(+)	+++	0	+++
Vessel wall						
Thickness	+++	+	++	+++	0	+
Integrity	++(+)	+	++	++	+	−
Vessel lumen	+++	+	++(+)	+++	0	+++
Flow pattern	+++	+	++(+)	+	0	++

+++, Excellent; ++, good; +, average; −, poor; 0, not possible.
[a] Intracoronary echo-Doppler.

Table 15.2. Further required improvements in cardiac MR

1. Real-time imaging
2. Improvements in spatial and temporal resolution
3. Prediction of cardiac events by in vivo characterization of atheromatous plaques
4. Faster and automated postprocessing techniques
5. Cardiac-dedicated MR systems
6. Further developments of tissue-specific and intravascular contrast agents
7. Analysis of myocardial strain-stress relationship
8. In vivo myocardial spectroscopy
9. High-resolution 3D MR coronary angiography in combination with quantification of the coronary flow in basal and stress conditions
10. Improvements in interventional capabilities, also in vessels such as the coronaries

which involves both a structural and a functional analysis. The best solution to this problem seems to be improved cooperation between the specialties. Finally, there is still limited interest of industry in cardiovascular MR, which explains, for instance, the absence of fast and dedicated postprocessing facilities which would markedly improve the clinical use of cardiac MR. Nevertheless, despite these limitations, cardiac MR has a bright future and will further mature toward becoming an "adult" technique. Improvements, as summarized in Table 15.2, will help cardiac MR to take its legitimate place in the cardiovascular arena.

Subject Index

List of Contributors

JAN BOGAERT, MD, PhD
Department of Radiology
University Hospitals Gasthuisberg
Catholic University of Leuven
Herestraat 49
B-3000 Leuven
Belgium

HILDE BOSMANS, PhD
Department of Radiology
University Hospitals Gasthuisberg
Catholic University of Leuven
Herestraat 49
B-3000 Leuven
Belgium

PIERRE CROISILLE, MD
Department de Radiologie
Hôpital Cardiovasculaire et Pneumologique
L. Pradel
BP Lyon Montchat
F-69394 Lyon Cedex 03
France

JÖRG F. DEBATIN, MD
Department of Diagnostic Radiology
Zurich University Hospital
Rämistrasse 100
CH-8091 Zürich
Switzerland

ALBERT DE ROOS, MD, PhD
Professor of Radiology
Department of Diagnostic Radiology
Leiden University Medical Center
Albinusdreef 2
P.O. Box 9600
NL-2300 RC Leiden
The Netherlands

ANDRÉ J. DUERINCKX, MD, PhD
Radiology Service, MRI-Bld #507
West Los Angeles Veterans Affairs Medical Center
11301 Wilshire Blvd.
Los Angeles, CA 90073
USA

STEVEN DYMARKOWSKI, MD
Department of Radiology
University Hospitals Gasthuisberg
Catholic University of Leuven
Herestraat 49
B-3000 Leuven
Belgium

GEORGE G. HARTNELL, FRCR, FACC
Department of Radiology
Beth Israel Deaconess Medical Center,
West Campus
and Associate Professor of Radiology
Harvard Medical School
One Deaconess Road
Boston, MA 02215
USA

WILLEM A. HELBING, MD, PhD
Department of Pediatrics
(Division of Pediatric Cardiology)
Leiden University Medical Center
Albinusdreef 2, P.O. Box 9600
NL-2300 RC Leiden
The Netherlands

STEFAN NEUBAUER, MD
Medizinische Universitätsklinik Würzburg
Josef-Schneider-Strasse 2
D-97080 Würzburg
Germany

Yicheng Ni, MD, PhD
Department of Radiology
University Hospitals Gasthuisberg
Catholic University of Leuven
Herestraat 49
B-3000 Leuven
Belgium

R. André Niezen, MD
Department of Diagnostic Radiology
Leiden University Medical Center
Albinusdreef 2, P.O. Box 9600
NL-2300 RC Leiden
The Netherlands

Dudley J. Pennell, MD, FRCP, FACC, FESC
Clinical Director
Magnetic Resonance Unit
Royal Brompton Hospital
Sydney Street
London SW3 6NP
UK

Thomas Pfammatter, MD
Department of Diagnostic Radiology
Zurich University Hospital
Rämistrasse 100
CH-8091 Zürich
Switzerland

Frank E. Rademakers, MD, PhD
Department of Cardiology
University Hospitals Gasthuisberg
Catholic University of Leuven
Herestraat 49
B-3000 Leuven
Belgium

Didier Revel, MD
Department de Radiologie
Hôpital Cardiovasculaire et Pneumologique
L. Pradel
BP Lyon Montchat
F-69394 Lyon Cedex 03
France

Andrew M. Taylor, MA, MRCP
Research Fellow
Magnetic Resonance Unit
Royal Brompton Hospital
Sydney Street
London SW3 6NP
UK

Simon Wildermuth, MD
Department of Diagnostic Radiology
Zurich University Hospital
Rämistrasse 100
CH-8091 Zürich
Switzerland

MEDICAL RADIOLOGY
Diagnostic Imaging and Radiation Oncology

Titles in the series already published

MEDICAL RADIOLOGY
Diagnostic Imaging and Radiation Oncology

Titles in the series already published

Springer
and the
environment

At Springer we firmly believe that an international science publisher has a special obligation to the environment, and our corporate policies consistently reflect this conviction.

We also expect our business partners – paper mills, printers, packaging manufacturers, etc. – to commit themselves to using materials and production processes that do not harm the environment. The paper in this book is made from low- or no-chlorine pulp and is acid free, in conformance with international standards for paper permanency.

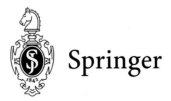 Springer

Printing and binding: Druckerei Triltsch, Würzburg